Brain Organization
of Language and
Cognitive Processes

Critical Issues in Neuropsychology

A Continuation Order Plan is available for this series. A continuation order will bring delivery of each new volume immediately upon publication. Volumes are billed only upon actual shipment. For further information please contact the publisher.

Brain Organization of Language and Cognitive Processes

Edited by

ALFREDO ARDILA

Miami Institute of Psychology
Miami, Florida

and
FEGGY OSTROSKY-SOLIS

National Autonomous University of Mexico
Mexico D.F., Mexico

Plenum Press • New York and London

Library of Congress Cataloging in Publication Data

Brain organization of language and cognitive processes.

(Critical issues in neuropsychology)
Includes bibliographies and index.
1. Language disorders. 2. Brain damage. 3. Neuropsychology. 4. Cognition. I. Ardila, Alfredo. II. Ostrosky-Solis, Feggy. III. Series. [DNLM: 1. Brain Injuries—
physiopathology. 2. Cognition—physiology. 3. Language Disorders—physiopathology.
4. Neuropsychology. WL 103 B81453]
RC423.B657   1989   616.85'5   89-16051
ISBN 0-306-43169-6

© 1989 Plenum Press, New York
A Division of Plenum Publishing Corporation
233 Spring Street, New York, N.Y. 10013

Printed in the United States of America

In memoriam

A. R. Luria
Professor and friend

Contributors

ALFREDO ARDILA, Konrad Lorenz Foundation University, Bogotá, Colombia, and Miami Institute of Psychology, Miami, Florida 33166-6612

D. FRANK BENSON, The Neurobehavior Unit, West Los Angeles Veterans Administration Medical Center, Departments of Neurology and Psychiatry and Behavioral Sciences, UCLA School of Medicine, Los Angeles, California 90024

AMY M. BIHRLE, The Salk Institute for Biological Studies, University of California-San Diego, and San Diego State University, San Diego, California 92138

JASON W. BROWN, Department of Neurology, New York University Medical Center, New York, New York 10016

HUGH W. BUCKINGHAM, Program in Linguistics and Communication Disorders, Louisiana State University, Baton Rouge, Louisiana 70803

JEFFREY L. CUMMINGS, The Neurobehavior Unit, West Los Angeles Veterans Administration Medical Center, Departments of Neurology and Psychiatry and Behavioral Sciences, UCLA School of Medicine, Los Angeles, California 90024

DEAN C. DELIS, San Diego Veterans Administration Medical Center, Department of Psychiatry, University of California-San Diego, School of Medicine, San Diego, California 92161

RENE DRUCKER-COLIN, Department of Neurosciences, Institute of Cellular Physiology, National University of Mexico, Mexico D.F. 4510, Mexico

JORGE ESLAVA-COBOS, Department of Child Neurology, Neurological Institute of Colombia, Bogotá, Colombia

ROBERT E. HANLON, Department of Psychology, City College of the City University of New York, New York, New York 10031

ANDREW KERTESZ, University of Western Ontario, St. Joseph's Health Centre, London, Ontario N6A 4V2, Canada

MARIA VICTORIA LOPEZ, Colombian Association of Neuropsychology, Bogotá, Colombia

IGNACIO MADRAZO, Department of Neurosurgery, Specialties Hospital, Centro Medico "La Raza," IMSS, Mexico D.F. 02990, Mexico

LYDA MEJIA, Colombian School of Rehabilitation, University of Rosario, Bogotá, Colombia

FEGGY OSTROSKY-SOLIS, Department of Psychophysiology, Faculty of Psychology, National University of Mexico, Mexico D.F. 4510, Mexico

OSCAR PINZON, San Juan de Dios Hospital, National University of Colombia, Bogotá, Colombia

ROBERTO A. PRADO-ALCALÁ, Department of Physiology, Faculty of Medicine, National University of Mexico, Mexico D.F. 4510, Mexico

LUIS QUINTANAR, Department of Psychophysiology, Faculty of Psychology, National University of Mexico, Mexico D.F. 4510, Mexico

MONICA ROSSELLI, Konrad Lorenz Foundation University, Bogotá, Colombia, and Miami Institute of Psychology, Miami, Florida 33166-6612

SIDNEY J. SEGALOWITZ, Department of Psychology, Brock University, St. Catharines, Ontario L2S 3A1, Canada

EUGENIA SOLANO, Neurologic Institute of Colombia, Bogotá, Colombia

DONALD G. STEIN, Dean of the Graduate School and Associate Provost for Research, Rutgers University, Newark, New Jersey 07102

Preface

Neuropsychology has presented a particularly formidable array of developments during recent years. The number of methods, theoretical approaches, and publications has been steadily increasing, permitting a step-by-step approach to a deeper understanding of the tremendously complex relationships existing between brain and behavior.

This volume was planned as a collection of papers that, in one way or another, present new research and clinical perspectives or interpretations about brain–behavior relationships. Some chapters present new research in specific topics, others summarize the evidence for a particular theoretical position, and others simply review the area and suggest new perspectives of research. Consistent with the spirit in which the book was planned, the authors present and propose new avenues for developing neuropsychology and understanding the organization of cognitive activity.

Part I is devoted to basic theoretical and technical approaches in studying brain organization of cognitive processes. Hanlon and Brown ("Microgenesis: Historical Review and Current Studies") present an overview of some clinical and experimental work from the standpoint of microgenetic theory. Microgenesis is considered to be the structural development of a cognition through qualitatively different stages. The authors discuss the growing dissatisfaction with both the old center and pathway theories and the newer modular or componential accounts. They also explore how microgenesis can be extended to the interpretation of symptoms of brain damage in developing a structural model of hierarchic levels through which the process of cognitive function unfolds.

Delis and Bihrle ("Fractionation of Spatial Cognition following Focal and Diffuse Brain Damage") analyze visuospatial impairments that occur subsequent to brain damage. They emphasize that spatial cognition, like language, fractionates in precise ways following focal and diffuse brain damage, and that selective deficits in visual attention, perception, and visuoconstructional abilities can be distinguished.

Kertesz's chapter ("Anatomical and Physiological Correlations and Neuroimaging Techniques in Language Disorders") details some of the advantages and limitations of various localizing techniques and summarizes the findings of the relatively new science of *in vivo* localization. The author considers traditional (autopsy, head injury, surgical procedure, cortical stimulation, EEG) and modern (isotope localization, computerized axial tomography, cerebral blood flow, positron emission tomography, single-photon computerized tomography, magnetic resonance imaging) techniques for localizing lesions in an in-depth analysis focusing on the issue of the extent to which a function is localizable and the variables that influence its symptomatology.

Segalowitz ("ERPs and Advances in Neurolinguistics") presents a review of some event-related potentials (ERP) techniques and technical contributions directly related to questions of research in neurolinguistics. He examines the application of ERP in the area of lexical semantics, syntaxis, reading, and primary and secondary language acquisition, and in the study of patients with disorders of language resulting from brain damage. Segalowitz emphasizes the advantages of the latter paradigm as an alternative technique to supplement the traditional behavioral measures.

Part II deals with language development and dissolution. Eslava-Cobos and Mejia ("Disorders in Language Acquisition and Cerebral Maturation: A Neurophysiological Perspective") present a historical review of concepts of disorders in language acquisition. They discuss the embryologic development of the nervous system with regard to normal language acquisition. In addition, they review Latin American studies, especially those carried out by Quiros and Azcoaga, emphasizing Pavlov's theory of analyzers as applied to language by Bechtereva. The authors also discuss abnormal language organization, trying to support a system of neurophysiological classification.

Cummings and Benson ("Speech and Language Alterations in Dementia Syndromes") present a broad clinical study focusing on speech and language in Alzheimer's dementia, Parkinson's disease dementia, and multi-infarction dementia. They analyze distinguishing features for each dementia and discuss differential profiles of preserved and impaired functions in each dementia syndrome.

Part III deals with oral and written language disorders. Buckingham ("Mechanisms Underlying Aphasic Transformations") outlines a language production model based on normality, underlining the fact that, without some notion of how a normal linguistic productive system operates, there is little hope of understanding aphasic errors. He points out that aphasic breakdowns arise through derailments of computation errors that are corrected in normal language production but augmented and sustained in aphasics. The author emphasizes that only through models of normal language production is it possible to characterize mechanisms underlying aphasic transformations.

Ardila, Rosselli, and Pinzon ("Alexia and Agraphia in Spanish Speakers: CAT Correlations and Interlinguistic Analysis") present a large-scale study of a brain-damaged population with regard to alterations in reading and writing. The authors emphasize the necessity of developing new models of alexias and agraphias and the importance of considering particular characteristics of each language.

Ardila, Lopez, and Solano ("Semantic Aphasia Reconsidered"), in a departure from some clinical cases, analyze the so-called semantic aphasia, which was postulated by Head and systematized by Luria. They propose that semantic aphasia and Gerstmann's syndrome conform to a single syndrome and that underlying cognitive deficits are common.

Part IV is devoted to discussion of some relations of the basal ganglia of the brain to cognitive activity. Ostrosky-Solis, Madrazo, Drucker-Colin, and Quintanar ("Cognitive Effects of Adrenal Autografting in Parkinson's Disease") present neuropsychological findings in patients with Parkinson's disease who have undergone adrenal autograft in Mexico City; those patients had an extensive pre- and postoperatory cognitive evaluation. The authors examine the changes observed in these patients, the cognitive area in which modifications are observed, and the factors with which they are correlated, and propose some explanatory hypotheses for the results observed.

Prado-Alcala ("The Striatum as a Temporary Memory Store") proposes that long-term memory implies the participation of different neuroanatomical and neurochemical systems that may be sequentially involved. He discusses the view that the caudate nucleus and striatonigral GABA neurons play a major role in the process underlying recent memory.

Part V is devoted to recovery from brain damage. Stein ("Development and Plasticity in the Central Nervous System: Organismic and Environmental Influences") examines in detail some fundamental and theoretical problems with regard to plasticity of the nervous system and recovery from brain damage, and analyzes contextual and environmental factors influencing recovery. He focuses on the effect of different variables, such as the moment of the lesion, and individual differences in recovery from brain damage, as well as the concept of plasticity.

Although many different topics are considered in this volume, all of them in one way or another enlighten (from the conceptual, experimental, or clinical point of view) the problem of the complex set of relationships between language and cognitive organization of activity in the brain.

The main contemporary trends in neuropsychology are clearly reflected in this book: the emphasis on cognition and the necessity to carry out an analytical approach to normal and pathological cognitive activity under both normal and abnormal conditions; the effort to develop increasingly sophisticated technical procedures to study psychological processes; the interest in correlating neurological conditions with linguistic events in the development as well as the dissolution of language; the analysis and differential characteristics of dementia syndromes; the application of complex linguistic concepts to neuropsychological analysis; the emphasis on language similarities and differences when analyzing language disorders; the current interest in studying participation of subcortical structures in cognitive activity; the enormous interest in developing procedures to overcome brain dysfunction; and the myriad remaining conceptual and practical problems.

We sincerely hope this collection of papers will further our developing knowledge of the brain's cerebral organization of language and cognitive activity.

Alfredo Ardila
Feggy Ostrosky-Solis

Contents

Part II: DEVELOPMENT AND DISSOLUTION OF LANGUAGE

Chapter 5

Disorders in Language Acquisition and Cerebral Maturation: A
Neurophysiological Perspective 85

Lyda Mejia and Jorge Eslava-Cobos

Chapter 6

Speech and Language Alterations in Dementia Syndromes 107

Jeffrey L. Cummings and D. Frank Benson

Part III: ORAL AND WRITTEN LANGUAGE DISORDERS

Chapter 9

Alfredo Ardila, Maria Victoria Lopez, and Eugenia Solano

Part IV: BASAL GANGLIA AND COGNITIVE ACTIVITY

Chapter 10

Feggy Ostrosky-Solis, Ignacio Madrazo, Rene Drucker-Colin,
and Luis Quintanar

Chapter 11

Roberto A. Prado-Alcalá

Part V: RECOVERY FROM BRAIN DAMAGE

Chapter 12

Brain Organization
of Language and
Cognitive Processes

I

Theoretical and Technical Approaches

Microgenesis
Historical Review and Current Studies

ROBERT E. HANLON and JASON W. BROWN

Currently, there is renewed interest in process-oriented approaches to the study of mental phenomena. In this chapter we review one of the more established approaches of this type, that of microgenesis. Originating from assumptions on the structural development of thought by the early experimental psychologists of Würzburg and Leipzig, the fundamental principles of microgenesis have been progressively elaborated.

First, a definition of the term, or rather a set of definitions, to specify and delimit the process that this term denotes. Microgenesis refers to the structural development of a cognition (idea, percept, act) through qualitatively different stages. The temporal period of this development extends from the inception of the cognition to its final representation in consciousness or actualization (expression) in behavior. In theoretical work on microgenesis, two major schools of thought can be distinguished, in terms of experimental and quasi-experimental methods utilized to demonstrate this process. These two schools relate to the microgeny of thoughts and the microgeny of percepts. Flavell and Draguns (1957) noted this methodological division but cautioned against any assumptions regarding a functional dichotomy.

EARLY STUDIES

Approaches to the analysis of the microgenesis of thought predominantly entail the description and interpretation of the microtemporal se-

ROBERT E. HANLON • Department of Psychology, City College of the City University of New York, New York, New York 10031.   JASON W. BROWN • Department of Neurology, New York University Medical Center, New York, New York 10016.

ries of conceptual stages that unfold, following the presentation of a stimulus, to a behavioral response. This approach lends itself to clinical application and to the interpretation of thought disorders and cognitive disorganization in various pathological populations. Such microgenetic models have been explored by a small group of theorists including Brown (1977), Ey (1950), Schilder (1951, 1953), and Werner (1956). Werner, in fact, is credited with coining the term *microgenesis* in translation of the German word *Aktualgenese*. The microprocessing approach of these clinicians incorporates the Jacksonian principle of hierarchical organization within the stage model of microgenetic progression. Investigations in perceptual microgenesis have been conducted in a very different manner with a stronger emphasis on stimulus properties and control. The classic experimental paradigm consists in the repeated presentation of a stimulus after an initially obscured or fragmented stage, through subsequent stages of increasing clarity, until the stimulus becomes clearly differentiated and complete. Draguns (1984, p. 5) notes that this approach "involves progressions of stimuli from maximal or pronounced information deprivation to the presentation of adequate or optimal amounts of information for the response or the decision at hand." While this methodological design was originally developed by Sander (1928), later experimentalists who have utilized and expanded on this technique with normals and pathological groups include Draguns (1967), Draguns and Multari (1961), Flavell (1956), Froelich (1978, 1984), Kragh (1955), and Smith (1956, 1984).

   This discussion will begin with a review of the historical development of microgenetic theory and experimentation (see also Brown, 1972, 1977, 1988a; Flavell & Draguns, 1957). Despite the methodological drawbacks of the introspective approach to the study of psychological processes, the work of the Würzburg group around the turn of the century produced the conceptual precursors of microgenesis. Humphrey (1963) reviewed in detail early experiments by Mayer and Orth (1901) and Marbe (1901). Though crude, these experiments led to the description of a nonsensory or imageless event or state of consciousness immediately following the presentation of a stimulus that could not be analyzed, termed the *Bewusstseinslage*. In an attempt to elucidate the *Bewusstseinslage* of meaning, Messer (1906) delineated a tripartite model of meaning from subjects' responses following the presentation of a word. According to Messer, the *Bewusstseinslage* constituted an intermediate or transitional stage between the initial direct derivation of the word's meaning from its presentation and the accessory image of meaning.

   Ach (1905) expanded the Würzburg doctrine through studies on awareness or the experience of knowing (*Wissen*). Through elaborate experiments on sensory reactions, Ach proposed a second stage of imageless knowing, which he termed *Bewusstheit*. This stage of awareness and expectation represented a phase in the process characterized by willed and directed thought. In other words, following the impalpable *Bewusstseins-*

lage, during which there occurred only the mere apprehension of a thought, the process advances to the *Bewusstheit,* at which point there is a distinct, yet vague, awareness, which constitutes a state of imageless knowing.

Following these early Würzburger proposals on the dynamic nature of imageless thought and particularly the transitional stages of thought formation, Pick (1913) and Jung (1919) presented theoretical models of thought development based on temporal hierarchies. From clinical experience in aphasia, Pick delineated four hypothetical stages through which thought develops in the process of language production. The first of the two pre-linguistic stages consisted of the initial formulation of the thought as a loose structural assembly of components. A stage of structural thought then emerges during which the predicative aspects are arranged. The third stage involves the development of the pattern for the utterance, and finally, word choice in conformity with this pattern (see De Bleser, 1987).

Jung's hierarchical model developed in relation to work on word associations. According to Jung, in the "apperceptive" process cognition progressed from an immediate superficial response that is ordinarily suppressed, through a contextual stage such as that of the phrase, and finally to a semantic level of denotative and connotative response. Pick (1931) described a comparable three-stage model, the first stage consisting of the initial recognition of the physical attributes of the word, the second of access to the word's "meaning sphere" or its position in conceptual space, and third, the determination of its grammatical character.

PERCEPTGENESIS

Until this time, process-oriented studies and theories were concerned with the microdevelopment of thought and language. The influence of the Gestalt movement, however, gave rise to experiments on the temporal development of percepts. Sander (1928) presented a theory of perception in which this perceptual microdevelopment was referred to as *Aktualgenese* (momentary genesis). The basic premise of this theory was that the process of perception consisted of several phases, which develop from an initial stage of a diffuse, undifferentiated percept through subsequent stages of differentiation and discrimination, leading to a distinct configuration. Sander described four discrete phases of perceptual microdevelopment. Initially, there is a stage of an amorphous undifferentiated percept. Next, the percept achieves course figure-ground properties. The third stage is pre-Gestalt (*Vorgestalt*), or preconfigurational, and is viewed as a labile, preparatory phase for the subsequent derivation of a veridical object. This stage is accompanied by a transient unpleasant anticipation of structural completion.

Sander was instrumental in the development and application of experimental techniques to demonstrate microgenetic phenomena. These paradigms involved the presentation of a stimulus under obstructive or inadequate conditions (e.g., brief tachistoscopic exposure, poor illumination, peripheral location). The initial presentation was followed by a series of presentations in which there was a successive increase in clarity, distinctiveness, and/or complexity. As a result of experimental evidence provided by the Sander group, clinicians again began to theorize on pathology within a microgenetic framework. Two pathological conditions that received considerable attention were aphasia and schizophrenia.

CLINICAL APPLICATIONS

Building primarily on the findings of Sander, Conrad (1947) presented a microgenetic interpretation of aphasia. In accordance with Sander's four-phase progression in perceptual microgeny, Conrad described four levels of disorder that can appear in aphasia. Aphasic symptoms, particularly word-finding difficulty, represented an arrest in the Gestalt formation process. The highest level of disorder in this process resulted in a fully developed end-Gestalt that was qualitatively distorted. The second level, which coincides with Sander's *Vorgestalt*, consisted of incomplete structural differentiation. Next is a level of blurred figure-ground discrimination, while the lowest level is characterized by an absence of formative processing. Conrad argued that cognition is a double-edged process of differentiation and integration, and either one or both of these components are disrupted in aphasia.

Arguably the most imaginitive microgenetic framework for thought formation was provided by Schilder (1951), who drew heavily on the work of the Würzburgers, particularly Ach and Messer, and studies of imageless thought. Schilder's theory was derived from studies of psychopathology, particularly schizophrenia and the effects of brain damage. He insisted that thought disorders "can all be understood as abortive formations produced in the course of the differentiation-process of thought" (p. 513). This notion is based on the idea that a "presentation" or a vague content is progressively incorporated within the developing thought structure. On this view, thought originates in a diffuse concept of the direction the thought is to take in its structural development. The determination of this directionality conforms to the overall goal of the thought development, which is roughly established at the moment of conception. Following the establishment of a goal and the determination of the direction that must be taken in order to reach this goal, the thought develops through a series of preliminary stages, constituting the preparatory phase of thought. During this preparatory phase, mental contents—presentations—impinge on and influence the thought formation. These presentations, which may take the form of images or ideas, then function to aid in the process of constructing the thought.

Though not explicit as to the manner in which some presentations influence and are integrated in the process of thought development while others are discarded, Schilder maintained that the dual processes of similarity and contiguity play a governing role—that is, "a presentation evolves through other presentations which are associated with it by similarity and contiguity, primarily by clang and external associations" (p. 499). The idea of inclusion versus exclusion entails that presentations holding a logical relevance to the developing thought will be incorporated into its structure, while those without a logical relationship fade into the background or periphery.

One of the more intriguing aspects of Schilder's work is the contention that these early, primitive presentations that contribute to the developing thought are symbolic images that aid in the apprehension of meaning. Moreover, these preparatory presentations have a tendency to fuse with associated presentations, as well as the capacity for alteration and transformation in response to emotional influences.

The direction of this process is a progressive evolvement toward object-directed, reality-oriented thought. Two major phases were differentiated within this unidirectional process, along with the primary determinants of the progression within each phase. Subjective, wish-determined symbolic images of the preparatory stages were referred to as the sphere. The thought structures that arise from this sphere show a progressive striving for objectivity in a manner that increasingly conforms to the rules of logic and the nature of reality. In this way the structure finally achieves the form of a concept. This conceptual phase represents the elaboration and structuration of the symbolic images of the sphere toward objectivity, resulting in the clear realization of the meaning content of the thought.

As mentioned, Schilder's theory of microgenesis is vast and encompassing, especially with regard to the interpretation of different forms of impaired cognitive processing in various pathological conditions. A fundamental idea in his writings is that the process of thought development recapitulates the phyloontogeny of cognition. In addition, and in keeping with the Jacksonian idea of hierarchical organization, Schilder (1953) concludes that this developmental progression occurs through the psychic "energy-exchanges" between the neural levels in the hierarchy. Schizophrenic thought disorders, expressive and receptive aphasia, the cognitive impairments such as dementia, agnosia, apraxia—essentially the entire realm of neuropsychology—reflects an incomplete development through the microgenetic levels of cognition.

Another major microgenetic theorist was Werner (1956), who set forth two basic assumptions: "First, the functions underlying abnormal behavior are in their essence not different from those underlying normal

behavior. Second, any human activity such as perceiving, thinking, act-
ing, etc., is an unfolding process, and this unfolding of microgenesis,
whether it takes seconds or hours or days, occurs in developmental sequence" (p. 347). Drawing on the work of Pick and Schilder, as well as his
own experiments, he described the semantic spheres through which linguistic processes develop in microgenetic progression. In early tachistoscopic experiments, subjects reported that verbal stimuli aroused feelings
of meanings or experiences of the semantic sphere of a stimulus prior to
the articulation of the word. Werner elaborated on the dynamic character
of this sphere of cognition in terms of "organismic involvement."

These organismic factors were revealed during the genesis of a percept—perceptgenesis—prior to actual word recognition. One such factor
involves a vague awareness or impression of the meaning sphere of
words, such as the feeling of warmth aroused by the initial, brief tachistoscopic exposure of the stimulus "gentle wind." Aspects of direc-
tional or intensity properties of the stimulus word then follow. Contextual
or situational aspects of the experience of word meaning may also develop prior to full realization and discrimination of word form.

Werner extended these microdevelopmental findings in normals on
the word recognition paradigm to aphasics in confrontation naming. He
noted that "in many instances, aphasic cognitions emerge in form of
organismic-bodily reactions which seem to be comparable to the responses of our normal subjects" (p. 349). Responses reflecting these organismic-bodily factors entailed verbalizations consistent with the action
sphere of the stimulus item (i.e., "blowing" in response to the picture of a
trumpet). Similarly, the impression of a direction or vector generated in
normals on word recognition were also formed in aphasics in object naming. While unable to generate the accurate name, aphasics were able to
access and describe the "vectorial-physiognomonic" character of the
word. In accordance with the third feature of spheric cognition demonstrated in the percept-genetic studies—the achievement of "atmospheric-
contextual" properties of words—a comparable picture was seen in aphasics. In Werner's view this feature was exemplified by the achievement of
the categorical sphere to which the object belonged. Further, depending
on task requirements, the contextual nature of the stimulus words may
appear in production of either the semantic or the grammatical category of
the item. In addition, he believed that the form of a given paraphasia
reflects the spheric character at which derailment in the microdevelopmental progression occurred.

In studies of perceptual disorders such as agnosia, Pötzl (1960) noted
the recurrence (intrusion) of unreported elements in subsequent object
descriptions. For example, a green asparagus stalk that was not reported
on one task might recur in confabulatory form as a green tie, in the description of a person a few moments later. Pötzl confirmed this effect in

normal subjects with tachistoscopic methods. He briefly presented scenes to subjects and found that unreported fragments were integrated into dreams and could be recovered in morning dream reports. Fisher (1960) confirmed these subliminal effects. The implications of these findings, that subconscious residues are linked to early stages in object perception, and that the symptoms of object breakdown can be reproduced through experiments in percept formation, were a major theme in Pötzl's writings (see Brown, 1988b) and played a prominent role in subsequent research on perceptgenesis.

The organodynamic theory of Ey (1950) represents another process model based on the idea of evolutionary levels of cognition. Symptomatic manifestations of psychosis and dementia reflect various levels of disorganization of consciousness. Evans (1972) contributed a detailed summary of Ey's theory. Drawing on the work of Jackson and Freud, Ey incorporates their concepts into an organodynamic theory of consciousness. The concept of dissolution of function as the basis of psychopathological symptomatology was derived from H. Jackson and Herbert Spencer. The process of dissolution entails both evolution and hierarchic order. Ey took the concept of repression from psychoanalytic theory but considered it conscious activity necessary for the organization of actuality. Ey believed consciousness to be a dynamic, nonlocalized activity in which the various cognitive processes participate, not merely an end result of this evolutionary progression. Rather, it is the actualization of the collective contribution of each level within this hierarchical process.

> The structure of consciousness represents a power of legislation, of control, of order and direction. The pathology of mental illness is a process of regression. But the process is an organically determined one in the same way that the symbolic elaboration of dreams occurs in and by sleep. Symptomatology merely indicates the level of dissolution at one point in time and to consider a symptom in isolation from the pathological process clouds the issue. (Evans, 1972, p. 418)

Ey elaborated three levels of disorganization of consciousness in psychosis that, together with the clinical expression of their respective disorders, conform to a hierarchical gradient of conscious organization. The highest level of psychotic disorganization within this model, the manic-depressive level, represents a breakdown in the temporal structure of consciousness. The development of control over psychological time is the most recent ontogenetic acquisition of consciousness. The next level in the hierarchy, that of delusion and hallucination, represents a dissolution of spatial orientation within the field of consciousness. This spatial component refers to existential space or the manner in which one represents the world. This conscious representation of the world develops through the structural process of thought formation that is based on the construction and incorporation of reality-oriented images. When this representational process breaks down, the subjective and objective components of imagery become confused. Delusions and hallucinations reflect the eruption of subjective imaginal components into the field of consciousness and a general disorganization of existential space. There is a detachment and projection of the content of thought.

Ey's lowest level of disorganization of consciousness is the confusional, oneiroid level. Consciousness is no longer constructed into a phenomenal field and is unable to represent a world of reality. Oneirism, the pathological dream state, is therefore a manifestation of the deepest level of conscious disorganization, which may be characterized as a disruption at a very primitive stage of thought formation. The structural components of developing consciousness are undifferentiated and fragmented, resulting in a miasma of confusing images.

More recently, Brown (see 1988a) has extended the microgenetic concept to the interpretation of symptoms of brain damage in developing a structural model of hierarchic levels through which the process of cognitive formation unfolds. In this model, the microgeny of acts and percepts is held to be identical to that for language, or affect, while other cognitive functions, such as thought or memory, are interpreted in fundamentally the same way. A basic assumption is that the symptoms of brain damage, like those of psychopathology, represent a premature exposure of preliminary levels in the microstructure of cognition that are normally transformed. On this view, symptoms take on a new meaning; they are not aberrations of brain injury but pieces of preliminary mentation that can be used to reconstruct the sequence of normal cognitive processing. Another assumption is that cognitions unfold in a vertical, unidirectional (bottom-up) manner over distributed anatomical systems, and that the sequence of this unfolding is the same as that in which the anatomical systems appeared in the course of forebrain evolution. In other words, microgeny retraces the phyletic history of brain development. The significance of this work is that it provides a neurological framework for what has been to date largely a psychological theory, and attempts to fill in the detail of level-to-level transformation using the clinical material as a guide to the processing that is taking place.

EXPERIMENTAL STUDIES

Returning to experimental psychology and the classic microgenetic methods handed down from Sander, there was comparatively little work on perceptgenesis from the 1930s through the mid-1950s. This lack of microgenetic and other process-oriented approaches was due chiefly to the predominance of behaviorism throughout this time. However, with renewed interest in information processing and mediational activity, there has been a modest renewal of microgenetic research (Draguns, 1984). Still, there are only a limited number of researchers actively involved in microgenetic experimentation. This research continues to be conducted mainly in Europe, most notably by Froelich and his group at the University of Mainz, Smith at Lund University, and Kragh at the University of Oslo.

Except for Werner's comparative-developmental studies (1948) at Clark University, Dragun's continuation of earlier work with Flavell (Flavell & Draguns, 1957), and Rimoldi's (1960, 1967) work on problem solving, experimental techniques and microgenetic theory have not found a firm foothold in America.

Froelich (1984) addressed the functional frame of reference for microgenetic procedures with respect to objectives and alternative methods. As outlined, the standard method of stimulus presentation entails the presentation of a patterned stimulus in a manner that provides for a sequential (trial-to-trial) increase in clarity, distinctiveness, or complexity. The subject must cope with an obscured, obstructed, too brief, or fragmented informational pattern that delays the formation of a stable cognitive response. Froelich (1978) proposed that the motivational force underlying the microdevelopment may be conceptualized as "effort after coping with ambiguity." In terms of information processing, these conditions induce a fractionated evolvement through a series of qualitatively different stages. With respect to information processing, one can distinguish two main experimental procedures. Merogenetic techniques entail a progression of stimulus presentations from figural fragmentation to an intact configurational whole. This procedure elicits imaginal activity, guessing and hypothesizing through the process of sequential comparison. Hologenetic techniques are based on a progressive change in the energy level of presentation of a figurally intact stimulus (i.e., luminosity, exposure time, clarity). These procedures reveal the evolvement of figure-ground discriminations through the stages of meaning assessment (Froelich, 1984).

In Scandinavia, primarily through the work of the Lund group (Kragh, 1955; Kragh & Smith, 1970; Smith & Danielsson, 1982), microgenetic research has progressed within the domain of percept-genetic approaches to personality. Kragh (1955) described changes in thematic content on merogenetic procedures from a psychodynamic perspective. These changes were consistent with microgenetic stages progressing from ambiguity to stabilization. More recently, Smith and his group have employed experimental procedures based on microgenetic principles in the assessment and differentiation of various psychopathological populations within a psychoanalytic frame of reference. Experimentation with serial afterimages (Smith, Fries, Andersson, & Reid, 1971; Smith & Kragh, 1967) demonstrated that successive change in the size of microgenetic afterimage serials could discriminate schizophrenia, depression, and anxiety states. Two tachistoscopic procedures, the Meta-Contrast Technique (MCT; Kragh & Smith, 1970) and the Defense Mechanism Test (DMT; Kragh, 1969; Westerlundh, 1976, 1984), in which incongruent and/or threatening stimuli are successively presented in order to induce anxiety and perceptual defenses, have been utilized in the assessment of normal and psychopathological personality organization.

Smith and Danielsson (1982) have applied these experimental techniques in percept-genetic studies of defensive strategies in Swedish schoolchildren. Incorporating psychoanalytic concepts and Piagetian ideas on cognitive development within a "dynamic-developmental perspective," they revealed "a series of transitions in anxiety manifestations and defensive strategies from early preschool age to adolescence" (p. 190). Johanson, Risberg, Silfverskiold, and Smith (1986) have also used MCT anxiety responses as activation stimuli during rCBF measures in patients with anxiety neurosis. Anxiety provocation resulted in a significant increase in regional blood flow in the left frontoorbital area.

Cegalis and colleagues at Syracuse (Cegalis, 1973; Cegalis & Leen, 1977; Cegalis & Young, 1974) studied the role of conflict in microgenesis. On the assumption that "disequilibration is a necessary condition for extended microgenetic development" (Cegalis, 1984, p. 108), Cegalis has utilized different types of stimulus distortions as disequilibrating situations in the demonstration of individual differences in the reactions to conflict.

CONCLUSION

This is a brief overview of some clinical and experimental work from a microgenetic perspective. Currently, there is little work from this theoretical angle but there is considerable interest in its applicability, provoked in large part by such findings as those of "blindsight," early semantic activation, behavior without awareness, and so on, which cannot easily be resolved within existing models. One also senses a growing dissatisfaction with old center and pathway theories and the newer modular or componential accounts to which they have given rise, for these also cannot deal with the richness and variety of normal and abnormal behavior, and they are fatally uncoupled from evolutionary and other process-oriented studies of brain function. In the final analysis, however, the test of the microgenetic model will rest on brain-imaging, electrical, magnetoencephalographic, or other studies that have the capacity to record the sequence of entrainment or engagement of specific brain systems in a brief creative or behavioral performance. This is an important goal for future research.

Ultimately, our concept of the mind is linked to our concept of the world around us. This is no less true for cognitivist or AI theories of mind than for the microgenetic theory. Thus, microgenesis entails that objects in the world are the end products of a chain of events in the mind, not a starting point in a piecemeal constructive process. In this sense, the microgenetic idea seems to be bound up with an idealist stand on the nature of externality. Microgenesis takes a strong position with regard to this question, so that the data supporting microgenetic theory can be taken as evidence for the correctness of its epistemological basis.

Similarly, the notion that representations develop out of subsurface stages, levels beneath awareness, has implications for our understanding of what a mental representation is. What it definitely is not is its propositional or perceptual content, for this is only the tip of its structure. On the microgenetic view, conscious representations are not the instigators of behavior but are rather outcomes of the processing rising from below. This clearly has profound consequences for our views on volition and agency. In fact, current physiological work lends support to the idea that actions develop prior to our awareness of them, and that the sense of volition does not stand behind and direct behavior but is given to awareness on the heels of the action development. These philosophical issues, and their admittedly somewhat unpalatable solutions, are deeply woven into the fabric of microgenetic thinking, perhaps accounting for some of the resistance to this concept. But the very fact that our idea of what the world is depends so importantly on our theory of mind and brain is precisely the reason why this theory is worth a closer look.

REFERENCES

Ach, N. (1905). *Über die Willenstatigheit und das Denken*. Gottingen: Vandenhoeck and Ruprecht.

Brown, J. W. (1972). *Aphasia, apraxia and agnosia: Clinical and theoretical aspects*. Springfield, IL: Thomas.

Brown, J. W. (1977). *Mind, brain, and consciousness*. New York: Academic Press.

Brown, J. W. (1988a). *The life of the mind: Selected papers*. Hillsdale, NJ: Erlbaum.

Brown, J. W. (1988b). *Classics in neuropsychology: Selected papers on agnosia and apraxia*. Hillsdale, NJ: Erlbaum.

Cegalis, J. A. (1973). Prism distortion and accommodtive change. *Perception and Psychophysics, 13*, 494–498.

Cegalis, J. A. (1984). On the role of conflict in microgenesis. In W. Froehlich, G. Smith, J. Draguns, & U. Hentschel (Eds.), *Psychological processes in cognition and personality*. Washington, DC: Hemisphere.

Cegalis, J. A., & Leen, D. (1977). Individual differences in responses to induced perceptual conflict. *Perceptual and Motor Skills, 44*, 991–998.

Cegalis, J. A., & Young, R. (1974). The effect of inversion-induced conflict on field-dependence. *Journal of Abnormal Psychology, 83*, 373–379.

Conrad, K. (1947). Über den Begriff der Vorgestalt und seine Bedeutung für die Hirnpathologie. *Nervenarzt, 18*, 289–293.

De Bleser, R. (1987). From agrammatism to paragrammatism: German aphasiological traditions and grammatical disturbances. *Cognitive Neuropsychology, 4,* 187–256.

Draguns, J. (1967). Affective meaning of reduced stimulus input: A study by means of the semantic differential. *Canadian Journal of Psychology, 21,* 231–241.

Draguns, J. (1984). Microgenesis by any other name . . . In W. Froehlich, G. Smith, J. Draguns, & U. Hentschel (Eds.), *Psychological processes in cognition and personality.* Washington, DC: Hemisphere.

Draguns, J., & Multari, G. (1961). Recognition of perceptually ambiguous stimuli in grade school children. *Child Development, 32,* 541–550.

Evans, P. (1972). Henri Ey's concepts of the organization of consciousness and its disorganization: An extension of Jacksonian theory. *Brain, 95,* 413–440.

Ey, H. (1950–1954). *Études psychiatriques* (Vols. 1–3). Paris: Desclée de Brouwer.

Fisher, C. (1960). Introduction: Preconscious stimulation in dreams, associations, and images. *Psychological Issues, 2,* 1–40.

Flavell, J. H. (1956). Abstract thinking and social behavior in schizophrenia. *Journal of Abnormal Social Psychology, 52,* 208–211.

Flavell, J. H., & Draguns, J. (1957). A microgenetic approach to perception and thought. *Psychological Bulletin, 54,* 197–217.

Froehlich, W. D. (1978). Stress, anxiety, and the control of attention: A psychophysiological approach. In C. D. Spielberger & I. G. Sarason (Eds.), *Stress and anxiety* (Vol. 5). Washington, DC: Hemisphere.

Froehlich, W. D. (1984). Microgenesis as a functional approach to information processing through search. In W. Froehlich, G. Smith, J. Draguns, & U. Hentschel (Eds.), *Psychological processes in cognition and personality.* Washington, DC: Hemisphere.

Humphrey, G. (1963). *Thinking: An introduction to its experimental psychology.* New York: Wiley.

Johanson, A. M., Risberg, J., Silfverskiold, P., & Smith, G. (1986). Regional changes in cerebral blood flow during increased anxiety in patients with anxiety neurosis. In U. Hentschel, G. Smith, & J. G. Draguns (Eds.), *The roots of perception.* Amsterdam: Elsevier North-Holland.

Jung, C. G. (1919). *Studies in word association* (M. D. Eder, Trans.). New York: Moffat.

Kragh, U. (1955). *The actual-genetic model of perception-personality.* Lund: Gleerup; Copenhagen: Munksgaard.

Kragh, U. (1969). *DMT-defense mechanism test.* Stockholm: Skandinaviska Testforlaget.

Kragh, U., & Smith, G. J. W. (Eds.). (1970). *Percept-genetic analysis.* Lund: Gleerup.

Marbe, K. (1901). *Experimentell-psychologische Untersuchungen über das Urteil.* Leipzig: Engelmann.

Mayer, A., & Orth, J. (1901). *Zeitschrift für Psychologie und Physiologie der Sinnesorgan, 26.*

Messer, A. (1906). *Archives Gesamte Psychologie, 8,* 1–224.

Pick, A. (1913). *Die agrammatischen Sprachstorungen.* Berlin: Springer.

Pick, A. (1931). Aphasie. In A. Bethe & G. von Bergmann (Eds.), *Handbuch der normalen und pathologischen Physiologie* (Vol. 15). Berlin: Springer.

Pötzl, O. (1960). The relationship between experimentally induced dream images and indirect vision. *Psychological Issues, 2,* 41–120.

Rimoldi, H. J. A. (1960). Problem solving as a process. *Educational and Psychological Measurement, 20,* 249–260.

Rimoldi, H. J. A. (1967). Thinking and language. *Archives of General Psychiatry, 17,* 568–576.

Sander, F. (1928). Experimentelle Ergebnisse der Gestaltpsychologie. In E. Becher (Ed.), *10 Kongres bericht experimentelle Psychologie.* Jena: Fischer.

Schilder, P. (1951). On the development of thoughts. In D. Rapaport (Ed.), *Organization and pathology of thought.* New York: Columbia University Press.

Schilder, P. (1953). *Medical psychology*. New York: International Universities Press.

Smith, G. J. W. (1956). Review of U. Kragh's "The actual-genetic model of perception-personality." *Theoria, 22,* 61–69.

Smith, G. J. W. (1984). Stabilization and automatization of perceptual activity over time. In W. Froelich, G. Smith, J. Draguns, & U. Hentschel (Eds.), *Psychological processes in cognition and personality*. Washington, DC: Hemisphere.

Smith, G. J. W., & Danielsson, A. (1982). *Anxiety and defensive strategies in childhood and adolescence*. New York: International Universities Press.

Smith, G. J. W., Fries, I., Andersson, A. L., & Reid, J. (1971). Diagnostic exploitation of visual after-effect measures in a moderately depressive patient group. *Scandinavian Journal of Psychology, 12,* 67–79.

Smith, G. J. W., & Kragh, U. (1967). A serial afterimage experiment in clinical diagnostics. *Scandinavian Journal of Psychology, 8,* 52–64.

Werner, H. (1948). *Comparative psychology of mental development* (2nd ed.). New York: International Universities Press.

Werner, H. (1956). Microgenesis and aphasia. *Journal of Abnormal Social Psychology, 52,* 347–353.

Westerlundh, B. (1976). *Aggression, anxiety and defense*. Lund: Gleerup.

Westerlundh, B. (1984). Perceptgenesis and the experimental study of conflict and defense. In W. Froehlich, G. Smith, J. Draguns, & U. Hentschel (Eds.), *Psychological processes in cognition and personality*. Washington, DC: Hemisphere.

2

Fractionation of Spatial Cognition following Focal and Diffuse Brain Damage

DEAN C. DELIS and AMY M. BIHRLE

Visuospatial dysfunction denotes a constellation of perceptual and constructional deficits in which the ability to organize visual features into perceptual wholes is lost or impaired. Despite the high incidence of visuospatial deficits following brain damage, there have been relatively few neuropsychological investigations of visuospatial dysfunction relative to the large number of studies of aphasia. Several reasons may underlie this disparity. While the structure of language is discrete and readily observable (Luria, 1966), the structure of visuospatial cognition is much more elusive. Visuospatial structure, unlike linguistic structure, does not contain temporally discrete entities, such as phonemes and words, but must be inferred from perceptual judgments and visuospatial constructions. This diffuse quality hinders the development of a grammar of visuospatial thinking (Chomsky, 1965; Fillmore, 1971). Additionally, specific brain lesions often interrupt aspects of linguistic processes in well-defined ways, enabling the development of reliable taxonomies of aphasias (Geschwind, 1970; Goodglass & Kaplan, 1972). In contrast, when visuospatial abilities are disrupted by brain damage, the nature of the impairment is difficult to characterize in a precise manner. Not surprisingly, one rarely refers to visuospatial syndromes resulting from specific brain lesions; instead, difficulties on visuospatial tasks tend to be amalgamated

DEAN C. DELIS • San Diego Veterans Administration Medical Center, Department of Psychiatry, University of California-San Diego, School of Medicine, San Diego, California 92161.   AMY M. BIHRLE • The Salk Institute for Biological Studies, University of California-San Diego, and San Diego State University, San Diego, California 92138.

into one category and referred to as "visuospatial dysfunction," "constructional apraxia," or "constructional difficulties."

HISTORICAL PERSPECTIVE

Visuospatial difficulties in neurological patients were first noted by Hughlings Jackson in 1876. He coined the term *imperception* to refer to a wide range of spatial deficits, including the inability to recognize familiar faces, find one's way around the environment, and dress oneself. Jackson implicated the posterior region of the right hemisphere in spatial processing. In 1934 Kleist introduced the term *constructional apraxia*, which, he posited, resulted from a disconnection between the perceptual and motor regions of the cortex. The term *constructional apraxia* was later extended beyond its original meaning of disconnection to include any visuospatial impairment. Critchley (1953), for example, defined constructional apraxia as "an executive defect within a visuospatial domain." Benson and Barton (1970) later cautioned against the misapplication of the term and proposed that *constructional disability* be used as the more general term for visuospatial disorders, with *constructional apraxia* being reserved for cases in which a disconnection exists between preserved perceptual and motor skills. More recently, Benton (1982) proposed a classificatory schema based on tasks used to clinically assess different aspects of spatial cognitive processing (e.g., visuospatial, visuoconstructive).

Extensive studies of visuospatial dysfunction did not emerge until as late as the 1960s. Initial studies concluded that the right hemisphere subserved nonverbal, visuospatial processing while the left hemisphere was specialized for language processing. This dichotomy was bolstered by studies demonstrating that right-hemisphere-damaged (RHD) patients performed poorly on tests of perceptual closure (Benton & Van Allen, 1968; Newcombe & Russell, 1969; Warrington & James, 1967), visual localization (Hannay, Varney, & Benton, 1976; Warrington & Rabin, 1970), and line perception (Benton, Hannay, & Varney, 1975), whereas patients with left-hemisphere damage (LHD) performed at the same level as neurologically intact normal control subjects. Other investigations, however, challenged the simple verbal/nonverbal dichotomy for hemispheric specialization. These studies found that LHD patients were also impaired on visuospatial tasks, though not as severely or as frequently as RHD patients, suggesting that both hemispheres have visuospatial capabilities, with the right hemisphere commanding the superior role (De Renzi, 1982). This conclusion was consistent with studies suggesting that the right hemisphere is involved in aspects of language functioning, including, for example, comprehension of nonliteral language such as metaphor (Gardner, Brownell, Wapner, & Michelow, 1983).

Until recently, few neuropsychological studies utilized constructs developed in cognitive psychology to characterize visuospatial dysfunction following brain damage. Within the past few years, however, an increasing number of researchers have begun to investigate whether focal brain lesions disrupt specific aspects of visuospatial functioning in a predictable manner. The continued development of sophisticated theories of normal cognitive processes has assisted neuropsychologists in more precisely delineating the neural substrate of cognitive operations. Concurrently, findings in neuropsychology have provided support for theories of normal cognition (Cermak & Butters, 1972) and have provided evidence for the independence of component processes by their "separability" in the brain.

VISUAL ATTENTION

Visual attention, one aspect of visuospatial processing, has been the subject of intensive study by Posner and his colleagues. Visual detection experiments with normal subjects have demonstrated that attention can be dissociated from eye movements (Posner, 1980). Furthermore, Posner and his colleagues have provided evidence for different operations underlying attention. For example, detection of a target in the periphery is facilitated if the target is preceded by a peripheral cue; however, if no target occurs in the periphery following the peripheral cue and the subject must then detect a target at the original fixation point, an inhibition of detection occurs (Posner & Cohen, 1984). Because different aspects of attention can be facilitated or inhibited, Posner and Cohen have posited specific elementary operations in normal attention, such as moving toward a target and disengaging from a target in order to move toward a new target.

With this model as a guide, the attentional capacities of patients with unilateral parietal lobe lesions have been investigated (Posner, Walker, Friedrich, & Rafal, 1984, 1987). In earlier neuropsychological investigations, attention was regarded as a unitary function that was either spared or impaired. Posner and his colleagues provided convincing evidence that attention is disrupted in a highly selective manner following parietal lobe lesions. The parietal lobe patients' difficulty in detecting targets was not in moving toward initial target sites but in disengaging from one site in order to detect another target. Furthermore, this deficit was most apparent when the patients were cued to attend to a target on the same side of the lesion (ipsilesion) and then were presented with a target on the opposite side (contralesion). If these studies had found that all the proposed elementary operations of visual attention were equally impaired following parietal lobe lesions, then one might have concluded that attention is disrupted in a unitary manner, a result that would have been of little theoretical import for cognitive psychologists. However, the findings in the Posner et al. (1984, 1987) studies give a neuropsychological reality to the notion of separate operations in normal visual attention. In addition, these findings enhance our understanding of neuroanatomical correlates of attentional processes by more precisely describing the role of the parietal lobe in the operations of visual attention.

PARTS AND WHOLES

Historically, visuospatial dysfunction has resisted fractionation into meaningful spared and impaired components (Newcombe, 1985). A distinction between processing of parts and wholes, however, has been a central focus of theories of normal perception. The possibility that the brain has evolved to differentially process parts or details versus wholes or configurations in different cerebral regions was initially proposed in the 1940s (Patterson & Zangwill, 1944). Subsequent research with split-brain patients following commissurotomy, unilateral brain-damaged patients, and neurologically intact subjects in laterality experiments has produced convergent evidence indicating that the two cerebral hemispheres represent a division of labor in processing parts and wholes (Levy-Agristi & Sperry, 1968; Sergent & Bindra, 1982; Warrington, James, & Kinsbourne, 1966). For example, Kaplan (1983) has reported that the drawings of LHD patients often lack internal details, whereas the drawings of RHD patients frequently have omitted or distorted outer configurations. Similarly, on the Block Design subtest of the WAIS-R, Kaplan (1983) reports that LHD patients have difficulty orienting individual blocks, frequently making internal, single-block rotational errors but maintaining the outer square configuration. RHD patients, in contrast, often break the two by two or three by three square configuration of the designs. These studies have concluded that both hemispheres are essential for successful performance on visuospatial tasks, with each hemisphere contributing qualitatively different processes. In short, the left hemisphere is superior for detailed, "analytic" processing, whereas the right hemisphere is superior for configural, "holistic processing" (see Bradshaw & Nettleton, 1981, for a review).

Despite the heuristic appeal of the analytic/holistic theory of hemispheric specialization, this distinction has been criticized for both methodological and theoretical reasons (see Brownell & Gardner, 1981; Delis, Robertson, & Efron, 1986; Moscovitch, 1979). A major weakness of the distinction is that "detailed and analytic" and "configural and holistic" are imprecisely and vaguely defined. Researchers tend to infer that a particular task involves more analytic or holistic processing without explicitly operationalizing these constructs. Furthermore, investigations with both unilateral brain-damaged and split-brain patients typically use stimuli (e.g., block designs, incomplete figures, facial stimuli; see critiques by Brownell & Gardner, 1981; De Renzi, 1982; Moscovitch, 1979) in which the boundary between features perceived as "parts" and "wholes" is unclear.

Recent investigations, however, have begun to provide a more precise characterization of hemispheric asymmetry for visuospatial processing by adopting paradigms from cognitive psychology. These studies suggest that the two hemispheres are differentially specialized for processing of different structural levels of visual hierarchical stimuli. A key feature of a series of studies that we have conducted is the use of visual hierarchical stimuli that have explicit demarcation between features perceived as "parts" and "wholes." These hierarchical stimuli consist of a large (higher-level) letter or shape constructed from numerous smaller (lower-level) letters and shapes. These two-leveled stimuli are methodologically superior to those traditionally used in visuospatial studies because (1) the two levels of structure are explicitly demarcated and (2) the same type of form (letter or shape) can exist at different levels of hierarchical structure, enabling a tightly controlled test of differential response at the two levels. Studies in which these stimuli were presented centrally to normal subjects have found evidence for cognitive operations differentially sensitive to higher- and lower-level analysis (Kinchla & Wolfe, 1979; Navon, 1977). They have also found that it is relative rather than absolute size that determines whether stimuli are analyzed as higher- or lower-level forms (Navon, 1977). The use of these stimuli with brain-damaged patients is particularly important in that the ability to organize visual features into perceptual wholes is a critical aspect of perception.

STUDIES OF VISUOSPATIAL PROCESSING USING HIERARCHICAL STIMULI

In one of our first studies (Delis *et al.*, 1986), we presented visual hierarchical stimuli consisting of a large (global) form made up of numerous smaller (local) forms to unilateral brain-damaged patients and normal control subjects. Stimuli were presented individually for 2 seconds to the central visual field, followed by a 15-second distractor task. Immediately after the distractor task, a forced-choice recognition test was given by presenting four alternative hierarchical stimuli (see Figure 1). The results indicated that RHD patients were selectively impaired in recognizing forms at the global structural level, whereas LHD patients were selectively defective at recognizing forms at the local level (see Figure 2). These findings are consonant with hemispheric asymmetries reported in two

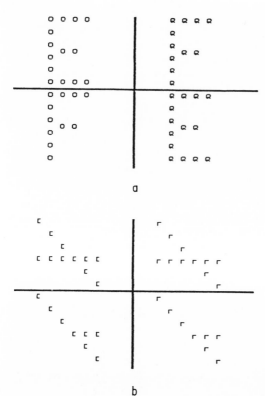

a

b

FIGURE 1. Examples of (a) linguistic hierarchical stimulus set and (b) non-linguistic hierarchical stimulus set used in the experiment.

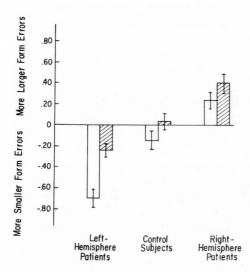

FIGURE 2. Error analysis in recognizing larger and smaller forms for the three subject groups. The LHD patients made more errors in recognizing smaller forms relative to larger forms, whereas the RHD patients made more errors in recognizing larger forms relative to smaller forms.

studies with normal subjects in which visual hierarchical stimuli were presented tachistoscopically to their visual half-fields (Martin, 1979; Sergent, 1982). For example, Sergent (1982) presented hierarchical letter stimuli to the visual half-fields of normal subjects and found a left visual-field advantage (putatively, a right-hemisphere superiority) for identification of the global letter, and a right visual-field advantage (putatively, a left-hemisphere superiority) for identification of the local level.

In a subsequent investigation (Delis, Kiefner, & Fridlund, 1988), we explored whether or not differential deficits in hierarchical processing following unilateral brain damage occur on a *constructional* task. This study was designed to tap impairments in both hierarchical and hemispatial processing within the same task across a broad range of stimuli. Deficits in hemispatial processing are common sequelae of brain damage, and other investigations have demonstrated consistently that unilateral brain damage impairs processing of visual stimuli presented in contralateral hemispace (Benton, Levin, & Van Allen, 1974; De Renzi, Faglioni, & Scotti, 1970; Heilman, Watson, & Valenstein, 1985; Samuels, Butters, & Goodglass, 1970). Three types of stimuli were used at the global and local levels: letters, shapes with established names, and shapes without established names. The stimuli pair were presented simultaneously in left and right hemispace to investigate the interaction between hierarchical and hemispatial processing. Unilateral brain-damaged patients and normal control subjects were first asked to draw the pairs of stimuli from immediate memory, and then to copy them. The findings revealed a pronounced dissociation: The RHD patients were selectively impaired in recalling the global forms relative to the local forms, whereas the LHD patients demonstrated the opposite pattern (see Figures 3 and 4). Although the unilateral brain-damaged patients were most impaired when drawing forms presented in the contralateral hemispace, the interaction between hierarchical level (global vs. local) and side of hemispace (right vs. left) was not significant, suggesting functional independence between these two aspects of visuospatial processing. Stimulus category did not differentiate the groups. This procedure thus revealed clear dissociations in global-local and hemispatial components of visuospatial processing. The results also suggest that for right-handers, the cerebral hemispheres may be functionally specialized to mediate global or local processing on both perceptual and constructive tasks.

The finding that the right hemisphere is specialized for global processing and the left for local processing has also been confirmed following commissurotomy. We had a rare opportunity (Delis, Kramer, & Kiefner, 1988) to administer hierarchical stimuli to a split-brain patient pre- and postcommissurotomy. Prior to surgery, the patient was able to represent both global and local forms in his drawings using either hand. After surgery, he was able to draw only local forms with his right hand (controlled

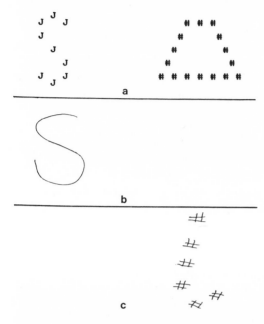

FIGURE 3. Examples of (a) pair of hierarchical stimuli, (b) drawing by an LHD patient illustrating correct construction of higher-level form presented in left hemispace, and (c) drawing by an RHD patient showing correct construction of lower-level forms presented in right hemispace.

primarily by his left hemisphere) and only global forms with his left hand (controlled primarily by his right hemisphere) (see Figures 5 and 6). His performance on a forced-choice recognition task was consistent with his drawing results: He was more accurate in recognizing global forms when pointing with his left hand and local forms when pointing with his right hand. These results strongly suggest that components of visuospatial processing can be disconnected in the same person following resection of the corpus callosum.

Up to this point, all of the procedures involved a memory or constructional component. We thus conducted a study to test whether the global–local dissociation is revealed on a purely perceptual task without memory or constructional demands (Robertson & Delis, 1986). In this experiment, a task developed by Palmer (1980) was presented to unilateral brain-damaged patients and normal control subjects. The subjects were asked to indicate in which direction an equilateral triangle appeared to point when it was either presented individually or aligned within other equilateral triangles or circles. This task enables an analysis of the influence of a more global reference frame (i.e., the aligned triangles) on the perception of more local elements (i.e., a single triangle). The procedure is well suited for brain-damaged populations because there is no time limit and it places minimal demand on motor manipulation and memory skills. The results of this experiment were consistent with our other findings: The RHD patients were influenced significantly less by the global alignment than the normal control subjects, whereas the LHD patients were influ-

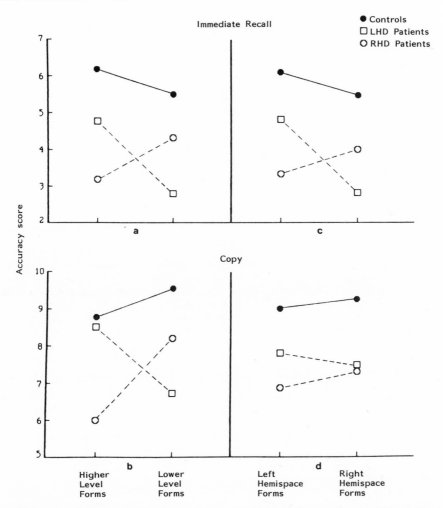

FIGURE 4. Drawing accuracy for (a and b) forms at higher and lower levels of hierarchical stimuli, and (c and d) forms presented in left and right hemispace, for controls (●), LHD patients (□), and RHD patients (○).

enced significantly more than the normal control subjects. These findings, in concert with other data, suggest that differential processing of levels of visual hierarchical structure has a biological basis in the brain.

FREQUENCY AND SEVERITY OF VISUOSPATIAL DEFICITS

Past investigations have been equivocal concerning the frequency and severity of visuospatial dysfunction following unilateral brain damage. As noted above, one group of studies reported that visuospatial im-

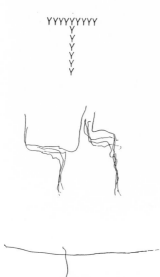

FIGURE 5. Examples of (a) target hierarchical stimulus, (b) drawing done with patient's right hand postcommissurotomy illustrating accurate representation of only the lower-level form, and (c) drawing done with his left hand postcommissurotomy illustrating accurate representation of only the higher-level form

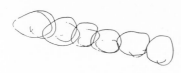

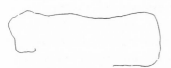

FIGURE 6. Examples of (a) target hierarchical stimulus, (b) drawing done with the patient's right hand postcommissurotomy illustrating accurate representation of only the lower-level form, and (c) drawing done with his left hand postcommissurotomy illustrating accurate representation of only the higher-level form.

pairment occurs primarily after RHD (Arrigoni & De Renzi, 1964; Benton, 1967; Benton & Fogel, 1962; De Renzi and Faglioni, 1967; Hannay et al., 1976; Piercy & Smyth, 1962), whereas others have concluded that damage to either hemisphere results in equivalent visuospatial dysfunction (Benton, 1973; Benson & Barton, 1970; Black & Strub, 1976; Colombo, De Renzi, & Faglioni, 1976). These contradictory findings have raised the question of whether visuospatial functioning is subserved primarily by the right hemisphere or both hemispheres (Benton, 1985; De Renzi, 1982).

Delis, Kiefner, and Fridlund (1988) investigated severity of drawing impairment and found that RHD and LHD patients were equally impaired when the results were collapsed across global and local level forms presented in right and left hemispace. However, when drawing performance was analyzed in terms of hierarchical levels and sides of hemispace, the results clearly indicated that both hemispheres contribute qualitatively different and complementary processes to visuospatial functioning (see also Kaplan, 1983; Levy, 1974; Nebes, 1973; Sergent, 1982). At least two reasons may account for past reports of greater visuospatial dysfunction in RHD patients: (1) Impaired global processing may be manifested more saliently than deficient local processing, especially when studies employ visual stimuli that have minimal or no internal details (e.g., the outline of a geometric shape); and (2) RHD is associated with defective processing in both sides of hemispace, whereas LHD is associated with impaired processing primarily in contralateral hemispace (Heilman et al., 1985).

Further evidence indicating that both hemispheres mediate qualitatively different visuospatial processes comes from studies of facial perception. Traditionally it was thought that the right hemisphere is superior for facial processing (Benton & Van Allen, 1968). It has recently been demonstrated that the right hemisphere is superior only when holistic aspects of faces must be considered. When individual featural aspects of faces are important to the task, the left hemisphere is dominant (Parkin & Williamson, 1987; Patterson & Bradshaw, 1975; Sergent, 1982). Thus it appears that facial processing may be either primarily a right- or a left-hemisphere function, depending on the task demands.

INTRAHEMISPHERIC DISSOCIATIONS IN VISUOSPATIAL PROCESSING

Up to this point, we have discussed dissociations in visuospatial processing between the two hemispheres. Visuospatial dissociations, however, have also been reported following lesions within the right hemisphere. Newcombe and colleagues found that patients with focal damage involving either a superior occipital-parietal or inferior occipital-tem-

poral pathway within the right hemisphere demonstrated different profiles of scores on clinical visuoperceptual and visuospatial tasks (Newcombe, Ratcliff, & Damasio, 1987; Newcombe & Russell, 1969).
Specifically, patients with superior occipital-parietal damage were impaired on some visuospatial tasks (e.g., maze learning) but not on others
(e.g., Mooneys visual closure task). Conversely, patients with inferior oc-
cipital-temporal damage demonstrated the opposite profile. An important
next step will be to characterize explicitly the component processes associated with these performance differences on clinical tests. Newcombe's
findings are consistent with physiological data based on ablation studies
in monkeys (Ungerleider & Mishkin, 1982) suggesting two cortical visual
processing pathways. Ungerleider and Mishkin (1982) proposed that the
function of the inferior temporal pathway is visual discrimination and
thus is chiefly concerned with the shape of the visual stimulus. In contrast, the function of the superior parietal pathway is analysis of spatial
relations and the location of objects in space.

TOWARD AN INTEGRATION OF INTRA- AND INTERHEMISPHERIC DISSOCIATIONS IN VISUOSPATIAL PROCESSING

Robertson, Lamb, and Knight (in press) have recently conducted an
important study aimed at integrating findings in the neuropsychological
and cognitive literatures on visuospatial processing. As noted earlier, it
has been well established that unilateral brain damage results in a dissociation between global and local processing, with RHD disrupting
global processing and LHD disrupting local processing. Furthermore, the
posterior parietal region plays a major role in attention (Posner et al.,
1984) and spatial relations, while temporal lobe damage disrupts one's
ability to identify objects (Newcombe et al., 1987; Newcombe & Russell,
1969). The relative contribution of attentional and/or perceptual mechanisms to the global–local dissociation found following unilateral right-
and left-hemisphere damage has heretofore been unexplored.

Robertson et al. (in press) employed a procedure developed by
Kinchla and his colleagues (Kinchla, Solis-Macias, & Hoffman, 1983) to
test whether the global–local dissociation in unilateral brain-damaged
patients could be attributed to controlled attentional processes, passive
perceptual processes, or both. The type of attention examined in this
study was defined as "controlled distribution of attention over the visual
field," and perceptual processing was defined as "direct automatic encoding of stimulus features." In this investigation, unilateral brain-
damaged patients and normal control subjects were presented with hierarchical stimuli and asked to identify one of two targets presented at

either the global or local levels. Stimuli were presented in three experimental conditions: a No Bias condition in which there was an equal probability of the target's appearing at either the global or the local level, a Local Bias condition in which there was a 75% probability of the target's appearing at the local level, and a Global Bias condition in which there was a 75% probability of the target's appearing at the global level. Predictably, subjects who are able to distribute attention between the global and local levels should show improved performance in the biasing conditions. The unilateral brain-damaged patients included a group with damage restricted to the right temporal-parietal region (RTP) and two groups of left-hemisphere-damaged patients with lesions in either the superior temporal gyrus (LSTG) or the rostral inferior parietal lobule (LIPL) as determined by CT scan.

The authors report three important findings. First, attentional processes in the LIPL patients were disrupted; that is, their performance did not vary as a function of biasing condition. In contrast, the LSTG group did not demonstrate an attentional disturbance. This finding is consonant with studies indicating that the parietal region of higher primates and humans plays a special role in attention (Bushnell, Goldberg, & Robinson, 1981; Mountcastle, 1978; Posner et al., 1984). More specifically, the present study suggests that the inferior parietal region is critical for the controlled distribution of attention over the visual field and between hierarchical levels. Second, overall response times were significantly lower for both global and local forms in the LTPG group than for the LIPL group and normal control group, suggesting a deficit in visual discrimination associated with temporal damage. Such an interpretation is in accord with the functional roles attributed to the two visual pathways. Third, there was a global–local dissociation between LSTG and RTP groups, but not between LIPL and RTP groups. The LSTG group showed a strong baseline advantage in identifying targets at the global level, whereas the RTP group demonstrated the opposite pattern. This finding suggests that the glocal–local dissociation previously reported with unilateral brain-damaged patients is related to perceptual, rather than attentional, mechanisms. It is also now clear that the hemispheric asymmetry observed in hierarchical processing occurs in the first few hundred milliseconds of analyzing a stimulus.

FRACTIONATION OF SPATIAL COGNITION IN DIFFUSE BRAIN PATHOLOGY

Dissociations in spatial cognition are much rarer and infrequently reported in cases of diffuse, relative to focal, brain damage. Recently, however, we have encountered a striking exception to this pattern. We conducted a study of visuospatial processing in two groups of mentally retarded subjects between the ages of 9 and 18 years; children with Williams syndrome and with Down syndrome (Bihrle, Bellugi, Delis, & Marks, in press). Although these two groups perform comparably on global measures of intelligence (mean IQ of 57) and on clinical visuo-constructive tests (e.g., block design subtest of the WISC-R), the qualitative features of their constructions are quite distinct. The Williams syndrome subjects' drawings typically show excessive attention to the parts of an object with no integration of the parts to form a coherent whole. In contrast, the Down syndrome subjects' drawings represent the outer configuration of an object, but internal details are frequently lacking. These characterizations have been systematically substantiated in a study using hierarchical stimuli. In both memory and copy conditions, the Williams syndrome subjects, like unilateral RHD patients, were significantly more impaired in global relative to local analysis, producing local forms with no attempt at representing the global figure (see Figure 7). In contrast, the Down syndrome subjects, like unilateral LHD patients, frequently produced only the global figure using a solid line and omitted the local figures completely. Thus, the interaction between subject group and hierarchical level (global–local) was highly significant, although the two groups did not differ in overall performance collapsed across global and local conditions.

These robust findings are important for a number of reasons. First, they suggest that sharp dissociations in visuospatial processing can occur in cases of diffuse brain damage, just as they occur following unilateral focal lesions. Neuroradiologic studies do not suggest that Williams syndrome or Down syndrome results in unilateral focal lesions (Jernigan, Tallal, & Bellugi, 1988). Furthermore, although it is well known that clusters of spared and impaired components of cognition occur following damage to particular regions of the brain, such patterns are infrequently reported in cases of global deterioration and may be theoretically important. Unilateral RHD typically results in relatively preserved language functioning and a proclivity for local processing. Perhaps it is not coincidental that Williams syndrome, also characterized by selectively preserved language ability relative to other cognitive functioning (Bellugi, Marks, Bihrle, & Sabo, in press; Bennett, LaVeck, & Sells, 1978; Udwin, Yule & Martin, 1986; von Armin & Engel, 1964), shows a local processing bias. In contrast, unilateral LHD is associated with language dysfunction and relatively preserved global processing. Down syndrome, as well, is marked by language ability disproportionately impaired relative to other cognitive functions (Fowler, in press) and a propensity for global processing. Further exploration of these neuropsychological profiles may aid us in understanding the interrelationship between spatial and language processing and their representation in the brain.

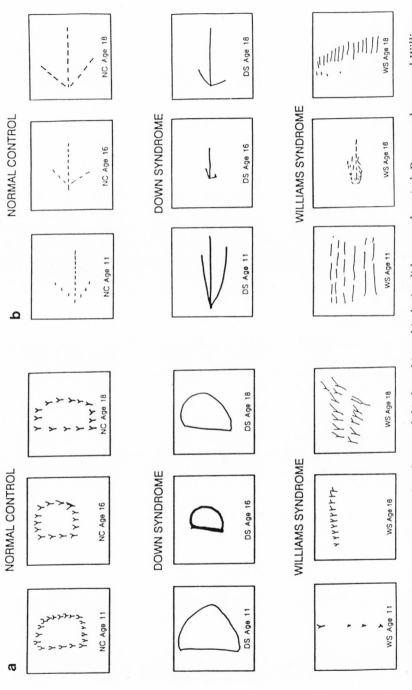

FIGURE 7. Examples of drawings of (a) letter and (b) shape hierarchical stimuli by normal control, Down syndrome, and Williams syndrome subjects in the memory condition.

Results from a pilot study we recently conducted suggest that asymmetric visuospatial profiles may also occur in some patients with Alzheimer disease. We administered the same global–local task used in the study cited above to six Alzheimer patients who showed lateralized cognitive deficits on other clinical tests. Five patients displayed normal performance on the Boston Naming Test and impaired performance on the WAIS-R Block Design subtest, whereas the other patient showed the opposite pattern. The Alzheimer patients with normal naming recalled primarily local forms, a performance similar to unilateral right CVA patients (Delis et al., 1988). In contrast, the patient with normal block constructions recalled only global forms, a performance similar to left CVA patients. These results are consistent with the finding that Alzheimer patients show significantly more lateral asymmetry of brain glucose metabolism than age-matched normal subjects (Haxby, Duara, Grady, Cutler, & Rapoport, 1985). A third group of Alzheimer patients who were impaired in both naming and block construction (but matched with the other patients in overall dementia severity; Mattis, 1976) showed less discrepancy in their recall of global and local forms with no global–local dissociation. Our results suggest that even in some cases of diffuse pathology, distinct visuospatial profiles may emerge.

CONCLUSION

Although it is difficult to characterize different aspects of visuospatial impairments, the studies cited in this chapter have been able to demonstrate selective deficits in visual attention, perception, and visuoconstruction. Recent research in neuropsychology, guided by work in cognitive psychology, has suggested that spatial cognition, like language, fractionates in precise ways following focal and diffuse brain damage.

ACKNOWLEDGMENT

This research was supported by the Medical Research Service of the Veterans Administration.

REFERENCES

Arrigoni, G., & De Renzi, E. (1964). Constructional apraxia and hemispheric locus of lesion. Cortex, 1, 180–197.
Bellugi, U., Marks, S., Bihrle, A., & Sabo, H. (in press). Dissociation between language and cognitive functions in Williams syndrome. In K. Mogford & D. Bishop (Eds.), Language development in exceptional circumstances. London: Churchill Livingstone.
Bennett, F. C., LaVeck, B., & Sells, C. J. (1978). The Williams elfin facies syndrome: The psychological profile as an aid in syndrome identification. Pediatrics, 61, 303–305.
Benson, D. F., & Barton, M. I. (1970). Disturbances in constructional ability. Cortex, 6, 19–46.

Benton, A. L. (1967). Constructional apraxia and the minor hemisphere. *Confinia Neurologica, 19,* 1–16.

Benton, A. L. (1973). Visuoconstructive disability in patients with cerebral disease: Its relationship to side of lesion and aphasic disorder. *Documenta Opthal. 34,* 67–706.

Benton, A. L. (1982). Spatial thinking in neurological patients: Historical aspects. In M. Potegal (Ed.), *Spatial abilities: Development and physiological foundations.* New York: Academic Press.

Benton, A. L. (1985). Visuoperceptual, visuospatial, and visuoconstructive disorders. In K. M. Heilman & E. Valenstein (Eds.), *Clinical neuropsychology.* New York: Oxford.

Benton, A. L., & Fogel, M. L. (1962). Three-dimensional constructional praxis. *Archives of Neurology, 7,* 347–354.

Benton, A. L., Hannay, J., & Varney, N. R. (1975). Visual perception of line direction in patients with unilateral brain disease. *Neurology, 25,* 907–910.

Benton, A. L., Levin, H. S., & Van Allen, M. W. (1974). Geographic orientation in patients with unilateral cerebral disease. *Neuropsychologia, 12,* 183–191.

Benton, A. L., & Van Allen, M. W. (1968). Impairment in facial recognition in patients with cerebral disease. *Cortex, 4,* 344–358.

Bihrle, A. M., Bellugi, U., Delis, D. C., & Marks, S. (in press). Seeing either the forest or the trees: Dissociations in visuospatial dysfunction. *Brain and cognition.*

Black, F. W., & Strub, R. L. (1976). Constructional apraxia in patients with discrete missile wounds of the brain. *Cortex, 12,* 212–220.

Bradshaw, J. L., & Nettleton, N. C. (1981). The nature of hemispheric specialization in man. *Behavioral and Brain Sciences, 4,* 51–91.

Brownell, H. H., & Gardner, H. (1981). Hemispheric specialization: Definitions, not incantations. *Behavioral and Brain Sciences, 4,* 64–65.

Bushnell, M. C., Goldberg, M. E., & Robinson, D. L. (1981). Behavioral enhancement of visual responses in monkey cerebral cortex. I. Modulation in posterior parietal cortex related to selected visual attention. *Journal of Neurophysiology, 46,* 755–772.

Cermak, L. S., & Butters, N. (1972). The role of interference and encoding in the short-term memory deficits of Korsakoff patients. *Neuropsychologia, 10,* 89–95.

Chomsky, N. A. (1965). *Aspects of the theory of syntax.* Cambridge, MA: M.I.T. Press.

Colombo, A., De Renzi, E., & Faglioni, P. (1976). The occurrence of visual neglect in patients with unilateral cerebral disease. *Cortex, 12,* 221–231.

Critcheley, M. (1953). *The parietal lobes.* London: Edward Arnold.

Delis, D. C., Kiefner, M., & Fridlund, A. J. (1988). Visuospatial dysfunction following unilateral brain damage: Dissociations in hierarchical and hemispatial analysis. *Journal of Clinical and Experimental Neuropsychology, 10,* 421–431.

Delis, D. C., Kramer, J. H., & Kiefner, M. G. (1988). Visuospatial functioning before and after commissurotomy: Disconnection in hierarchical processing. *Archives of Neurology, 45,* 123–130.

Delis, D. C., Robertson, L. C., & Efron, R. (1986). Hemispheric specialization of memory for visual hierarchical stimuli. *Neuropsychologia, 24,* 205–214.

De Renzi, E. (1982). *Disorders of spatial exploration and cognition.* New York: Wiley.

De Renzi, E., & Faglioni, P. (1967). The relationship between visuospatial impairment and constructional apraxia. *Cortex, 3,* 327–342.

De Renzi, E., Faglioni, P., & Scotti, G. (1970). Hemispheric contribution to exploration of space through the visual tactile modality. *Cortex, 6,* 191–203.

Fillmore, C. J. (1971). Types of lexical information, In D. D. Steinberg & L. A. Jakobouits (Eds.), *Semantics: An interdisciplinary reader in philosophy, linguistics, and psychology.* Cambridge: Cambridge University Press.

Fowler, A. E. (in press). The development of language structure in children with Down syndrome. In D. Cicchetti & M. Beeghly (Eds.), *Down syndrome: The developmental perspective.* New York: Cambridge University Press.

Gardner, H., Brownell, H. H., Wapner, W., & Michelow, D. (1983). Missing the point: The role of the right hemisphere in the processing of complex linguistic materials. In E. Perecman (Ed.), *Cognitive processes in the right hemisphere*. (pp. 169–191). New York: Academic Press.

Geschwind, N. (1970). The organization of language and the brain. *Science, 170*, 940–944.

Goodglass, H., & Kaplan, E. (1972). *The assessment of aphasia and related disorders*. Philadelphia: Lea & Febiger.

Hannay, H. J., Varney, N. R., & Benton, A. L. (1976). Visual localization in patients with unilateral brain disease. *Journal of Neurology, Neurosurgery and Psychiatry, 39*, 307–313.

Haxby, J. V., Duara, R., Grady, C. L., Cutler, N. R., & Rapoport, S. I. (1985). Relations between neuropsychological and cerebral metabolic asymmetries in early Alzheimer's disease. *Journal of Cerebral Blood Flow and Metabolism, 5*, 193–200.

Heilman, K. M., Watson, R. T., & Valenstein, E. (1985). Neglect and related disorders. In K. M. Heilman & E. Valenstein (Eds.), *Clinical neuropsychology*. New York: Oxford University Press.

Jackson, J. H. (1876). Case of large cerebral tumour without optic neuritis and with left hemiplegia and imperception. *Royal Opthalmological Hospital Reports, 8*, 434–444.

Jernigan, T., Tallal, P., & Bellugi, U. (1988). *Cerebral morphology of magnetic resonance imaging (MRI) in developmental cognitive disorders*. Paper presented at the International Neuropsychological Society annual meeting, New Orleans, LA.

Kaplan, E. (1983). Process and achievement revisited. In S. Wapner & B. Kaplan (Eds.), *Toward a holistic developmental psychology*. Hillsdale, NJ: Erlbaum.

Kinchla, R. A., Solis-Macias, V., & Hoffman, J. (1983). Attending to different levels of structure in a visual image. *Perception and Psychophysics, 33*, 1–10.

Kinchla, R. A., & Wolfe, J. M. (1979). The order of visual processing: Top-down, bottom-up, or middle-out. *Perception and Psychophysics, 25*, 225–231.

Kleist, K. (1934). *Gehirnpathologie*. Leipzig: Barth.

Levy, J. (1974). Cerebral asymmetries as manifested in split-brain man. In M. Kinsbourne & W. L. Smith (Eds.), *Hemispheric disconnection and cerebral function*. Springfield, IL: Thomas.

Levy-Agristi, J., & Sperry, R. W. (1968). Differential perceptual capacities in major and minor hemispheres. *Proceedings of the National Academy of Sciences, 61*, 1151.

Luria, A. R. (1966). *Higher cortical functions in man*. New York: Basic Books.

Martin, M. (1979). Local and global processing: The role of sparsity. *Memory and Cognition, 6*, 476–484.

Mattis, S. (1976). Mental status examination for organic mental syndrome in the elderly patient. In L. Bellack & T. B. Karusu (Eds.), *Geriatric psychiatry*. New York: Grune & Stratton.

Moscovitch, M. (1979). Information processing and the cerebral hemispheres. In M. S. Gazzaniga (Ed.), *The handbook of behavioral neurobiology*. New York: Plenum Press.

Mountcastle, V. B. (1978). Brain mechanisms for directed attention. *Journal of the Royal Society of Medicine, 71*, 14–28.

Navon, D. (1977). Forest before trees: The precedence of global features in visual perception. *Cognitive Psychology, 9*, 353–383.

Nebes, R. D. (1973). Perception of spatial relationships by the right and left hemispheres of commisurotomized man. *Neuropsychologia, 11*, 285–289.

Newcombe, F. (1985). Neuropsychology qua interface. *Journal of Clinical and Experimental Neuropsychology, 7*, 663–681.

Newcombe, F., Ratcliff, G., & Damasio, H. (1987). Dissociable impairments of visual and spatial processing following right posterior cerebral lesions: Clinical, neuropsychological, and anatomic evidence. *Neuropsychologia, 25*, 149–161.

Newcombe, F., & Russell, W. R. (1969). Dissociated visual perceptual and spatial deficits in focal lesions of the right hemisphere. *Journal of Neurology, Neurosurgery and Psychiatry, 32,* 73–81.

Palmer, S. E. (1980). What makes triangles point: Local and global effects in configuration of ambiguous triangles. *Cognitive Psychology, 12,* 285–305.

Parkin, A. J., & Williamson, P. (1987). Cerebral lateralisation at different stages of facial processing. *Cortex, 23,* 99–110.

Patterson, K., & Bradshaw, J. L. (1975). Differential hemispheric mediation of nonverbal stimuli. *Journal of Psychology: Human Perception and Performance, 1,* 246–252.

Patterson, A., & Zangwill, O. L. (1944). Disorders of visual space perception associated with lesions of the right cerebral hemisphere. *Brain, 67,* 331–358.

Piercy, M., & Smith, V. O. G. (1962). Right hemisphere dominance for certain nonverbal intellectual skills. *Brain, 85,* 775–790.

Posner, M. I. (1980). Orienting of attention. *Quarterly Journal of Experimental Psychology, 32,* 3–25.

Posner, M. I., & Cohen, Y. (1984). Components of visual orienting. In H. Bouma & D. Bowhuis (Eds.), *Attention and performance.* Hillsdale, NJ: Erlbaum.

Posner, M. I., Walker, J. A., Friedrich, F. J., & Rafal, R. D. (1984). Effects of parietal injury on covert orienting of visual attention. *Journal of Neuroscience, 4,* 1863–1874.

Posner, M. I., Walker, J. A., Friedrich, F. J., & Rafal, R. D. (1987). How do the parietal lobes direct covert attention? *Neuropsychologia, 25,* 135–147.

Robertson, L. C., & Delis, D. C. (1986). "Part-whole" processing in unilateral brain damaged patients: Dysfunction of hierarchical organization. *Neuropsychologia, 24,* 363–370.

Robertson, L. C., Lamb, M. R., & Knight, R. T. (in press). Effects of lesions of temporal-parietal junction on perceptual and attentional processing in humans. *Journal of Neuroscience,*

Samuels, I., Butters, N., & Goodglass, H. (1970). Visual memory deficits following cortical and limbic lesions: Effect of field of presentation. *Neuropsychologia, 6,* 447–452.

Sergent, J. (1982). The cerebral balance of power; Confrontation or cooperation? *Journal of Experimental Psychology: Human Perception and Performance, 8,* 253–272.

Sergent, J., & Bindra, D. (1982). Differential hemispheric processing of faces: Methodological considerations and reinterpretation. *Psychological Bulletin, 89,* 541–554.

Udwin, O., Yule, W., & Martin, N. D. T. (1986). Age at diagnosis and abilities in idiopathic hypercalcemia. *Archives of Disease in Childhood, 61,* 1164–1167.

Ungerleider, L. G., & Mishkin, M. (1982). Two cortical visual pathways. In D. J. Ingle, M. A. Goodale, & R. J. W. Mansfield (Eds.), *Analysis of visual behavior,* (pp. 549–585). Cambridge, MA: M.I.T. Press.

Von Armin, G., & Engel, P. (1964). Mental retardation related to hypercalcemia. *Developmental Medicine and Child Neurology, 6,* 366–377.

Warrington, E. K., & James, M. (1967). An experimental investigation of facial recognition in patients with unilateral lesions. *Cortex, 3,* 317–326.

Warrington, E. K., James, M., & Kinsbourne, M. (1966). Drawing disability in relation to laterality of cerebral lesion. *Brain, 89,* 53–82.

Warrington, E. K., & Rabin, P. (1970). Perceptual matching in patients with cerebral lesions. *Neuropsychologia, 8,* 475–487.

3

Anatomical and Physiological Correlations and Neuroimaging Techniques in Language Disorders

ANDREW KERTESZ

Localization of brain lesions has undergone a revolutionary development in the last 10 years, yet some workers in cognitive science ignore the wealth of new information that has direct bearing on brain function. The most important achievement is the appearance of *in vivo* techniques of localization, which allows the collection of localizing information, at the same time as the neuropsychological examination of the brain-damaged patient, in a prospective, planned detail. For nearly 100 years since Broca's epoch-making clinicopathological correlation, neurological scientists relied on the rarely available postmortem examination of patients who were assessed during life, often long before they came to autopsy. In this chapter, I intend to detail some of the advantages and limitations of various localizing techniques and summarize the findings of the relatively new science of *in vivo* localization.

AUTOPSY LOCALIZATION

This oldest of techniques has been further perfected by the discovery of fixative and staining techniques, as well as optical enlarging and photographic instruments. Initially, alcohol fixation allowed the dissection of fiber tracts (Gall & Spurtzheim, 1810; Reil, 1809). Formalin fixation, and myelin and neuronal staining, around the turn of this century, resulted in

ANDREW KERTESZ • University of Western Ontario, St. Joseph's Health Centre, London, Ontario N6A 4V2, Canada.

the creation of cortical maps based on cellular differentiation (Brodmann, 1909; Economo & Koskinas, 1925). The study of human cytoarchitectonics and myeloarchitectonics diminished considerably after the 1920s in favor of experimental neuroanatomy in animals bolstered by autoradiography and axonal tracers, such a horseradish peroxidase (HRP). Recent advances in pigment cytoarchitectonics and the application of silver stains to antegrade and retrograde degeneration of tracts in human lesions opened new opportunities to study human cerebral connectivity and cortical organization (Galaburda & Mesulam, 1983; Sanides, 1962).

The accuracy of postmortem localization makes the method the standard with which others are compared. Autopsy examination of the human brain allows topographical localization of gyral and sulcal structures, and fiber tracts and the accurate determination of the extent of lesions. In addition to gross photography, the myelin and cellular stains allow microscopic analysis of neuronal structures and lesions. Economo and Koskinas (1925) standardized the nomenclature of the sulcal patterns and described the common variations in conjunction with cytoarchitectonic maps. Very little information has been accumulated since then concerning the extent of variations in surface geography. Recently, integration of anatomical landmarks with the vascular territories of the brain has been achieved (Talairach & Szikla, 1967; von Keyserlingk, De Bleser, & Poeck, 1983).

The description of the etiology of lesions and the surrounding tissue changes allows conclusions to be drawn about the possible effects of these changes on the brain at the time of clinical observation.

The major disadvantage of the autopsy method is that the brain usually becomes available only long after the patient has been examined clinically. Only occasionally is it possible to have the postmortem examination of the brain shortly after detailed, clinical examination was performed. Patients who die after a cerebral event are usually so severely affected that they could not be examined in the acute premortem illness in any detail. If they die after a downhill course, such as in the case of a brain tumor, by the time they come to autopsy the brain is severely distorted and will not reflect the clinical state that was previously studied.

Although many circumscribed lesions have come to autopsy, the corresponding clinical examinations have often been scanty and incomplete. Unfortunately, the reverse is also true. When the clinical examination has been conducted in great length, the patient often recovers; when death eventually occurs for some other reason, permission to carry out a postmortem examination is not granted or the patient dies in another location and the opportunity to establish correlation is lost.

The occasional situation where detailed examination is followed by an autopsy report fresh after the clinical observations remains a very important method of localization, even though it will provide only a random and rare opportunity for single cases and precludes the collection of groups for generalizations to be made. Attempts to collect a large number of postmortem examinations correlated with clinical observations have been made in the early 20th century, but they are plagued with the heterogenity of the material and the lack of reliable detail in the neurological and psychological examinations. Especially prominent are the works of Moutier (1908), who wrote a monograph on Broca's aphasia and associated syndromes. He described a systematic aphasia examination as an appendix to his book. He borrowed many cases, especially from Bernheim (1900), and this method of collecting cases from the literature to augment a few new descriptions became popular and is widely used even today. It is not unusual to trace a case description through several series (sometimes losing quite a bit in translation). Marie and Moutier (his pupil) entered a vigorous debate concerning the localization of lesions in Broca's aphasia and singled out the "quadrilateral space" central to the insula as crucial for language, opposing Dejerine and his anatomist wife, Klumpke, who favored the frontal operculum, also on the basis of autopsy evidence. The most monumental collection of autopsy material is that of Henschen (1922), who in seven large volumes collected 1,337 cases with descriptions and illustrated more than 300 of them, often including myelin-stained sections and photographs of specimens. The turn of the century autopsy studies not only described the anatomy of lesions but drew elaborate diagrams (resembling at times the more recent processing models) to illustrate their particular theory of language production as inferred from the lesion evidence. This activity was dampened by the criticism of Henry Head, who derided the "diagram makers." Von Monakow's (1914) influential work pointed out the problems of distant effects of tumors and the effects of depression of surrounding or functionally connected structures with acute stroke diaschisis. Nielson (1946) and Kleist (1962) wrote more recent monographs on postmortem examinations and clinical pathological correlation with language function and cognition. They espoused rather extreme views of equating specific anatomy with function. Since then, mostly single case reports have appeared with a variable quality of clinical and psychological detail.

Improvements in autopsy studies may come about by the systematic examination of stroke populations with the more sophisticated cytoarchitectonic and connectivity techniques described above. Stroke registries established at several centers allow more careful follow-up of patients. The topographical analysis of the brain regions has been limited largely to sulcal and gyral patterns, but cytoarchitectonic methods may correspond more to functional differentiation. Our knowledge of functional differences between children and adults, left and right hemispheres, sexes, handedness, and cultural influences on cerebral organization may further improve the sophistication of interpretations.

LOCALIZATION THROUGH HEAD INJURIES

The first group studies of live patients with neuropsychological deficits were carried out using localization information provided by the radiographs or surgical explorations of head-injured patients. Most of these head injury studies relied on a postwar population. Marie and Foix (1917), in France, used the overlap method of estimating the extent of injuries in various types of aphasia, distinguishing five syndromes with distinct localizations, contradicting somewhat Marie's earlier dogma of the unitary nature of the aphasic syndrome. Even Henry Head (1926) constructed an elaborate wire grid to localize the lesions from radiographs based on anatomical specimens. After World War II, Schiller (1947), in Germany, provided anatomical overlaps in a well-studied population based on skull X rays. Further large series were carried out by Luria (1970), in Russia, and Russell and Espir (1961), in England.

The major disadvantage of this method is that penetrating head injuries often cause damage distant from the entry wound, and radiographs of the skull defects are too inaccurate to draw reliable conclusions as to the exact location and depth of the damage. Nonpenetrating head traumas, even though they are more common in peacetime, are not usable because they cause diffuse, shearing injuries and widespread disconnection in the brain, as well as severe hemorrhage and destruction, with edematous brain tissue that is, at times, infarcted irreversibly. Unfortunately, diffuse head injury is often added to penetrating trauma, further detracting from the information about localization. An advantage of the head injury population is their relative youth and freedom from cerebral atrophy or repeated vascular insults.

SURGICAL LOCALIZATION

Neurosurgical resection of tumors and surgery for epilepsy, and at times operation on penetrating head injuries, provide a variable measure of localization. Tumor resection is not the most suitable material because slowly growing tumors compress the brain in an insidious fashion and often there is a great deal of compensation for the slowly incurred deficit. In fact, this may result in false negative conclusions concerning the role of certain areas in the brain. Malignant tumors infiltrate the brain tissue beyond resection, and it is often difficult to determine how far they actually exert their influence. The distant effects of edema, vascular insufficiency, and displacement of the tissues are difficult to quantitate on surgical explorations. Epilepsy surgery is often performed in scarred brains and the removed tissue may not be functional at all. The extent of the excision is difficult to judge because of the limitation of the exposure and the variability of the surface anatomy.

Burkhardt (1891) removed Broca's area and posterior T¹ and T² without permanent aphasia. Dandy (1931), after three cases, concluded that Broca's area is where Broca described it, except that it may be a little more posterior. He also said that visual speech (reading) is distinct, and that it is impaired by occipital lobectomy including the angular and supramarginal excisions. Mettler (1949) reported that bilateral removal of Broca's area did not produce aphasia, but the actual areas were not identified by stimulation or autopsy, and detailed language examination was lacking. Penfield and Roberts (1959) described language impairment in 581 left-hemisphere operations, and limited removal was compatible with recovery even in Broca's area. Persistent defects were associated with larger lesions. In a study of 214 surgically verified cases of mostly tumor and trauma, Hecaen and Angelergues (1964) found that disturbances of fluency, articulation, and naming were related to temporal lesions.

Hemispherectomies have been used to eradicate malignant tumors in adults (Smith, 1966) and for the excision of severely scarred epileptogenic tissue in infants and children. Some of these were extensively studied. Left hemispherectomies in adults produced global aphasia, but they retained emotional and automatic utterances, articulated even at a sentence level, and some comprehension of single nouns. The limitations on studying adult hemispherectomies are the rarity of the operation (most surgeons do not consider it worthwhile) and the usually relentless spread of the neoplasm into the other hemisphere. Infantile hemispherectomies have been well studied, indicating almost complete recovery of function on either side. However, sophisticated language measures have indicated less than normal development in verbal IQ and in grammatical competence in children who had left hemispherectomy in their infancy.

Sections of the corpus callosum performed for intractable epilepsy provides an opportunity to study the function of each hemisphere (Sperry, Gazzaniga, & Bogen, 1969). In this respect, the method is not a surgical resection but a disconnection of two functional areas. The results have illuminated many right-hemisphere functions, including a certain capacity for comprehending language. (A more detailed review can be found in Gazzaniga, 1970.) Some of the operations have been less than complete, as recent MRI studies have indicated, and this may have led to some false conclusions concerning function.

CORTICAL STIMULATION

Cortical stimulation developed for epilepsy surgery is a major contribution to cerebral localization. Initially it was used by physiologists to map the function of the cerebral cortex in animals, and subsequently neurosurgeons, such as Otto Foerster in the 1920s, have tried to identify cortical function with stimulation in preparation for their excisions. Sensory, motor, and language areas can be spared using this technique. Penfield and Roberts (1959) mapped the language areas and Van Buren, Fedio, and Frederick (1978), Ojemann and Whitaker (1978), and Ojemann and Mateer (1979) have added further information concerning cortical localization.

The advantage of the method is that it can be applied in the awake, cooperative patient who can perform selected functions during stimulation. In this respect, it resembles other so-called functional methods of localization, such as cerebral blood flow (CBF) and positron emission tomography (PET). However, stimulation interferes with functions, interrupts or alters them, and, less frequently, elicits positive phenomena. In this respect, it is more like the lesion method, but stimulation involves a much smaller area, allowing a greater resolution for mapping. Several functions can be examined by repeated stimulation of the same area.

Limitations of the technique include the logistics of a lengthy surgical procedure, difficulty reproducing the stimulation on the same spot, and the brevity of tasks that can be employed during the short period of stimulation (maximum about 12 seconds). The subjects usually have epilepsy or tumors with reorganized brains, and the conclusions may not always be generalizable.

The results of cortical stimulation reveal a striking discreteness of function that is different from the conclusions drawn from lesion studies. Naming, for example, may be affected over one gyrus, but not a few millimeters next to it. On the other hand, naming errors could be elicited from a wide variety of cortical areas. The most consistent area to produce speech arrest was in Broca's area, the posterior inferior frontal cortex, in front of the face motor cortex (Ojemann & Whitaker, 1978). The posterior superior temporal cortex seemed to be the next most important area involved in language. Cortical mapping in bilingual patients showed sites where one language was impaired but not the other. Naming in the less competent and more recently acquired language was disrupted from a wider area of stimulation. Some dissociations were also observed between oral and sign language. When multiple language functions are tested over the same site, only one may be involved. Grammar, semantics, and articulation seem to be dissociated in a highly variable fashion across patients. Grammatical errors often occurred in the frontal lobe without articulatory deficit. Semantic errors were from more widely distributed sites of stimulation. Memory-related sites surround the perisylvian (usually parietal) cortex at some distance from it. Individual variability may be related to anatomical and educational differences and IQ (Mateer, 1983).

The localization of nonverbal functions in the nondominant hemisphere was also studied with cortical stimulation using line orientation, face-matching, and facial recognition tasks. Perceptual errors were observed at the parietooccipital and also at the frontal sites. Recognition errors occured in the posterior portion of the superior temporal gyrus and parietal lobe. The different spatial tasks, such as face matching and line orientation, were affected at similar sites, but dissociation was observed between the sites for perception and recognition (Mateer, 1983). The tentative conclusion reached was that visuospatial functions in the nondominant hemisphere appeared to be as discretely localized as verbal functions in the dominant hemisphere. This is somewhat contrary to the conclusions drawn from lesion studies by Semmes, Weinstein, Ghent, and Teuber (1960) and Kertesz and Dobrowolski (1981).

ELECTROENCEPHALOGRAPHY AND EVOKED POTENTIALS

This physiological method of localization utilizes the small electric potentials generated by neuronal activity that can be detected by surface electrodes on the scalp or on the brain surface during operations. Electroencephalograms have been used for more than 50 years. However, the method suffers from relatively low specificities, since the electric potential changes often present a summation of remote effects. The localization of cognitive function in aphasia with EEG has been reported by Marinesco, Sager, and Kreindler (1936) and Tikofsky, Kooi, and Thomas (1960). Galin and Ornstein (1972) observed suppression of the alpha rhythm in the dominant hemisphere during verbal tasks and in the nondominant side during spatial tasks. An attempt to assess intercortical connections was made by measuring the degree of correlation between pairs of electrodes, called cortical coupling (Callaway & Harris, 1974).

The introduction of signal-averaging computers allowed the measurement of event-related potentials (ERP) by averaging out the background EEG activity. Differences in ERP lateralization were observed by using verbal and nonverbal stimuli (Buchsbaum & Fedio, 1970), words versus nonsense syllables (Shelburne, 1972), and contextual meaning (Brown, Marsh, & Smith, 1973; Teyler et al., 1973). Long-latency ERPs are sensitive to task relevance and expectancy. The 300-msec positive component is called P300, which is considered endogenous and less dependent on stimulus characteristics. A potential that precedes movement or cognition is called the contingent negative variation (CNV). This has been correlated with hemispheric dominance and has been useful in various cognitive studies (Low, Wada, & Fox, 1973). Another example of negative potentials associated with processing is the N400 potential, which is related to the occurrence of context incongruity in serial semantic tasks (Kutas & Hillyard, 1980; Nevill, Kutas, & Schmidt, 1982).

Cerebral event-related potentials are technically difficult because of the many artifacts that interfere with the study. Some of these technical difficulties have been discussed by Desmedt (1977). Another problem with the method is the time restriction on the stimuli. The stimulation has to be very short and have a definite onset, duration, and offset, in order to be connected with cerebral event. In a way, it is the opposite to cerebral blood flow studies (see below), which require more sustained cerebral activity to be analyzed. The major advantage of the technique is that it reflects a physiological event connected with actual cerebral processing, although the resolution of localization is poor and the potentials are usually over a large area of the scalp and the brain. The origin and the generation of evoked potentials are often obscure, and their interpretation is often subject to argument and to change over the course of years. For instance, P300 potentials, which were initially interpreted as reflecting cerebral perceptual processing, are now considered a postdecisional potential, signifying the closure of the perceptual process and target selection. Since the method is noninvasive and is becoming relatively less expensive, future expansion of the technique can be expected. Its major requirement and, at the same time, limiting factor is the necessity of having a trained electrophysiologist who devotes full time to this activity.

ISOTOPE LOCALIZATION OF LESIONS

Isotope scanning made it possible to outline lesions with considerable accuracy for the first time in patients who could be tested coincidentally. Many radioisotopes will not penetrate the blood brain barrier, unless there is some pathology. First, it was obvious that brain tumors and vascular lesions could be seen and the extent of the lesion could be estimated quite adequately. Subsequently, it became evident that cerebral infarcts will also take up the isotopes approximately a week after the stroke and continue to do so for about a month. Therefore, the technique is particularly applicable for the localization of acute lesions and the differentiation of acute from chronic lesions. For example, an infarct on a CT scan would appear as an area of decreased density that would be the same in the acute or the chronic state. Enhancement after contrast injection on the CT scan may help to clarify the problem, but a radioisotope scan can still be used as a confirmatory evidence for an acute stroke.

Initial radioisotope localization of aphasias demonstrated a clear anterior–posterior dichotomy (Benson, 1967). An isotope study confirmed that transcortical motor aphasia was seen with lesions of the supplementary motor area and also of Broca's area (Rubens, 1976). An objective method of tracing a series of radioisotope lesions and correlating them with aphasic syndromes defined by cognitive scores was a forerunner of subsequent CT studies (Kertesz, Lesk, & McCabe, 1977). Maximum overlap for Broca's aphasia was over Broca's area and at the foot of the rolandic fissure. Wernicke's aphasia involved the posterior superior temporal gyrus and the posterior perisylvian region, and conduction aphasia involved a smaller and somewhat more anterior region between Wernicke's and Broca's area. Lesions causing conduction aphasia appeared to cluster bimodally into anterior and posterior groups. Lesions of anomic aphasics were widely scattered, and transcortical aphasics were outside the perisylvian speech area. Transcortical motor aphasics overlapped in the supplementary motor area in the superior frontal lobe, and transcortical sensory aphasics were posterior to Wernicke's area. The severity of aphasia as measured with a standardized test correlated inversely with lesion size.

The major disadvantage of isotope scanning is that the normal landmarks are few, so that accurate anatomical localization is difficult and depends on inference. The edges of the lesions are somewhat indistinct and can be subject to misinterpretation. A certain portion of the lesions is missed because the scan is undertaken either too early or too late. This restriction in time is often a disadvantage and excludes localization in many patients studied chronically. However, as discussed above, the specific interval during which the scan will be positive makes it useful as a diagnostic tool. This method has been eclipsed by the CT scan and subsequently by MRI scanning. However, there are still conditions where this method is superior to all others, such as in the localization of herpes simplex encephalitis, where, in several examples, the CT scan was negative while the radioisotope study showed a clear-cut uptake in both temporal lobes. Another continuing advantage of the method is its relatively high availability in just about every hospital and its relatively low expense.

COMPUTERIZED TOMOGRAPHIC (CT) LESION LOCALIZATION

CT scanning is a significant breakthrough in radiological diagnosis and has also become the most important method in localizing lesions in the brain. The technique combines X-ray technology and computerization. Modern CT scanners provide fairly accurate bony detail and delineation of CSF spaces. The latest generation scanners also show some gray and white matter differentiation and allow us to see changes in density, such as brain edema. The technique utilizes a rotating X-ray beam, which circles the head rapidly with a paired detector; the computer calculates the densities of the tissue being imaged. Contrast enhancement with radio-opaque material, such as organic iodine, increases the visualization of vascular structures and the increased vascularity around an acute infarct. CT shows lesions earlier than radioisotope scans, but not as early as MRI scans, and the early changes tend to be not as distinct as the ones obtained after about 3 weeks. One of the reasons for negative localization with a clear-cut clinical syndrome could be related to the timing of the CT scan. Alteration in tissue density, 1 to 2 weeks after the infarct, sometimes produces a decrease in contrast, so-called fogging, and occasionally even a temporary disappearance of the lesion. Contrast enhancement and isotope study may be helpful to visualize infarcts at that stage. Hemorrhages are quite dramatic, and brain tumors are also shown superiorly on CT scans. Old infarcts are quite distinct, with sharp margins and lower densities than the surrounding brain, and enlargement of the ventricles and sulci also provide an accurate measurement of atrophy.

CT scanning has become the standard method of localization of lesions not only in clinical neurology but also in neuropsychology. The correlation of lesions with behavioral studies began soon after the CT equipment became available. These studies differ in the quality of the scans, the sophistication of localization, the number of patients included, the actual neuropsychological measurements used, and the definition of the syndromes. One of the most important considerations, which is missing from some of the studies, is the time from onset. Some patients with large lesions may have recovered considerably, and this may lead to the conclusion that the area involved plays no role in a function. It is especially misleading to mix acute and chronic patients. CT studies, nevertheless, have contributed a great deal to our knowledge about localization of lesions in syndromes of language and cognitive impairment.

Severe persisting Broca's aphasia is associated with large lesions that include not only Broca's area but also the inferior parietal and often the anterior temporal region (Kertesz, 1979; Mohr, 1976). Small lesions involving Broca's area only are compatible with good recovery. Small Broca's area lesions often produce a minor motor aphasia (called "cortical motor aphasia," "pure motor aphasia," or "verbal apraxia") (Kertesz, 1979; Mohr, 1976). Although both acute and chronic Broca's aphasia is associated with Broca's area lesion (Kertesz, Harlock, & Coates, 1979), Levine and Mohr (1979) presented autopsy evidence in favor of the inferior precentral gyrus. Pure motor aphasia or verbal apraxia has been associated with anterior subcortical as well as cortical lesions (Kertesz, 1983). Subcortical lesions produce atypical aphasias that may vary clinically, depending on their anterior posterior location and the extent of involvement of various subcortical structures.

The study of lesions in fluent aphasia has revealed not only a cortical location but also thalamic involvement. Neologistic jargon output is associated with lesions of both the superior temporal and the inferior parietal region (Kertesz, 1979). Thalamic lesions, on the other hand, produce fluctuating jargon aphasia alternating with relatively nonfluent speech (Mohr, Watters, & Duncan, 1975). Repetition is often preserved (Cappa & Vignolo, 1979). Conduction aphasia is associated with lesions in the arcuate fasciculus, as well as in the insula (Damasio & Damasio, 1983). Transcortical sensory aphasia is associated with inferior temporooccipital lesions (Kertesz, Sheppard, & MacKenzie, 1982).

Right-hemisphere function appears to be much less well localized than that on the left side. This conclusion was first suggested from cortical excision studies by Semmes *et al.* (1960) and later received support from a CT study by Kertesz and Dobrowolski (1981). Line bisection drawing, block design, and Raven's scores were not significantly different among frontal, central, subcortical, parietal, and occipital lesions. Lesion size was certainly a contributing variable. In the study by Hier, Mondlock, and Caplan (1983) left neglect motor impersistence and anosognosia tended to occur with rather large lesions extending beyond the right parietal lobe. On a few occasions, small deep lesions also produced behavioral abnormalities comparable to the larger superficial cortical lesions.

The correlation of lesion size and recovery was found to be significant in overall group studies (Kertesz *et al.*, 1979; Yarnell, Monroe, & Sobol, 1976). Care must be taken to distinguish between outcome measures and recovery rates. Sometimes patients with a large lesion and greater initial severity show greater recovery rates because they have much more room to improve than those with smaller lesions and a higher level of initial deficit.

The major advantage of a CT scan is its ability to localize lesions with high anatomical resolution, especially in the late model scanners. CT scanning is especially useful in chronic lesions where the edges of infarcts are well outlined, and in horizontal cuts that are usually oriented 15 degrees above the orbitomeatal line. CT scans are now available in most major centers, and the method has become standard for neurological investigation. The scanning time is brief, and there is no discomfort associated with it.

Disadvantages are few. A clinical indication is needed for scanning because of radiation. Repeated, frequent exposures to X rays are considered harmful. Cortical landmarks are not usually seen, and one has to use ventricular and bony landmarks for anatomical orientation. Variations in head positioning, head size, ventricular size, extent of atrophy, and cerebral asymmetries are important to consider in accurate localization. The variation in the sulcal and gyral pattern and the depth of the cortex in the central portions of the brain is often underestimated in CT studies. Many of the "subcortical" lesions often involve insular cortex, for example. The initial appearance of a CT infarct may be negative, and it is in the chronic state that localization is most reliable. CT provides some image of dynamic changes around the edge of the infarct in the acute state if enhancement is used, but this is a somewhat more invasive method, involving the injection of iodinated contrast, which is not entirely without risks. The chronic state only shows the static structural damage.

In summary, CT remains the standard of *in vivo* localization with which all other localizing methods are compared. Because of its availability and easy administration, it will likely retain this position for considerable time to come. Much neuropsychological work has been done with CT and will continue to be relevant.

CEREBRAL BLOOD FLOW (CBF) LOCALIZATION

The CBF technique utilizes the physiological and pathological alterations in regional blood supply that is measured in a resting state and can be related to functional alterations. The technique is based on measuring the clearance of radioactive isotopes from various regions of the brain through surface detectors. The values are expressed as percentages of the hemispheric average. Increase of blood flow are assumed to be associated with increased neuronal and, therefore, functional activity. A sustained repetitive task of at least 3 to 5 minutes' duration is required for activation.

The color-coded images of CBF have become popular in illustrating that the brain is activated in multiple locations when, for instance, a person reads or the right hemisphere also "lights" up when one speaks. The resting pattern shows precentral high and postcentral low flows (Ingvar & Schwartz, 1974). Simple repetitive movements of the mouth, hand, or foot augment CBF in the contralateral sensorimotor area, outlining the topography of the cortical homunculus.

Visual perceptual tasks increase CBF occipitally and in the frontal eye field. The posterior parietal regions are involved in shape discrimination. Tactile perception activates the anterior parietal (sensory) area. Auditory perceptual tasks increase regional blood flow to the temporal region verbal tasks on the left and nonverbal sound discrimination on the right. Verbal answers during the tests were also assumed to cause the increased flow to the frontal regions. A trimodality stimulation paradigm appears as a summation of the single modality activation, but in addition, the posterior superior frontal cortex, which is considered a supramodal processing area, is also activated. Widespread cortical systems, in addition to specific primary areas, show activation during complex processing (Lassen & Roland, 1983). The technique is also sensitive to general arousal, in addition to selective activation of local regions. A more detailed review of the application of CBF in neuropsychology was reviewed by Wood (1980).

The important advantage of the technique is that it reflects physiological metabolic changes accompanying psychological function and it can be used to study normal processes. It must be remembered, however, that these changes are not directly measuring neuronal events. These techniques are best suited for the study of sustained repetitive acts of cognition. Lesions, such as infarcts producing a deficit, may appear as areas of low flow with an area of "luxury perfusion" of high flow surrounding them.

The major disadvantage is a relatively poor resolution of the noninvasive xenon inhalation method. It only measures blood flow on the surface. The more accurate intraarterial injection is rarely used because it is invasive and requires the indications of an angiogram. A more recent modification of the technique combines xenon-133 inhalation with computerized tomography, achieving three dimensional representations in slices similar to those in PET scanning (see SPECT section below).

POSITRON EMISSION TOMOGRAPHY (PET)

PET scanning measures oxygen and glucose metabolism by using a positron-emitting isotope and a computerized tomographic scanner. It can also be used to study regional blood flow. This complex and expensive technique is available only in a few centers equipped with a particle accelerator (cyclotron) and a team of nuclear physicists, radiopharmacists, computer experts, isotope specialists, clinicians, and experimental psychologists. The positron labeled metabolites, such as ^{18}F-desoxyglucose, must be given immediately at their source because of their short half-life. The nature of tracer kinetics require that the physiological activity studied has to be sustained for 20 to 40 minutes. Currently, a bolus administration of oxygen-15 shortens the period of observation and allows repeated measurements in the same subjects in one session (Raichle, Herscovitch, Mintun, Martin, & Power, 1984). A new device, the "super-PETT-1" is capable of a temporal resolution of less than 1 minute (Ter-Pogossian et al., 1984). This opens up the possibility of following brief physiological events in the brain in the future.

PET observations in normal volunteers showed hemispheric lateralization that varied with stimulus content in the visual and auditory systems, and with the response strategy of subjects. Particularly interesting were metabolic asymmetries (left greater than right) in sensory deprivation and also on auditory stimulation (Mazziotta & Phelps, 1984). Bilateral activation of the thalamus was observed in auditory verbal stimulation. Ambient test conditions influenced the results considerably, and caution must be exercised in interpreting all PET results because of that.

After a stroke, two phases of "luxury perfusion" are seen surrounding an area of hypometabolism. PET studies showed prominent hypometabolism of the ipsilateral subcortical regions and the basal ganglia in cortical focal lesions even though these structures remained intact on the CT scan (Metter, Wasterlain, Kuhl, Hanson, & Phelps, 1981). There are often much larger areas of hypometabolism around a lesion on PET than the decreased densities seen on CT. Following subcortical lesions, cortical activation is also decreased, possibly because of lowered metabolic demand. Future applications of the PET technique may reveal areas in the brain that play a role in functional compensation for structural lesions. So far, contralateral homologous structures have been implicated. In epilepsy, cortical zones considered responsible for seizures were hypometabolic without a structural lesion being demonstrated. In Huntington's disease, a decrease in metabolism was seen in the caudate and putamen early, preceding bulk tissue loss. PET studies of Alzheimer's disease show widespread cortical hypometabolism. Elderly normals also show a significant decrease in cerebral glucose metabolism (Benson, Metter, Kuhl, & Phelps, 1983).

The major advantage of PET is that it measures cerebral metabolism, therefore function, in normals and in disease. The major disadvantages are large expense and general unavailability, poor anatomical resolution, uncertainties between the temporal sequence of cerebral events and the isotope kinetics in time, and the influence of unrelated cerebral activity.

SINGLE-PHOTON COMPUTERIZED TOMOGRAPHY (SPECT)

Regional blood flow can also be estimated by using a single-photon technique that is much cheaper than PET scanning (Hill, 1980). This is the latest of the functional localizing methods, but experience is rapidly accumulating because it is more generally available than PET. Single-photon tracers can be used to measure blood flow, blood volume, and also blood brain barrier integrity. Disadvantages are that large amounts of costly xenon gas (in nearly anesthetic doses) or iodinated isopropyl amphetamine (IMP) are needed. Sequential scans at each level mean repeated exposure to X rays. The exact positioning is crucial, and this restricts the study to cooperative subjects. In brain damage, IMP is not only a blood flow tracer but also an index of impaired cellular function. It has a longer biological half-life (13 hours) than xenon, which is inert. Studies in neuropsychology with SPECT are just beginning to appear (Tikofsky et al., 1984).

MAGNETIC RESONANCE IMAGER (MRI)

MRI is the latest imaging modality, and it shows the greatest promise in accurate localization of lesions without invasive radiation. The technique uses the inherent magnetic properties of spinning atomic nuclei by placing the structure to be imaged in a large magnet and applying shortwave radiofrequency pulses to produce a resonance signal that can be quantified and computerized (Doyle et al., 1981). Superior anatomical detail can be achieved with excellent gray and white matter differentiation and an accurate outline of the edge of the brain from CSF spaces. The brain can be imaged in coronal and sagittal sections, in addition to the horizontal ones, which is the usual plane obtained in other modalities. This imaging flexibility, combined with anatomical accuracy, has already established MRI as a useful clinical and research tool. The apparent lack of biohazard allows it to be used to study normals without clinical indications, as well as a more frequent repetition of imaging in patients than is possible in other modalities that use ionizing radiation.

Various pulse sequences can be used to probe the metabolic and molecular environment of various regions of the brain, and this makes the technique much more dynamic than the CT scan. Currently, two major pulse sequences are used. One called "inversion recovery" emphasizes gray and white matter differences and provides excellent anatomical detail. The second, called "spin echo," is utilized to detect edema and other metabolic changes associated with lesions. Spin echo sequences are often superior to CT scanning in the early detection of cerebral infarct, thus reducing the false negative rate obtained on CT in the first 2 or 3 days of a stroke. The technique is particularly suited to detect demyelinating plaques and some other degenerative diseases in addition to early strokes. The evolution of an infarct follows a regular pattern, with a gradual clearing of the central portion on the spin echo image that leaves a ring of increased signal intensity around the infarct in the chronic state. This ring appears to extend beyond the hypodensity seen on CT. The selection of various repetition times and pulse sequences permits a differentiated visualization of brain tissues, such as the CSF versus the brain, by altering the influence of various tissue properties. The inversion recovery sequence emphasizes the T1 or longitudinal relaxation time, which is the return of the spinning nuclei to their original axis in the large magnetic field. The spin echo sequences are weighted for the T2 relaxation time, which depends on the interaction of the spinning nuclei with each other.

MRI is a new technology that is currently in a relatively unstable state of development. The expense is somewhat greater than that of scanners for most prototype equipment. Recently, this modality has become available to most major centers. It will likely not displace, but will complement CT scanning. Clinical imaging can be accomplished in 15 minutes, but for research purposes the pulse sequences can take an hour. Lesions are well outlined, and the dynamic changes around or in the lesions can be followed over time. Variations in the images are dependent on the molecular environment and water density of the tissues. Actual functional changes or psychological states cannot be examined with the current equipment.

Neuropsychological studies with MRI include the localization of lesions in aphasia and a study of anatomical asymmetries utilizing the excellent anatomical detail on the inversion recovery scan, which allows the direct visualization of the opercular sulci in the planum temporale (Kertesz & Black, 1983; Kertesz, Black, & Howell, 1984). In the future, with improved technology, it is likely that metabolic alterations such as changes in high energy phosphates can be imaged and that physiological, in addition to structural, changes in the brain can be investigated.

DISCUSSION AND CONCLUSION

The integration of structural alterations with functional changes presents a challenge that is at its greatest in the central nervous system. Cognitive behavior and language in man is, to a large extent, tied to localizable brain structures, and the purpose of this chapter was to summarize the methods of localization. Any attempt to correlate function with lesions must cope with a multitude of theoretical and practical problems. These issues in localization have undergone considerable change in the last few years, not only because of revolutionary new technology in localization but also because of our increasing sophistication and knowledge of neuropsychological phenomena.

One of the most important issues in localization is the extent to which function is localizable. Primary sensory and motor areas in the brain are clearly related to well-defined functions. Such a relationship is exemplified by the recent physiological studies exploring the relationship of columnar organization of cerebral cortex to visual feature analysis (Hubel & Wiesel, 1965). Secondary and tertiary areas of the brain that are associated with elaboration of cognitive and language function are much less clearly localizable. Language appears to take an intermediate position among cognitive processes in that it is well localized to the left side, in most instances, and there exists a dichotomy of output and articulation, and input and comprehension, in relation to the different structures involved. There are similar dichotomies in agrammatism and paragrammatism, phonemic and semantic paraphasias, and various dissociations in reading and writing that may be related to differential localization. Other cognitive processes, such as semantic elaboration and retrieval, and multiple modality associations, appear to occupy a much less localizable network that can be impaired from lesions in many areas of the left hemisphere. Memory function also represents a less localizable component of cognition, even though recent memory deficits are clearly related to lesions of the limbic lobe, which itself is a widely distributed but localizable network. The diffuse reticular activating system and thalamocortical projections underlie the widespread activation involved in attention and in the performance of many cognitive tasks. Visuospatial functions are elaborated, mainly by the right hemisphere, although some components are clearly related to left-hemisphere function as well. Recent studies have confirmed the right-hemisphere dominance for directed attention and visuospatial function. Most of these functions are complex enough that bilateral hemispheric integration is necessary for their performance.

The definition of what constitutes a function is often dynamic and arbitrary. Complex alternative theories are offered analyzing certain functions. A great deal of fractionation and the reduction of complex behaviors to its elements risks the loss of meaning and biological significance to the organism. Some psychological concepts of functions may not be appropriate to describe the brain function as we know it from the structural point of view. On the other hand, some structural alterations cannot be correlated with function, but only with the deficit syndrome that is seen after a lesion. The behavior observed after a lesion may not be analyzable in terms of normal function. This often prevents any direct conclusion about normal mechanisms that is based on structural and pathological observations. However, this does not diminish the usefulness of the clinicopathological correlations. The analysis of behavior after a lesion should be complemented by studies of function in normals. The function lost after a circumscribed area of brain damage is clearly better analyzed if the components of the function are known and can be identified to be missing.

A major objection to relating lesions to function is that the observed function after a lesion is related not to the area damaged but to other areas or structures that take over function or become reorganized to substitute for it. At times after a lesion, not only do deficit symptoms appear but new behavior or positive symptoms can also be observed. These may represent elements of neural activity that had been suppressed by the structure that is destroyed by the lesion. This argument pertains not only to lesions but to other methods as well, such as electrical stimulation or the recording of single units, because these are all connected to the remaining system. This consideration is important for the interpretation of any method, but it should not eliminate them from the correlation of function with structure.

Most functions are represented in the brain as a network of interconnected sites. It is also likely that these networks overlap and therefore lesions of a certain cortical area are going to produce multiple deficits (syndromes). Since some of the components of a certain function remain intact when only one circumscribed area is damaged, recovery often occurs by reorganization of the residual network. A severe and lasting impairment of a function requires the multiple involvement of several components, usually the majority of them. Some of the functional networks are more widely distributed than others, and therefore the same function can be impaired from several cortical areas that may be quite far from each other.

The variability of deficits following similar lesions in the brain are partly related to problems of localization that are corrected by improvement in the techniques of localization itself. However, some factors are related to the effect of recovery or reorganization in the nervous system. Therefore, in all attempts to correlate deficit with lesion, the time from the onset is crucial. Failure to consider this variable is a major source of confusion in neuropsychology. The extent of substitution and reorganization in the central nervous system is considerable, far beyond that which can be attributed to anatomical regeneration. This, of course, complicates efforts to localize function in any part of the nervous system.

The interconnection of functional networks results in distance effects in sudden lesions, which is known as "diaschisis" (von Monakow, 1914). This principle, in essence, explains the initial effect of a lesion on a function that produces a more severe deficit, which eventually recovers as the rest of the network becomes reorganized. This explains much of the observed recovery and plasticity in central nervous system lesions. On the other hand, slowly growing lesions produce relatively little functional deficit. Therefore, the etiology of the lesion is a very important variable in considering lesion localization. For instance, transcortical sensory aphasia or Wernicke's aphasia may appear with Alzheimer's disease, associated with diffuse neuronal degeneration that is not localizable with our present methods to the same extent as a focal infarct causing those deficits.

Differences between individuals are also factors that need to be taken into consideration in the interpretation of the localization of function. The plasticity of the young brain allows for greater compensation by homologous structures of the other hemisphere. There may be differences in the distribution of the function between the left and right hemispheres in individuals with various degrees of handedness or some other factor that influences lateralization. Gender differences have also been postulated concerning the functional organization of language and visuospatial function.

The various methods of correlating cerebral function with structure are summarized in Table 1. This table indicates the major characteristics of the methods, such as their accuracy, relation to function, expense, availability, and the various advantages and disadvantages. Table 2 summarizes the areas of application of each method. This indicates the work that has been done with the technique, as well as the suitability for future studies. The investigator must have a great deal of familiarity with each technology if the appropriate experiments or study paradiagms are to be designed with these methods. However, a considerable amount of general knowledge is needed also for those who want to evaluate the information obtained with these complex techniques, which are ever increasing in number.

TABLE 1. Localization Techniques

	Anatomical resolution	Availability	Relation to function	Performance duration	Invasiveness	Expense	Advantages	Disadvantages
Autopsy	The ultimate in accuracy	Restricted to some cases	Indirect remote	Only in the past	Postmortem	Moderate	Accuracy	Retrospective
Skull wounds	Poor, only an approximation	Restricted group	Indirect	Unlimited after lesion	Penetrating injury	Minor	In *vivo* exam	Inaccurate
Neurosurgery	Accurate	Restricted group	Indirect	Unlimited after lesion	Neurosurgery	Moderate	In *vivo* exam	Altered tissue
Cortical stimulation	Accurate surface only	Restricted to a few	Indirect	12 sec and control	Neurosurgery	Moderate to expensive	Small areas	Limited testing
EEG, evoked potentials	Poor (lobar only)	Limited to physiologists	Expectations, attention	Minutes and milliseconds	Noninvasive	Moderate	Physiological	Low specificity
Isotope scans	Poor (outline only)	Everywhere	Indirect	Unlimited acute stage	Noninvasive	Minor	In *vivo* exam	Poor resolution
CT scans	Accurate to a degree	Almost everywhere	Indirect	Unlimited after lesion	Minor radiation	Moderate	In *vivo* exam	Limited landmarks
CBF scans	Poor, better arterially	Restricted to stroke centers	Closely related	5 min	Minor (more if arterial)	Moderate to expensive	Related to function	Poor resolution
PET scans	Poor but improving	Only few	Direct (metabolic)	20–60 min <1 min in future	Minor radiation	Very expensive	Directly functional	Resolution, expense
SPECT scans	Poor but improving	Restricted to few centers	Closely related	5–20 min	Minor radiation	Moderate to expensive	CBF in slices	Resolution, expense
MRI scans	Accurate	Expanding major centers	Indirect	Unlimited after lesion	Noninvasive	Moderate to expensive	Best resolution	Not yet available

TABLE 2. The Areas of Application

Autopsy	Aphasias, apraxias, agnosias, memory, neglect, constructional and visuospatial syndromes
Skull wounds	Frontal lobe syndromes, aphasias, visual field defects, memory
Neurosurgery	Temporal, frontal, and occipital lobe function; memory; callosal disconnection
Cortical stimulation	Naming, articulation, grammar, semantics, gesture, polyglots, face matching
EEG and ERP	Cerebral lateralization, attention, expectation, task relevance, central processing
Isotope scans	Aphasias, agnosias, memory, neglect, superior for herpes encephalitis
CT scans	All lesion localization; superior for hemorrhages, tumors, and chronic stroke
CBF scans	Resting activity, normal physiology, perceptual functions, lateralization, integrative processes
PET scans	Perceptual activation, lateralization, distance effects of lesions, epilepsy, subcortical lesions
SPECT scans	Lateralization, processing, perceptual activation, lesion effect
MRI scans	All lesion localization, superior for demyelination and early strokes, anatomical studies

REFERENCES

Benson, D. F. (1967). Fluency in aphasia: Correlation with radioactive scan localization. Cortex, 3, 373–394.

Benson, D. F., Metter, E. J., Kuhl, D. E., & Phelps, M. (1983). Positron-computed tomography in neurobehavioral problems. In A. Kertesz (Ed.), Localization in neuropsychology. New York: Academic Press.

Bernheim, F. (1900). De l'aphasie motrice. Paris: Carre et Naud.

Brodmann, K. (1909). Vergleichende Lokalisationslehre der Grosshirnrinde. Leipzig: Barth.

Brown, W. S., Marsh, J. T., & Smith, J. C. (1973). Contextual meaning effects on speech-evoked potentials. Behavioral Biology, 9, 755–761.

Buchsbaum, M., & Fedio, P. (1970). Hemispheric differences in evoked potentials to verbal and nonverbal stimuli in the left and right visual fields. Physiology and Behavior, 5, 207–210.

Burkhardt, G. (1891). Ueber Rindenexcisionen, als Beitrag zur operativen Therapie der Psychosen. Allgemeine Zeitschrift für Psychiatrie, 47, 463–548.

Callaway, E., & Harris, P. R. (1974). Coupling between cortical potentials from different areas. Science, 183, 873–875.

Cappa, S. F., & Vignolo, L. A. (1979). "Transcortical" features of aphasia following left thalamic hemorrhage. Cortex, 15, 121–130.

Damasio, A. R., & Damasio, H. (1983). Localization of lesions in achromatopsia and prosopagnosia. In A. Kertesz (Ed.), Localization in neuropsychology. New York: Academic Press.

Dandy, W. (1931). The effect of total removal of the left temporal lobe in a right handed individual: Localization of areas of the brain concerned with speech. Journal of Nervous and Mental Disease, 74, 739–742.

Desmedt, J. E. (1977). Some observations on the methodology of cerebral evoked potentials in man. In J. E. Desmedt (Ed.), *Attention, voluntary contraction and event-related cerebral potentials*, Progress in Clinical Neuropsychology (Vol. 1). Basel: Karger.

Doyle, F. H., Gore, J. C., Pennock, J. M., Bydder, G. M., Orr, J. S., Steiner, R. E., Young, I. R., Burl, M., Clow, H., Gilderdale, D. J., Bailes, D. R., & Walters, P. E. (1981). Imaging of the brain by NMR. *Lancet, 8237*, 53–57.

Economo, C., & Koskinas, G. N. (1925). *Die Cytoarchitektonik der Hirnrinde des erwachsenen Menschen.* Berlin: Springer-Verlag.

Galaburda, A. M., & Mesulam, M. M. (1983). Neuroanatomical aspects of cerebral localization. In A. Kertesz (Ed.), *Localization in neuropsychology.* New York: Academic Press.

Galin, D., & Ornstein, R. (1972). Lateral specialization of cognitive mode: An EEG study. *Psychophysiology, 9*, 412–418.

Gall, F. J., & Spurtzheim, G. (1810). *Anatomie et physiologie du systeme nerveux en general et du cerveau en particulier* (Vol. 1). Paris: F. Schoell.

Gazzaniga, M. S. (1970). *The bisected brain.* New York: Appleton-Century-Crofts.

Head, H. (1926). *Aphasia and kindred disorders of speech.* Cambridge: Cambridge University Press.

Hecaen, A., & Angelergues, R. (1964). Localization of symptoms in aphasia. In A. De Reuck & M. O'Connor (Eds.), *Disorders of language.* London: Churchill.

Henschen, S. E. (1922). *Klinische und anatomische Beitrage zur Pathologie des Gehirns* (Vols. 5–7) Stockholm: Nordiska Bokhandel.

Hier, D. B., Mondlock, J., & Caplan, L. R. (1983). Behavioral abnormalities after right hemisphere stroke. *Neurology, 33*, 337–344.

Hill, T. C. (1980). Single-photon emission computed tomography to study cerebral function in man. *Journal of Nuclear Medicine, 21*, 1197–1199.

Hubel, D., & Wiesel, T. (1965). Receptive fields and functional architecture in two nonstriate visual areas (18 and 19) of the cat. *Journal of Neurophysiology, 28*, 229–289.

Ingvar, D. H., & Schwartz, M. S. (1974). Blood flow patterns induced in the dominant hemisphere by speech and reading. *Brain, 97*, 273–288.

Kertesz, A. (1979). *Aphasia and associated disorders: Taxonomy, localization and recovery.* New York: Grune & Stratton.

Kertesz, A. (1983). *Localization in neuropsychology.* New York: Academic Press.

Kertesz, A., & Black, S. E. (1983). *Lesion localization in aphasia.* Paper presented at the Academy of Aphasia meeting, Minneapolis.

Kertesz, A., Black, S. E., & Howell, J. (1984). *Anatomical asymmetries on nuclear magnetic resonance: Correlation with dissection and functional lateralization.* Paper presented at the Academy of Aphasia meeting, Los Angeles.

Kertesz, A., & Dobrowolski, S. (1981). Right hemisphere deficits, lesion size and location. *Journal of Clinical Neuropsychology, 4*, 283–299.

Kertesz, A., Harlock, W., & Coates, R. (1979). Computer tomographic localization, lesion size and prognosis in aphasia. *Brain and Language, 8*, 34–50.

Kertesz, A., Lesk, D., & McCabe, P. (1977). Isotope localization of infarcts in aphasia. *Brain, 100*, 1–18.

Kertesz, A., Sheppard, A., & MacKenzie, R. A. (1982). Localization in transcortical sensory aphasia. *Archives of Neurology, 39*, 475–478.

Kleist, K. (1962). Sensory aphasia and amusia. In F. J. Fish & J. B. Stanton (Eds.), *The myeloarchitectonic basis.* Oxford: Pergamon Press.

Kutas, M., & Hillyard, S. A. (1980). Reading between the lines: Event-related brain potentials during natural sentence processing. *Brain and Language, 11*, 354–373.

Lassen, N. A., & Roland, P. R. (1983). Localization of cognitive function with cerebral blood flow. In A. Kertesz (Ed.), *Localization in neuropsychology.* New York: Academic Press.

Levine, D., & Mohr, J. (1979). Language after bilateral cerebral infarctions: Role of the minor hemisphere in speech. Neurology, 29, 297–338.

Low, W., Wada, J. A., & Fox, M. (1973). Electroencephalographic localization of the conative aspects of language production in the human brain. Transactions of American Neurological Association, 98, 129–133.

Luria, A. R. (1970). Traumatic aphasia. The Hague: Mouton.

Marie, P., & Foix, C. (1917). Les aphasies de guerre. Revue Neurologique, 24, 53–87.

Marinesco, G., Sager, O., & Kreindler, A. (1936). Etudes électroencephalographiques; électroencephalogrammes dans l'aphasie. Bulletin of the Academy of Medicine of Paris, 116, 182.

Mateer, C. (1983). Localization of language and visuospatial functions by electrical stimulation. In A. Kertesz (Ed.), Localization in neuropsychology. New York: Academic Press.

Mazziotta, J. C., & Phelps, M. E. (1984). Human sensory stimulation and deprivation: Positron emission tomographic results and strategies. Neurology, 14, 50–60.

Metter, E. J., Wasterlain, C. G., Kuhl, D. E., Hanson, W. R., & Phelps, M. E. (1981). 18 FDG positron emission computed tomography in a study of aphasia. Annals of Neurology, 10, 173–183.

Mettler, R. (1949). Selective partial ablation of the frontal cortex: A correlative study of the effects of the human psychotic subjects. New York: Hoeber.

Mohr, J. P. (1976). Broca's area and Broca's aphasia. In H. Whitaker & H. A. Whitaker (Eds.), Studies in neurolinguistics (Vol. 1). New York: Academic Press.

Mohr, J. P., Watters, W. C., & Duncan, G. W. (1975). Thalamic hemorrhage and aphasia. Brain and Language, 2, 3–17.

Moutier, F. (1908). L'aphasie de Broca. Paris: Steinheil.

Neville, H. J., Kutas, M., & Schmidt, A. (1982). Event-related potential studies of cerebral specialization during reading. I. Studies of normal adults. Brain and Language, 16, 300–315.

Nielsen, J. M. (1946). Agnosia, apraxia, aphasia. New York: Hoeber.

Ojemann, G. A., & Mateer, C. (1979). Human language cortex: Localization of memory, syntax and sequential motor-phoneme identification systems. Science, 250, 1401–1403.

Ojemann, G. A., & Whitaker, H. A. (1978). Language localization and variability. Brain and Language, 6, 239–260.

Penfield, W., & Roberts, L. (1959). Speech and brain mechanisms. Princeton, NJ: Princeton University Press.

Raichle, M. E., Herscovitch, P., Mintun, A. M., Martin, W. R. W., & Power, W. (1984). Dynamic measurements of local blood flow and metabolism in the study of higher cortical function in humans with positron emission tomography. Neurology, 14, 48–49.

Reil, J. C. (1809). Untersuchungen über den Bau des grossen Gehirns im Menschen. Archiv für Anatomie und Physiologie, 9, 136–524.

Rubens, A. B. (1976). Transcortical motor aphasia. In H. Whitaker & H. A. Whitaker (Eds.), Studies in neurolinguistics (Vol. 1). New York: Academic Press.

Russell, W. R., & Espir, M. L. E. (1961). Traumatic aphasia. London: Oxford University Press.

Sanides, F. (1962). Die architektonik des menschlichen Stirnhirns. Berlin: Springer-Verlag.

Schiller, F. (1947). Aphasia studied in patients with missile wounds. Journal of Neurology, Neurosurgery and Psychiatry, 10, 183.

Semmes, J., Weinstein, S., Ghent, L., & Teuber, H. L. (1960). Somatosensory changes after penetrating brain wounds in man. Cambridge, MA: Harvard University Press.

Shelburne, S. A. (1972). Visual evoked responses to word and nonsense syllable stimuli. Cortex, 12, 325–336.

Smith, A. (1966). Speech and other functions after left (dominant) hemispherectomy. Journal of Neurology, Neurosurgery and Psychiatry, 29, 467–471.

Sperry, R. W., Gazzaniga, M. S., & Bogen, J. E. (1969). Interhemispheric relationship: The neocortical commissures; syndromes of hemispheric disconnection. In P. J. Vinken & G. W. Bruyn (Eds.), Handbook of clinical neurology (Vol. 4). Amsterdam: North-Holland.

Talairach, J., & Szikla, G. (1967). Atlas of stereotaxic anatomy of the telencephalon. Paris: Masson.

Ter-Pogossian, M. M., Ficke, D. C., Mintun, M. A., Herscovitch, P., Fox, P. T., & Raichle, M. E. (1984). Dynamic cerebral positron emission tomographic studies. Neurology, 15, 46–47.

Teyler, T. J., Roemer, R. A., Harrison, T. F., et al. (1973). Human scalp-recorded evoked-potential correlates of linguistic stimuli. Bulletin of the Psychonomic Society, 1, 333–324.

Tikofsky, R. S., Collier, B. D., Saxena, V. K., Hellman, R. S., Zielonka, J. A., & Palmer, D. W. (1984). I-123 iodoamphetamine (IMP) single photon emission computerized tomography (SPECT) imaging in normals and aphasics. Paper presented at the Academy of Aphasia meeting, Los Angeles.

Tikofsky, R. S., Kooi, K. A., & Thomas, M. H. (1960). Electroencephalographic findings and recovery from aphasia. Neurology, 10, 154–156.

Van Buren, J., Fedio, P., & Frederick, G. (1978). Mechanism and localization of speech in the parietotemporal cortex. Neurosurgery, 2, 233–239.

Von Keyserlingk, D. G., De Bleser, R., & Poeck, K. (1983). Stereographic reconstruction of human brain CT series. Acta Anatomique, 115, 336–344.

Von Monakow, C. (1914). Die Lokalisation im Grosshirn und der Abbau der Funktionen durch corticale Herde. Wiesbaden: Bergmann.

Wood, F. (1980). Theoretical, methodological, and statistical implications of the inhalation rCBF technique for the study of brain-behavior relationships. Brain and Language, 9, 1–8.

Yarnell, P. R., Monroe, M. A., & Sobel, L. (1976). Aphasia outcome in stroke: A clinical and neuroradiological correlation. Stroke, 7, 516–522.

4

ERPs and Advances in Neurolinguistics

SIDNEY J. SEGALOWITZ

Neurolinguistics is the study of the brain correlates of language, and the methods used have been drawn from experimental and clinical neuropsychology as well as from experimental and descriptive linguistics. Traditionally, the database has drawn from clinical aphasiology (Caplan, 1987; Lecours, Lhermitte, & Bryans, 1983), but experimental neuropsychology has added a number of research paradigms that neurolinguists have found useful (Beaumont, 1982; Bryden, 1982; Hannay, 1986).

The event-related potential (ERP) technique is beginning to prove very useful in neurolinguistics, providing another metric with which to attack some long-standing questions. In this chapter, I will summarize some of the ways the ERP technique may prove useful in addressing neurolinguistics research questions and have focused on neurolinguistic issues that I think are amenable for use with the ERP paradigm. The idiosyncratic mix for research questions reflects both current issues in the field and my own particular interests. I will begin, however, with a review of some ERP techniques and technical controversies that relate directly to the research questions of interest.

OVERVIEW OF ERP METHODOLOGY

There are a great many reviews of ERP techniques for those intending to set up an ERP laboratory (e.g., Callaway, Tueting, & Koslow, 1978; Gaillard & Ritter, 1983). In this section, rather than outline these details, I

SIDNEY J. SEGALOWITZ • Department of Psychology, Brock University, St. Catharines, Ontario L2S 3A1, Canada.

will describe in rough terms the philosophy underlying this methodology for cognitive neuropsychology.

The basic assumption behind the measuring of event-related electrical potential shifts on the scalp is that these shifts are sensitive to the cognitive activity of the brain. As obvious as this assumption is, it is useful to examine it in some detail to explicitly state its limitations and its strengths. For example, this sensitivity is a mixed blessing, since the resultant EEG wave form during any particular event is a reflection of the many information processes and nervous system activities occurring during the event. Most of these processes are not of interest to our research question, especially those relating to movements idiosyncratic to the particular event. The way to eliminate the effects of these activities is, of course, to average the EEG wave form over many trials with appropriate control conditions, effectively averaging out any random nonevent-related potential shifts and summating those that are truly event-linked. Because of restrictions designed to help eliminate the unwanted noise factors, we find that the ERP paradigm is not as ideally suited to measuring brain events as we might like. More on this later.

ERP versus Reaction Time

One of the strengths of the cognitive experimental paradigm is the imaginative ways that reaction times (RTs) can be used to examine component processes of a task. For example, if we find that subjects consistently require more time to solve Task A than Task B, we can safely conclude that the tasks require different cognitive or motor resources. This paradigm has been elaborated to a high degree of sophistication (Posner, 1986). It is difficult, however, to rely on RT (or error-score) paradigms when we have reason to believe that the cognitive processes are not additive, or when we are interested in examining processing that occurs during the event and not just as a result of its completion. The ERP paradigm is especially useful here since the wave form is a reflection of ongoing activity.

A second advantage of the ERP over the RT paradigm in neurolinguistic research relates to issue of brain localization of function. There are limits to how much visual half-field or dichotic listening paradigms will aid our determining even hemispheric asymmetries of processing. In these cases, we once again are limited by the response reflecting only the finished product, as well by the attendant problem of the artifacts peculiar to these paradigms (Bryden, 1982). Now, there are considerable limits on the localizing potential of most ERP paradigms, but there are also reasonable conclusions that can be made from information on brain localization of the signals.

FIGURE 1. Averaged ERP results from Segalowitz and MacGregor (1987) illustrating a common configuration of peaks. In this case, the subjects were presented with English words on a CRT screen to read aloud, one at a time. The ERP duration is 500 msec. The similarity across the hemispheres indicates that functional asymmetries contribute very little variance to the ERP, although this variance can be consistent (see Figure 3).

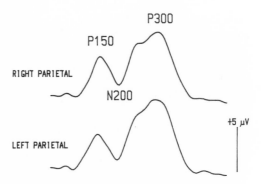

Methods of Analysis

Rather than outline the evidence in favor of and against interpretations of the various wave peaks that have been propounded, I would like to focus on the aspects of wave analysis that pertain to neurolinguistics specifically. The first question we must address in cognitive electrophysiology is whether the effect we find is attributable to the specific cognitive processes of interest or to general attentional processes. For example, the early negative (N100 and sometimes N200), late positive (P300), and later negative (N400) components seem to be sensitive to attentional aspects of the typical cognitive ERP paradigm, and the peaks have become quite famous in the ERP literature (see Figure 1 for a simple example). The size and latency of these components may vary depending on the stimuli or the processing task, allowing us to conclude that there are processing differentiations being made. For example, reading high-frequency words may produce values quite different from reading low-frequency words. As useful as these components are in cognitive electrophysiology (see Friedman, Simson, Ritter, & Rapin, 1975; Gaillard & Ritter, 1983; Kutas & Van Petten, 1988, for reviews), we can never be sure that the cognitive component we are interested in is reflected in these famous peaks, since the wave contains much information beyond these particular points.

An alternate approach is to compare the entire wave shape across the experimental conditions. This is done usually with one of two methods, either with what is known as the PCA-ANOVA technique (Donchin, 1966) or by using Pearson correlations in particular time frames across the wave. The former is a highly controversial technique that derives time-clustered components by which to parse the wave shape, and then compares the factor scores for these components across the independent variables. The factor scores essentially reflect amplitude differences associated with the independent variables. The controversy surrounds the issue of whether or

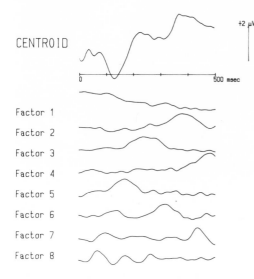

FIGURE 2. An example of a PCA output from an ERP experiment (Segalowitz & Cohen, 1988). The centroid is the averaged response over frontal, parietal, and temporal sites to a series of consonant-vowel speech sounds. The eight factors represent statistically orthogonal time clusters that together account for 93% of the variance in the raw data. See text for further discussion.

not the time-based components are true underlying factors in the makeup of the aggregate averaged ERP (Möcks, 1986; Möcks & Verleger, 1986; Wood & McCarthy, 1984). The true test of this technique is, like any other technique, in replication and generalization, which has been occasionally done (e.g., Molfese, 1978, vs. Segalowitz & Cohen, 1989), but much less often than for the more traditional analysis of wave peaks. This situation may be as much a product of the relatively few laboratories utilizing this complex technique as of the inherent complications in using it (Kramer & Donchin, 1987).

For example, one of the facets of this technique that deserves caution is that in a single study, the averaged ERPs are subjected to a principal components analysis that derives several factors, each representing some time clustering (see Figure 2). For each factor, the analysis produces factor scores for each combination of independent variables for each averaged ERP entering the analysis. These factor scores indicate the relative weight for the dependent measures—i.e. the cell in the design—leading to an analysis of variance for each factor. One may question the true Type I error when, say, 10 such ANOVAs are performed, not exactly on the same data set, but on scores derived from the same data set. We do not know whether this should be a concern, and perhaps the test of time will be an empirical one. For example, Segalowitz and Cohen (1988) tried to replicate Molfese's (1978) study of cerebral asymmetries in ERPs produced to certain phonological contrasts. The effect seemed to generalize well to the new stimuli, contexts, and electrode sites used by Segalowitz and Cohen, but the nagging problem of true alpha level remained. To test for this, they performed 100 repeated ANOVAs on the factor scores for the critical condition that replicated Molfese for each of eight factors, each time randomizing the factor score set. There were in this way nine chance replications of the original result. They concluded that the .025 level was more than safe as a level of Type I error to accept for the replication.

It may be that the strength of the PCA-ANOVA technique is not simply in finding differentiations in the ERPs that are very difficult to make from a visual scan of the data, but is to be found in the focusing of attention to a particular portion of the wave. As long as we accept the idea that the ERP is highly sensitive to all sorts of processing, we will be left with the problem of deciding which subtle fluctuation in the waves are reflections of our experimental design. To return to the example given from Segalowitz and Cohen, after verifying that the effect replicating Molfese was not a statistical quirk, they returned to the raw ERPs and examined the wave in the section indicated by the factor in question. If the factor had been an emergent statistical product, there should be no correspondence in the raw data. They found that the raw data produced the same interaction. It was unlikely, though, that they would have thought to look at that part of the wave if the PCA had not pointed to it, since it did not represent one of the famous peaks. Similarly, Brown, Marsh, and Smith (1979) found the same results using a PCA-ANOVA treatment of data reported earlier using ERP correlations (Brown, Marsh, & Smith, 1976).

A simpler method of comparing the overall wave shape that would be useful for neurolinguistic investigations is a straight correlational metric. For example, Brown, Marsh, and Smith (1973, 1976) found that the Pearson correlation of the ERPs for noun and verb forms of ambiguous words was higher over the right hemisphere than over the left hemisphere, and that this difference was especially found for the anterior sites. The beauty of this technique is that we do not have to interpret the specifics of the wave characteristics, only that the waves resemble each other across conditions over some sites and not over others. Refinement of this method involves restricting the time frame for the calculation of the ERP.

Is a Mental Chronometry Possible?

One of the benefits of the ERP paradigm in cognitive electrophysiology is that it allows us to examine ongoing processing. Does this really allow a "mental chronometry," a specification of what information is being processed when? Or barring that, does it at least allow us to say something about the timing of the thinking, as opposed to the response? An important demonstration that this may be the case is the classic study of McCarthy and Donchin (1981), where it was shown that the P300 is not simply a reflection of the impending motor response. That is, the P300 peak reflects in a systematic way something other than the preparation or execution of the response. Donchin et al. showed this by demonstrating that the latency of the P300 peak is not correlated with the RT response, and thus could not be simply due to some preparation to respond. This is important because, without being assured of this separation, we could conclude that the ERP did not reflect cognitive processes at all, but only motor responses. This would have been easy to accept since movement effects are very strong in the EEG record. Since, however, the P300 seems to reflect something in the decision-making process, we can entertain the possibility that the peaks in general reflect important steps in the cognitive requirements of the tasks.

Now, if we find that a change in processing requirement causes a prominent peak to lag or lead, we may wish to conclude that the processing change occurs at this point in the task. This is a reasonable hypothesis to form from such data, but are the data sufficient to conclude this? Clearly the processing must occur at some time before the evidence of it appears in the ERP. The difficulty is that we do not know, and perhaps cannot know, how much before. Thus, a mental chronometry is possible only in terms of "at least by the point" constructs.

More elaborate mental chronometries can be constructed from the PCA-ANOVA technique, since many research questions can be asked at the same time of the same data, each with a timing figure. For example, Segalowitz, Menna, and MacGregor (1987) presented the results of adult subjects' making matching judgments on pairs of words, which either (1) look similar and rhyme (e.g., *look, book*), (2) look similar and do not rhyme (e.g., *paid, said*), (3) rhyme but do not look similar (e.g., *make, ache*), or (4) do not rhyme or look similar (e.g., mind, wall), a paradigm used by Polich, McCarthy, Wang, and Donchin (1983). A factor peaking at 272 msec indicates that the left hemisphere has reacted differentially to the rhyme confusion list (list 3) compared with the two control lists (lists 1 and 4), whereas the right hemisphere does not. A factor at 370 msec shows that the left hemisphere is clearly differentiating both confusion lists (2 and 3) from the controls, while the right hemisphere is only differentiating the visual confusion list (list 2). By 490 msec, both hemispheres are sensitive to the two confusion lists. This simple story would be fine if we could be confident that these times really reflected the decision point in the mental progression in the task. Because of the difficulties mentioned earlier in verifying the objective reality of the component factors, it is important to replicate these sorts of specific findings. The use of the ERP technique to create a mental chronometry would certainly be a breakthrough for cognitive electrophysiology. Whether the techniques outlined will prove useful in the end is an empirical question.

There are, however, built-in limitations that should be acknowledged at the outset. First of all, the generalizability of the results across laboratories will always be difficult not because of instability of the results but because of differing amplification and filtering systems. Each set of amplifiers has to have some setting for the time constant (Duncan-Johnson & Donchin, 1981), and this time constant effectively sets the lower limit of the frequency response. Similarly, each laboratory must decide on the set of signal filters that it will use, these usually being analogue filters built into the amplifier system. Analogue filters, however, cause phase shifting. For example, the peaks of slow waves can be delayed by half a cycle with standard 30-Hz low pass filters, which can translate into as much as 50 msec or more. This shift can be easily measured for a pure signal, say a 10-Hz sine wave, but is unpredictable for an irregular wave such as an EEG signal. Since most laboratories use the upper cutoff of 30 Hz and a lower cutoff of under 1 Hz, there may be fairly good correspondence in the literature, but it does not mean that this will hold for all laboratories (cf. Kramer & Donchin, 1987).

A second difficulty with obtaining a fine chronometry is the inherent limitation of the filtered ERP signal. The usual 30-Hz band pass is used to reduce the higher frequencies that stem from muscle artifacts, and indeed, EEG signals filtered at 30 Hz are considerably cleaner to view. The difficulty is that at 30-Hz filtering, defining a peak takes 33 msec, which means that peaks cannot be fully resolved in a time period shorter than this, although with averaging, apparently higher frequencies can be obtained. Is 33 msec a long or a short time for cognitive processing? This clearly depends on the processing we are concerned with, but we can easily think of cases where much can be done in this time period. It is not surprising, then, that the major ERP peaks that have been tied to cognitive processing are separated by at least 100 msec. The technique as it is currently used limits the temporal resolution.

Is Cortical Localization Possible?

Can we localize cognitive processes using electrical signals? This is still a controversial issue. Gevins, Bressler, and Illes (1988), for example, recently argued that misleading conclusions are drawn from localizing attempts when too few electrodes are used. His illustrations involved at least 128 electrode sites. One can use mathematical interpolation to help localize the source of signal changes (Duffy, Burchfiel, & Lombroso, 1979). This is dependent, of course, on the degree of detail of the input. But what if we have far fewer sites than are needed for mathematical interpolation? The research question, in such a case, usually focuses on either the issue of anterior versus posterior location or that of left versus right hemisphere. There are cases of each where we can suspect difficulty with such localization. The recording at the scalp may be driven by a generator at some distance if the distant brain surface is oriented toward the recording site and the signal is well localized within that brain surface. For example, if care is not taken, the electrical response a visual stimulus delivered to the left hemisphere via the right visual half-field will be greater over the right hemisphere, especially if recorded at the 01 and 02 sites (Wood, 1982). This is because the visual signal registers in the mesial section of the occipital lobe, and the more centrally located the stimulus, the stronger this effect. One solution is to display stimuli laterally enough to have them represented on the lateral occipital surface; another is not to record occipitally when using visual stimuli. For example, Neville, Kutas, and Schmidt (1982a) find ERP asymmetries in temporal and frontal regions that are independent of the visual field of stimulus presentation. There have been no suggestions, though, that this problem of hemisphere differentiation arises from any cognitive activity outside of visual perception, although presumably mesial primary sensory cortex of the parietal lobe would produce similar results.

A similar situation holds for the N100 component of the ERP obtained in an auditory attention task. This negative wave is found maximally over the frontocentral areas of the scalp. Yet it has been shown to be generated in the auditory cortex of the temporal lobe (Scherg & Von Cramon, 1986). Notice that once again we are dealing with primary sensory cortex.

The Problem of Electrode Reference

Another issue reputedly leading to difficulty in localizing hemispheric asymmetries stems from the question of appropriate reference electrode. This problem has an interesting history, and no commonly acceptable solution. Katznelson (1981) has argued that using the usual linked-ear reference sites reduces lateral asymmetries electrically because of an equalizing of the potentials at the ears, and presumably linked mastoids produces a similar situation. Thus, if one temporal lobe is generating a signal, linking the ears will reduce this asymmetry at the scalp. Alternative reference sites can be complex (such as using a form of averaged site; Hjorth, 1982) or simple (such as using Cz), but then introduce vagaries of their own. The latter site itself is very highly responsive to cognitive processing and therefore is perhaps not a good reference location; the former method produces a result that is dependent on the particular electrode configuration used. Since different laboratories insist on using different site configurations, this is problematical. The original problem may be overstated by Katznelson, though. There have been many studies finding lateral asymmetries with linked ears or mastoids as references (e.g., Brown et al., 1973, 1976, discussed below; see Kutas & Van Petten, 1988; Molfese, 1983, for reviews). If Katznelson is correct, these findings are interesting for neurolinguistics in that they may reflect a relative lack of generators in the lateral temporal lobes, especially for linguistic material.

In summary, it may be that any attempt to localize cognitive components with only a few electrode sites will be hampered by various factors. However, simple laterality questions may be addressable still with modest ERP paradigms. Clearly, however, the trend will be toward more elaborate methods, with more elaborate data analysis.

ERPs AND SOME RESEARCH ISSUES IN NEUROLINGUISTICS

Neurolinguistics and psycholinguistics have burgeoned as fields of research in the past two decades. It is now well-nigh impossible to keep up with the books in the field, not to mention the proliferating journals. Many advances have been made, but some questions remain, perhaps clarified and sharpened by the attention they have received, but nonetheless available for further clarification. Some of the issues, on the other hand, seem to be unresolvable, given traditional research paradigms, and may have become more philosophical than empirical. The semantics/syntax distinction falls into this position. However, the new ERP technology will allow us to open up some of these questions again for empirical study in new ways and may help us sharpen once again the deep questions being posed. In this section, I will address several research areas in neurolinguistics that may benefit or have benefited from examination in the ERP paradigm.

Lexical Semantics

There has been a considerable increase in interest in the last few years on the issue of lexical semantics, which for the purposes of this chapter will be defined as the network of meaning relationships that is mediated through the linguistic system (cf. Job & Sartori, 1988). The increase in interest stems no doubt from both cognitive and neuropsychological sources. The development of semantic network systems over the past two decades (e.g., Collins & Loftus, 1975; Johnson-Laird, Hermann, & Chaffin, 1984) has spurred hope of understanding the structure of the web of meaning in the human mind. Until recently, however, the neurolinguistic issue remained fairly simple: Linguistic semantics is entirely a function of the left hemisphere, and the primary issue was whether or not there were semantic-syntactic disruptions in anterior versus posterior forms of aphasia (Zurif & Caramazza, 1976). Brown et al. (1973, 1976), for example, as mentioned earlier found that when subjects listen to a word that could be interpreted as a noun or a verb depending on the context (i.e., fire, duck, lead/led), ERPs over the left hemisphere, and the anterior presentation especially, differentiated the two grammatical forms.

More recently, however, patients with right-hemisphere damage have been documented to have subtle communicative dysfunctions that could be seen to involve lexical semantics. For example, Brownell, Potter, Michelow, and Gardner (1984) examined the sensitivity of left- and right-brain-damaged patients to connotative versus denotative facets of a word's meaning. They found a double dissociation linking the right hemisphere to connotation. Similarly, the right hemisphere has been linked in clinical studies to certain aspects of verbal humor (Brownell, Michel, Powelson, & Gardner, 1983), difficulty with negative sentences (D'Urso, Denes, Testa, & Senenza, 1986), difficulty with logicogrammatical relations (Hier & Kaplan, 1980), difficulty with organizing sentences into coherent paragraphs (Delis, Wapner, Gardner, & Moses, 1983), difficulty with two-term series problems, such as "Tom is taller than Fred. Who is shorter?" (Caramazza, Gordon, Zurif, & DeLuca, 1976), and difficulty in the acquisition of the meaning of new lexical items from context (Grossman & Carey, 1978). It would be interesting to see if ERP evidence of these processes patterns itself similarly since one can imagine complex interactions between the intact hemispheres such that the asymmetry model suggested above is not adequate (Gevins, 1986).

Similarly, the ERP paradigm may prove useful as a way of examining the semantic networks involved in the issues of polysemy, semantic priming, and activation. For example, Burgess and Simpson (1988) have proposed an interesting neurolinguistic hypothesis. They suggest that when a subject reads an ambiguous word, both major and minor meanings are invoked but the minor meaning is quickly suppressed. They then show by means of the visual half-field paradigm that this pattern is true for the left hemisphere only, and that the right hemisphere indeed promotes the subordinate meaning of the word, which they interpret as akin to the link between metaphorical thinking and right-hemisphere processing. Van Petten and Kutas (1987) conducted an analogous study using ERPs and conclude on the contrary that both meanings are not activated at the same time. Unfortunately, they did not utilize posterior lateral recording sites and so did not examine the lateralization hypothesis. Clearly, however, it would be interesting to examine the Burgess et al. finding more closely with an ERP paradigm that allows for more normal reading processes.

Semantics versus Syntax

Separating semantics from syntax has been a long-standing controversy in linguistics (Caplan, 1987; Crystal, 1988). The neurolinguistic aspect of this difficulty is seen in the controversy over whether it is possible for some aphasics to have a semantic deficit without concomitant syntactic losses, and vice versa. There are many aspects to this problem, and the traditional difficulty is that behavioral paradigms have usually not simultaneously addressed the semantic and syntactic components of the task. For example, Zurif and Caramazza (1976) concluded that there are grammatical competence disruptions in frontal aphasics; however, they do not claim to have assessed semantic comprehension. Similarly, in an ERP study, Brown et al. (1973, 1976) do demonstrate that the anterior areas of the brain are more sensitive to the distinction between verb and noun, but the task does not separate out semantic processing. However, Kutas and Hillyard (1983) have provided direct ERP evidence for some separation by comparing the N400 component to semantic versus syntactic anomalies (i.e., stimuli representing an inappropriate semantic category versus incorrect verb tense or number marking). They found that semantic anomalies produce the N400 deflection whereas the syntactic ones do not. Moreover, the degree of deflection varies with the unexpectedness of the anomaly (Kutas & Hillyard, 1984). They also found (in the 1983 study) that the open- versus closed-class distinction was associated with the more anterior sites. Garnsey (1985) also found that the ERPs were sensitive to open- versus closed-class words but not RT.

Reading in Normals

Can we discern component processes in reading and use ERPs to define them, time-track them, and localize them cerebrally? Current theories of reading focus on English, probably because most of the researchers in the field work in English-speaking countries (e.g., Coltheart, 1987; Coltheart, Patterson, & Marshall, 1980; Henderson, 1984). The models of reading English almost invariably include two routes: a phonologically based route, which involves the grapheme–phoneme correspondence (GPC) rules, and a so-called visual route, which makes use of visual information. The need for the two routes in English is clear (Patterson, 1982). The reading of new words is clearly first attempted by "sounding out," if the spelling seems to be regular, and often pronunciation errors are based on spelling-pronunciations. Visual information is also clearly used since English has many homophones that have distinct spellings (e.g., seas, seize, sees). Both these situations obtain in French as well (i.e., new words pronounced by GPC analogies to known words, and the existence of homonyms such as il LIE, le lit, je lis). The mapping of spelling onto sound and vice versa differs in interesting ways, however, and so the psycholinguistic processes in reading may differ across the two languages (N. S. Segalowitz, 1986). Languages with more regular GPC, such as Spanish, Italian, or Estonian, again may involve the reader with a different set of cognitive strategies. These interlanguage differences are only beginning to be studied (Patterson, Marshall, & Coltheart, 1985).

In any case, the existence of these two routes for English is well established in the neurolinguistic literature, especially in the acquired dyslexia domain (Marshall, 1985; Marshall & Newcombe, 1973). Some have stated that whereas the phonological route must be left-hemisphere-based, the visual route may involve right-hemisphere processes (Colt-heart, 1980), although there is actually very little or no empirical support for this neurolinguistic hypothesis. Visual half-field studies (Chiarello, 1985; Hatta, 1977, 1981; Leong, Wong, Wong, & Hiscock, 1985; Sasanuma, Itoh, Kobayashi, & Mori, 1980; Sasanuma, Itoh, Mori, & Kobayashi, 1977) suggest that the hemispheres may differ on the processes involved. The ERP paradigm enables us to examine ongoing processing with more normal reading (centrally presented, unlimited viewing). So, for example, Kramer and Donchin (1987) found that in a word-matching paradigm, a specific ERP component (N200) appears in response to an orthographic mismatch whether the subject is attending to orthography or not, while an N200 is elicited by a phonological mismatch only if phonology is task-relevant. That is, orthographic analysis is automatic while phonological is not. This may be relevant to the issue of pre- versus postlexical phonology in reading English.

Using this approach to examine the hemispheric specialization issue directly, Segalowitz et al. (1987) have found that with both nonword matching of letter strings and reading of real words, left/right-hemisphere asymmetries can be manipulated by varying the decoding route primarily used. This was done with nonword letter string matching (same/different judgment) by making the letter strings either pronounceable or unpronounceable. The pronounceable letter strings encouraged a phonological coding strategy, which is probably the more natural one for fluent readers (in this case, university undergraduates). The unpronounceable letter string discourages the phonological coding, and the subjects reported a visual strategy. The N1-P3 amplitude shift was significantly greater over the left hemisphere for the pronounceable lists and over the right hemisphere for the unpronounceable lists (see Figure 3).

Similarly, they asked university undergraduates to perform either a rhyme judgment or a visual-similarity judgment (as in Polich et al., 1983; Kramer & Donchin, 1987, discussed above) on word pairs that either rhymed and/or looked similar (i.e., looked as if they should rhyme). They compared the general amplitude shift of the averaged ERPs of the control nonrhyming, nonvisually similar list with the others. The visually confusing list (i.e., the ones that look similar without rhyming, such as *said* and *paid*) differentiated from the control list in sites over the right hemisphere, while the phonologically confusing list (e.g., *ache* and *make*) differentiated from the control list only after the left hemisphere. Thus, there appears to be support for different hemisphere sensitivities to the processes involved in the two decoding routes. No doubt the picture will be much more complex when considering reading in context.

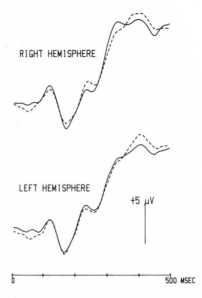

FIGURE 3. Averaged ERPs from left- and right-hemisphere sites taken to the second of a pair of letter strings (Segalowitz, Menna, & MacGregor, 1987). Subjects had to indicate by button press whether the two letter strings, which were either pronounceable (---) or un-pronounceable (—), were the same or different. These averages are for the "same" trials only, and illustrate the slight but consistent hemisphere by stimulus list interaction.

Development of Reading Skills

Perhaps it is a bit too cynical to suggest that children learn to read in spite of the pedagogical technique currently in vogue at the time they enter public school, but one is tempted to look for some cognitive strategies that children apply to the task whether the curriculum recommends "whole-word" or "phonic" methods. This controversy as to the most efficient technique for teaching reading may pertain more to the teaching of English than other languages. Indeed, the number of children who experience difficulty in phonic decoding is considerably higher in English-speaking countries than in those with more phonically regular writing systems, although it is hard to attribute the difference solely to the writing system since there are also differences in SES, cultural attitudes toward schooling, age at school entry, and so on (Taylor & Taylor, 1983). The acquisitions of English, then, may involve a subtle balance between the two decoding routes, as many specialists in the field have suggested (e.g., Boder, 1973; Ellis, 1984; Mitterer, 1982). It would be interesting to try to define these processes with ERP measurement techniques in children using paradigms similar to those described above, and to explore developmental shifts in how these processes are distributed.

Licht, Bakker, Kok, and Bouma (1988), for example, have collected ERPs from a group of children for 4 consecutive years beginning in kindergarten. The ERPs were to reading words in Dutch. The children were taught explicitly with a whole-word method initially, and proceeded to more phonic strategies later. The researchers performed a regression of

ERP variables onto reading performance scores at each age group. The finding relevant to the present discussion is that as the children got older, the amount of variance accounted for by the left temporal site increased dramatically while that for the parietal sites, especially the right, decreased. Thus, there is support, circumstantially at least, for the neurolinguistic right-to-left shift for reading. By the hypothesis given here, this relationship may not hold for those languages where phonics is the sole strategy used.

These researchers, however, suggest that the important issue here is not the application of GPC rules but of automaticity. Many theorists (Ellis, 1984) suggest that beginning readers first decode words element by element and gradually automatize the process so that larger groupings are apprehended. This chunking is necessary, of course, for rapid, fluent reading. Remaining research questions include, however, whether the advanced reader truly abandons the more elemental process and whether the automatized process represents a shift in cerebral functioning. Bakker and Licht (1986), for instance, report that normally, beginning reading children show a shift in greater ERP amplitude to reading words from the right hemisphere to the left hemisphere. Poor readers who remain slow at decoding seem to be stuck at the first element-by-element stage and do not show such a shift. Poor readers who read rapidly with many mistakes— that is, who seem to move to automatized reading before they have built up the processing chunks adequately—make this ERP amplitude shift sooner than normal. If these results are reliable, the neurolinguistic implications for reading and for automatized processes in general are considerable with pedagogical implications (Bakker, 1984).

Language Development

We expect that language acquisition, as a phonological guessing game, is primarily left-hemisphere-based. Molfese, Freeman, and Palermo (1975), in their classic study, found ERP hemisphere differentiation of speech sounds versus musical sounds in young infants. Many similar findings (Molfese & Betz, 1988; S. J. Segalowitz, 1983) have since reinforced the view that hemisphere specialization is congenital in most children and is not gradually developed during childhood, as was formerly thought (Lenneberg, 1967). ERPs have proved very useful for cognitive studies with young infants because there are few behavioral paradigms that will tap processing at such an early stage, especially in the auditory modality. Molfese and Betz list 11 ERP studies with infants demonstrating cerebral asymmetries. They then go on to describe their line of studies that focus on the mechanisms of such early functional asymmetries, again illustrating how the ERP paradigm is well suited for this research question. For example, they have shown not only that certain stop consonant distinctions are made from birth onward but that such data can be used to predict later delay in language acquisition (Molfese & Molfese, 1985). As well, they are using the ERP paradigm to examine the brain correlates of word acquisition by comparing the ERP response to arbitrarily paired nonsense syllables with a new object (Molfese et al., 1985) and to real known versus unknown words (Molfese, n.d.).

There are many other developmental neurolinguistic hypotheses worthy of investigation using this technique. For example, the development of lexical semantics is an area that has been well studied behaviorally over the last two decades. Meanwhile, neurolinguistic investigators have suggested that word acquisition requiring a new category distinction may especially entail right-hemisphere mechanisms (Grossman, 1981; Grossman & Carey, 1978). From a developmental neurolinguistic viewpoint, this is an important question, since we are still exploring the relationship between lexical and nonlexical semantics. Given that Molfese has shown that the ERP paradigm is sensitive to at least some aspect of word acquisition, it would be interesting to examine developmental data on these same parameters that were of interest in the adult lexical semantic studies.

Second-Language Acquisition

All of the research questions in lexical semantics and language acquisition have new aspects to them in studies of second-language acquisition. The study of the brain correlates of bilingualism is highly complex (Albert & Obler, 1978; Paradis, 1983; Vaid, 1983; Vaid & Genesee, 1980), and this is not the place to explore the details of the issues. However, it is easy to see that many of the neurolinguistic hypotheses outlined in various reviews (such as Vaid, 1983) are highly amenable to the ERP paradigm.

Another (admittedly more complex) twist to this issue is that of the acquisition of English as a second language by deaf individuals. For example, Neville, Kutas, & Schmidt (1982b) found ERP results (using the N400 paradigm) indicating a lack of asymmetry in congenitally deaf adults reading English, compared with the usual asymmetry found in normals. These results are fully compatible with current behavioral work examining the reading skills and strategies of deaf individuals (Gibson, 1988; Gibson & Segalowitz, 1986).

Issues in Clinical Neurolinguistics

Research in NL with clinical populations has utilized a variety of paradigms, deriving from various information-processing procedures (Beaumont, 1982; Hannay, 1986; Posner, 1986). It would be interesting to apply ERP techniques to some of these issues. There are a variety of obstacles, of course, making this application somewhat more problematic than for the issues outlined earlier. First of all, as with behavioral paradigms, there is the issue of compliance and consent. It is often the case that clinical patients are undergoing enough stress in their lives not to need or want the further stimulation of participating in basic research. In addition, those caring for this group may not be interested in the research questions enough to devote their own time to such projects.

Assuming, however, that these obstacles are overcome, there are research design technicalities that must be attended to. The electrical field configuration of the head may be altered among some clinical populations owing to physical damage to the skull. Nunez (1981) presents the physical problem that an irregularity, such as a break, in the skull theoretically alters the electric field properties of the scalp. However, Campbell and his colleagues (Campbell, Deacon-Eliott, & Proulx, 1986; Campbell, Deacon-Eliott, Suffield, & Proulx, 1987; Deacon-Eliott, Campbell, Suffield, & Proulx, 1987) report little difficulty in working with closed head injury (CHI) patients, although one could argue that, since they do find ERP differences between this group and normals, it is impossible to determine whether the effect is due to the physical alteration of the skull or to the consequences of CHI on the brain. Presumably, this is a testable hypothesis given the known condition of the subjects, using a quasi-case study design (Dywan & Segalowitz, 1986).

Neurolinguistic hypotheses involving populations with brain damage of whatever origin are critical to the field. For example, we may ask whether language recovery after severe left-hemisphere damage is done in the right hemisphere or in the residual tissue of the left hemisphere. This has been a long-debated issue, and the controversy continues. For example, much has been made of the residual ideogram-reading skills of some Japanese aphasics and of the semantic substitutions made by deep dyslexics to support the notion of a right-hemisphere reading capacity (Coltheart, 1980). To the extent that various ERP paradigms allow for lateral localization, we could address the issue. We could look for N400 asymmetries (with auditory presentation) to semantic incongruities in somewhat recovered aphasics. Papanicolaou, Levin, and Eisenberg (1984) used the ERP probe paradigm to test this hypothesis and indeed found support for a right-hemisphere basis for language in recovered aphasics.

Further work on subtle aspects of recovered language is possible. We may be interested in differences in the lexical semantics of patients who show left-hemisphere or right-hemisphere recovery of language. For example, Chapman, Bragdon, Chapman, and McCrary (1977) found ERP correlates of the semantic differential structure of nouns. Is this structure altered systematically in aphasics with differing symptoms (e.g., fluent vs.

nonfluent), in dementia patients, or in CHI patients who seem to have difficulty appreciating complexities in the world?

SUMMARY

The field of neurolinguistics is already well established and highly active. Many of the research questions derive from the clinic's using behavioral paradigms that have some inherent limitations. This chapter presents an outline of some of the advantages and disadvantages of the ERP paradigm as an alternate technology to supplement the traditional behavioral measures, and argues that a great many of the classic and new research questions in neurolinguistics could benefit from this paradigm.

REFERENCES

Albert, M., & Obler, L. (1978). The bilingual brain. New York: Academic Press.
Bakker, D. J. (1984). The brain as a dependent variable. Journal of Clinical Neuropsychology, 6, 1–16.
Bakker, D. J., & Licht, R. (1986). Learning to read: Changing horses in midstream. In G. Th. Pavlides & D. F. Fisher (Eds.), Dyslexia: Its neuropsychology and treatment. New York: Riley.
Beaumont, J. G. (Ed.). (1982). Divided visual field studies of cerebral organization. London: Academic Press.
Boder, E. (1973). Developmental dyslexia: A diagnostic approach based on three atypical reading-spelling patterns. Developmental Medicine and Child Neurology, 15, 663–687.
Brown, W. S., Marsh, J. T., & Smith, J. C. (1973). Contextual meaning effects on speech-evoked potentials. Behavioral Biology, 9, 755–761.
Brown, W. S., Marsh, J. T., & Smith, J. C. (1976). Evoked potential wave form differences produced by the perception of different meanings of an ambiguous phrase. Electroencephalography and Clinical Neurophysiology, 41, 113–123.
Brown, W. S., Marsh, J. T., & Smith, J. C. (1979). Principal component analysis of ERP differences related to the meaning of an ambiguous word. Electroencephalography and Clinical Neurophysiology, 46, 709–714.
Brownell, H. H., Michel, D., Powelson, J., & Gardner, H. (1983). Surprise but not coherence: Sensitivity to verbal humor in right-hemisphere patients. Brain and Language, 18, 20–27.
Brownell, H. H., Potter, H. H., Michelow, D., & Gardner, H. (1984). Sensitivity to lexical denotation and connotation in brain-damaged patients: A double dissociation? Brain and Language, 22, 253–265.
Bryden, M. P. (1982). Laterality: Functional asymmetry in the intact brain. New York: Academic Press.
Burgess, C., & Simpson, G. B. (1988). Cerebral hemisphere mechanisms in the retrieval of ambiguous word meanings. Brain and Language, 33, 86–103.
Callaway, E., Tueting, P., & Koslow, S. H. (1978). Event-related brain potentials in man. New York: Academic Press.
Campbell, K., Deacon-Elliott, D., & Proulx, G. (1986). Electrophysiological monitoring of

closed head injury, I. Basic principles and techniques. *Cognitive Rehabilitation, September–October,* 26–32.

Campbell, K., Deacon-Elliott, D., Suffield, J. B., & Proulx, G. B. (1987). Electrophysiological monitoring of closed head injury, II. Multimodal sensory evoked potentials. *Cognitive Rehabilitation, January–February,* 26–33.

Caplan, D. (1987). *Neurolinguistics and linguistic aphasiology: An introduction.* Cambridge: Cambridge University Press.

Caramazza, A., Gordon, J., Zurif, E. B., & DeLuca, D. (1976). Right-hemispheric damage and verbal problem solving behavior. *Brain and Language, 3,* 41–46.

Chapman, R. M., Bragdon, H. R., Chapman, J. A., & McCrary, J. W. (1977). Semantic meaning of words and averaged evoked potentials. In J. E. Desmedt (Ed.), *Recent developments in the psychobiology of language: The cerebral evoked potential approach.* London: Oxford University Press.

Chiarello, C. (1985). Hemisphere dynamics in lexical access: Automatic and controlled priming. *Brain and Language, 26,* 146–172.

Collins, A. M., & Loftus, E. F. (1975). A spreading-activation theory of semantic processing. *Psychological Review, 82,* 407–428.

Coltheart, M. (1980). Deep dyslexia: A right-hemisphere hypothesis. In M. Coltheart, K. Patterson, & J. C. Marshall (Eds.), *Deep dyslexia.* London: Routledge and Kegan Paul.

Coltheart, M. (1987). *The psychology of reading.* Hillsdale, NJ: Erlbaum.

Coltheart, M., Patterson, K., & Marshall, J. C. (1980). *Deep dyslexia.* London: Routledge and Kegan Paul.

Crystal, D. (1988). Linguistic levels in aphasia. In F. C. Rose, R. Whurr, & M. Ryke (Eds.), *Aphasia* (pp. 23–45). London: Whurr.

Deacan-Eliott, D., Campbell, K. B., Suffield, J. B., & Proulx, G. B. (1987). Electrophysiological monitoring of closed head injury. III. Cognitive evoked potentials. *Cognitive Rehabilitation,* 12–21.

Delis, D. C., Wapner, W., Gardner, H., & Moses, J. A. (1983). The contribution of the right hemisphere to the organization of paragraphs. *Cortex, 19,* 43–50.

Donchin, E. (1966). A multivariate approach to the analysis of averaged evoked potentials. *IEEE Transactions on Biomedical Engineering, BME-13*(3), 131–139.

Duffy, F. H., Burchfiel, J. L., & Lambroso, C. T. (1979). Brain electrical activity mapping (BEAM): A method for extending the clinical utility of EEG and evoked potential data. *Annals of Neurology, 5,* 309–321.

Duncan-Johnson, C. C., & Donchin, E. (1981). The time constant in P300 recording. *Psychophysiology, 16,* 53–55.

D'Urso, V., Denes, G., Testa, S., & Semenza, C. (1986). The role of the right hemisphere in processing negative sentences in context. *Neuropsychologia, 24,* 289–292.

Dywan, J., & Segalowitz, S. J. (1986). The role of the case study in neuropsychological research. In J. Valsiner (Ed.), *The individual subject and scientific psychology.* New York: Plenum Press.

Ellis, A. W. (1984). *Reading, writing and dyslexia: A cognitive analysis.* London: Erlbaum.

Friedman, D., Simson, R., Ritter, W., & Rapin, I. (1975). The late positive component (P300) and information processing in sentences. *Electroencephalography and Clinical Neurophysiology, 38,* 255–262.

Gaillard, A. W. K., & Ritter, W. (Eds.). (1983). *Tutorials in ERP research: Endogenous components.* Amsterdam: North-Holland.

Garnsey, S. (1985). Function words and context words: Reaction time and evoked potential measures of word recognition. *Cognitive Science Technical Report URCS-29,* University of Rochester, Rochester, New York.

Gevins, A. S. (1986). Quantitative human neurophysiology. In H. J. Hannay (Ed.), *Experi-*

mental techniques in human neuropsychology (pp. 419–456). New York: Oxford University Press.

Gevins, A. S., Bressler, S. L., & Illes, J. (1988, January 27–30). Effects of incipient fatigue on higher cortical function. Paper presented at the 16th Annual International Neuropsychological Society meeting, New Orleans.

Gibson, D. (1988). The impact of early developmental history on cerebral asymmetries: Implications for reading ability in deaf children. In D. L. Molfese & S. J. Segalowitz (Eds.), Developmental implications of brain lateralization. New York: Guilford Press.

Gibson, C., & Segalowitz, S. J. (1986). The impact of visual-spatial information on the development of reading proficiency in deaf children. In J. L. Nespoulous, P. Perron, & A. R. Lecours (Eds.), The biological foundations of gestures: Motor and semiotic aspects (pp. 215–227). Hillsdale, NJ: Erlbaum.

Grossman, M. (1981). A bird is a bird is a bird: Making reference within and without superordinate categories. Brain and Language, 12, 313–331.

Grossman, M., & Carey, S. (1978, October). Word-learning after brain damage. Paper presented to the Academy of Aphasia, Chicago.

Hannay, J. H. (1986). Experimental techniques in human neuropsychology. New York: Oxford University Press.

Hatta, T. (1977). Recognition of Japanese kaiji in the left and right visual fields. Neuropsychologia, 15, 605–688.

Hatta, T. (1981). Differential processing of kaiji and kana stimuli in Japanese people: Some implications from Stroop-test results. Neuropsychologia, 19, 87–93.

Henderson, L. (1984). Orthographies and readings: Perspectives from cognitive psychology. Hillsdale, NJ: Erlbaum.

Hier, D. B., & Kaplan, J. (1980). Verbal comprehension deficits after RH damage. Applied Psycholinguistics, 1, 279–294.

Hjorth, B. (1982). An adaptive EEG derivation technique. Electroencephalography and Clinical Neurophysiology, 54, 654–661.

Job, R., & Sartori, G. (1988). The cognitive neuropsychology of visual and semantic processing of concepts. Cognitive Neuropsychology, 5(1).

Johnson-Laird, P. N., Hermann, D. J., & Chaffin, R. (1984). Only connections: A critique of semantic networks. Psychological Bulletin, 96, 292–315.

Katznelson, R. D. (1981). EEG recording, electrode placement, and aspects of generator localization. In P. L. Nunez, Electrical fields of the brain. New York: Oxford University Press.

Kramer, A. F., & Donchin, E. (1987). Brain potentials as indices of orthographic and phonological interaction during word matching. Journal of Experimental Psychology: Learning, Memory and Cognition, 13, 76–86.

Kutas, M., & Hillyard, S. A. (1983). Event-related brain potentials to grammatical errors and semantic anomolies. Memory and Cognition, 11, 539–550.

Kutas, M., & Hillyard, S. A. (1984). Brain potentials during reading reflect word expectancy and semantic association. Nature, 307, 161–163.

Kutas, M., & Van Petten, C. (1988). Event-related brain potential studies of language. In P. K. Ackles, J. R. Jennings, & M. G. H. Close (Eds.), Advances in psychophysiology (139–187). Greenwich, CT: JAI Press.

Lecours, A. R., Lhermitte, F., & Bryans, B. (1983). Aphasiology. London: Balliere Tindall.

Lenneberg, E. H. (1967). Biological foundations of language. New York: Wiley.

Leong, C. K., Wong, S., Wong, A., & Hiscock, M. (1985). Differential cerebral involvement in perceiving Chinese characters: Levels of processing approach. Brain and language, 26, 131–145.

Licht, R., Bakker, D. J., Kok, A., & Bouma, A. (1988). The development of lateral event-related potentials (ERPs) related to word meaning: A four year longitudinal study. *Neuropsychologia, 26,* 327–340.

Marshall, J. C. (1985). On some relationships between acquired and developmental dyslexia. In F. H. Duffy & N. Geschwind (Eds.), *Dyslexia: A neuroscientific approach to clinical evaluation.* Boston: Little, Brown.

Marshall, J. C., & Newcombe, F. (1973). Patterns of paralexia: A psycholinguistic approach. *Journal of Psycholinguistic Research, 2,* 175–199.

McCarthy, G., & Donchin, E. (1981). A metric for thought: A comparison of P300 latency and reaction time. *Science, 211,* 77–80.

Mitterer, J. O. (1982). There are at least two kinds of poor readers: Whole-word poor readers and recoding poor readers. *Canadian Journal of Psychology, 36,* 445–461.

Möcks, J. (1986). The influence of latency jitter in principal component analysis of event-related potentials. *Psychophysiology, 23,* 480–484.

Möcks, J., & Verleger, R. (1986). Principal component analysis of event-related potentials: A note on misallocation of variance. *Electroencephalography and Clinical Neurophysiology, 65,* 393–398.

Molfese, D. L. (1978). Left and right hemisphere involvement in speech perception: Electrophysiological correlates. *Perception and Psychophysics, 23,* 237–243.

Molfese, D. M. (1983). Event related potentials and language processes. In A. W. K. Gaillard & W. Ritter (Eds.), *Tutorials in ERP research: Endogenous components* (pp. 345–367). Amsterdam: North Holland.

Molfese, D. M. (n.d.). *Electrophysiological correlates of word meanings in 14-month-old human infants.* (Mimeo)

Molfese, D. M., & Betz, J. C. (1988). Electrophysiological indices of the early development of lateralization for language and cognition and their implications for predicting later development. In D. M. Molfese & S. J. Segalowitz (Eds.), *Developmental implications of brain lateralization* (pp. 17–190). New York: Guilford Press.

Molfese, D., Freeman, R. B., & Palermo, D. S. (1975). The ontogeny of brain lateralization for speech and non-speech stimuli. *Brain and Language, 2,* 356–368.

Molfese, D. L., & Molfese, V. J. (1985). Electrophysiological indices of auditory discrimination in newborn infants: The bases for predicting later language development? *Infant Behavior and Development, 8,* 197–211.

Molfese, D. M., Wetzel, W. F., Linnville, S. E., Imbasciate, C., Leicht, D., Courtney, C., Baldwin, K., & Adams, C. A. (1985). *Word recognition in 16-month-old infants: Electrophysiological indices.* Paper presented at the 57th annual meetings of the Midwestern Psychological Association.

Neville, H. J., Kutas, M., & Schmidt, A. (1982a). Event-related potential studies of cerebral specialization during reading. I. Studies of normal adults. *Brain and Language, 16,* 300–315.

Neville, H. J., Kutas, M., & Schmidt, A. (1982b). Event-related potential studies of cerebral specialization during reading. II. Studies of congenitally deaf adults. *Brain and Language, 16,* 316–337.

Nunez, P. L. (1981). *Electric fields of the brain.* New York: Oxford University Press.

Papanicolaou, A. C., Levin, H. S., & Eisenbeg, H. (1984). Evoked potential correlates of recovery from aphasia after focal left hemisphere injury in adults. *Neurosurgery, 14,* 412–415.

Paradis, M. (Ed.). (1983). *Readings on aphasia in bilinguals and polyglots.* Montreal: Didier.

Patterson, K. E. (1982). The relation between reading and phonological coding: Further neuropsychological observations. In A. W. Ellis (Ed.), *Normality and pathology in cognitive functions* (pp. 77–111). London: Academic.

Patterson, K. E., Marshall, J. C., & Coltheart, M. (1985). *Surface dyslexia: Neuropsychological and cognitive studies of phonological reading.* Hillsdale, NJ: Erlbaum.

Polich, J., McCarthy, G., Wang, W. S., & Donchin, E. (1983). When words collide: Orthographic and phonological interference during word processing. *Biological Psychology,*
16, 155–180.
Posner, M. I. (1986). *Chronometric explorations of mind.* New York: Oxford University
Press.
Sasanuma, S., Itoh, M., Kobayashi, Y., & Mori, K. (1980). The nature of the task–stimulus
interaction in the tachistoscopic recognition of kana and kanji words. *Brain and Lan-*
guage, 9, 298–306.
Sasanuma, S., Itoh, M., Mori, K., & Kobayashi, Y. (1977). Tachistoscopic recognition of kane
and kanji words. *Neuropsychologia, 15,* 547–553.
Scherg, M., & Von Cramon, D. (1986). Evoked dipole source potentials of the human auditory
cortex. *Electroencephalography and Clinical Neurophysiology, 65,* 344–360.
Segalowitz, N. S. (1986). Skilled reading in the second language. In J. Vaid (Ed.), *Language*
processing in bilinguals: Psycholinguistic and neuropsychological perspectives. Hills-
dale, NJ: Erlbaum.
Segalowitz, S. J. (1983). Cerebral asymmetries for speech in infancy. In S. J. Segalowitz (Ed.),
Language functions and brain organization. New York: Academic Press.
Segalowitz, S. J., & Cohen, H. (1989). Right hemisphere EEG sensitivity to speech. *Brain and*
Language. (in press).
Segalowitz, S. J., & MacGregor, L. (1987, February 19–21). *ERP correlates of reading pho-*
nologically regular and non-regular English words. Paper presented at the International
Neuropsychological Society meeting, Washington, DC.
Segalowitz, S. J., Menna, R., & MacGregor, L. (1987, July 1–4). *Left and right hemispheric*
participation in normal adults' reading: Evidence from ERPs. Paper presented at the
European meeting of the International Neuropsychological Society, Barcelona, Spain.
Taylor, I., & Taylor, M. M. (1983). *The psychology of reading.* New York: Academic Press.
Vaid, J. (1983). Bilingualism and brain lateralization. In S. J. Segalowitz (Ed.), *Language*
functions and brain organization. New York: Academic Press.
Vaid, J., & Genesee, F. (1980). Neuropsychological approaches to bilingualism: A critical
review. *Canadian Journal of Psychology, 34,* 417–445.
Van Petten, C., & Kutas, M. (1987). Ambiguous words in context: An event-related potential
analysis of the time course of meaning activation. *Journal of Memory and Language, 26,*
188–208.
Wood, C. C. (1982). Application of dipole localization methods to source identification of
human evoked potentials. *Annals of the New York Academy of Sciences, 388,* 139–155.
Wood, C. C., & McCarthy, G. (1984). Principal component analysis of event-related potentials: Simulation studies demonstrate misallocation of variance across components.
Electroencephalography and Clinical Neurophysiology, 59, 249–260.
Zurif, E., & Caramazza, A. (1976). Psycholinguistic structures in aphasia: Studies in syntax
and semantics. In H. Whitaker & H. A. Whitaker (Eds.), *Studies in neurolinguistics* (Vol.
1). New York: Academic Press.

Development and Dissolution of Language

Disorders in Language Acquisition and Cerebral Maturation

A Neurophysiological Perspective

LYDA MEJIA and JORGE ESLAVA-COBOS

Since Broadbent (1872) described congenital aphasia in children with brain lesions, many authors have expanded on the same topic. Nevertheless, a considerable portion of the published material has centered on the discussion of the appropriate terminology more than on the basic mechanisms that account for delays or involution of language organization in children.

After Broadbent, Coën in 1886 for the first time used the expression *audiomutism*, which since then has been employed with such different meanings by various authors (Ajuriaguerra & Marcelli, 1982; Borel-Maisonny, 1979; Quiros *et al.*, 1971; Quiros & Della Cella, 1971) that one of them proposed it be abandoned until a consensus could be reached as to its exact meaning.

Referring to Broadbent's "congenital aphasia," Hadden (1891), Ucherman (1891), and Wyllie (1894) mentioned how brain lesions can produce congenital aphasia alone or associated with paralysis and other symptoms. Before 1900, however, Kerr (1897) disputed this hypothesis as he showed how "congenital aphasia" could develop without past history of brain lesion. In the late 1920s, Worster-Drought and Allen (1929) referred to "congenital auditory imperception" and emphasized how it could also appear in children without a past history of brain lesion but usually with other parents affected and male preponderance. They also

LYDA MEJIA • Colombian School of Rehabilitation, University of Rosario, Bogotá, Colombia.   JORGE ESLAVA-COBOS • Department of Child Neurology, Colombian Institute of Neurology, Bogotá, Colombia.

pointed out how these children usually had difficulties in learning certain skills.

Ley (1930) defined two types of difficulties in children's language. The first, which he considered a delay in the praxic functions in language, is one in which the child can pronounce sounds and syllables but has great difficulties in the synthesis of these elements, which nevertheless still allow an adequate expression of language. Interestingly enough, he described in this problem an alteration of abstract concepts, which he explained as due to the fact that they are acquired through the spoken word. The other clinical entity he called "hearing agnosia of evolution," characterized by impairment in the comprehension of words and of written material, which he considered due to difficulties in abstract thinking.

Worster-Drought (1943, 1968) returned to his analysis of "congenital auditory imperception" and further defined its characteristics as impossibility for the comprehension of language, poor expression (frequently as idioglossia), normal nonverbal IQ, and normal audiogram; some of these patients have a discrete hearing loss but not sufficiently severe as to explain their language difficulties. He defined four types of imperception, ranging from difficulty to comprehension of words to imperception of all sounds—a situation extremely difficult to differentiate from deafness. At the same time, he described delays in development of spoken language without any difficulty in comprehension, called by him "developmental executive aphasia."

Separating cases in which expression was impaired from those that affected comprehension, Morley (1957) described "developmental aphasia," distinguishing three subtypes of expression impairment: expression aphasia of evolution, evolutive dysarthria, and evolutive apraxia of expression.

In the early 1950s, Landau, Goldstein, and Kleffner (1954) described autopsy findings in a child whose language development started at age 6 and by the moment of his death—4 years later—was quite functional. They found extensive bilateral destruction of the perisylvian cortex in the area of the central sulcus and retrograde degeneration in both medial geniculate nuclei, and concluded that his language had developed through different connections from the usual primary thalamocortical projections. In a commentary to this case, Lenneberg (1967) says: "I cite this case to illustrate the enormous plasticity of the human brain (or the lack of cortical specialization) with respect to language during the first years of life" (p. 183).

In the mid-1950s and 1960s, the discussion frequently centered on terminology. Many rejected the term *aphasia*, because they felt it implied loss of something that children had not acquired, and preferred *dysphasia*. Others, Ajuriaguerra *et al.* (1969) among them, preferred the term *aphasia* for the most serious symtoms and *dysphasia* for "a population who presents a disturbance in the integration of language without sensory or phonatory disability and who can nevertheless express themselves verbally—although with difficulty—and whose mental level can be considered normal" (p. 119). He distinguished two groups of children: one who choose actions or gestures as means for communication, and the other who—in spite of their difficulties—still prefer language for communication. In this second category he recognized two subgroups: (1) the "economomensurates," who always communicate verbally, although with difficulty, and who he felt had a better prognosis, and (2) the "impertinents," children who speak abundantly with poor language and who are not interested in being understood.

In 1971 Quiros et al. published The So-called Aphasias of Childhood, where after a detailed revision of the literature they concluded that child aphasia is "a symptomatic label which tries to include all deficiencies of language of neurologic origin, once sensory, intellectual or psychic possible causes have been ruled out." They then proposed their own classification. For what had been called "sensory aphasia of childhood" they distinguished three syndromes: "aphasoidism," "auditive agnosia," and "troncular integrative deafness." For "mixed aphasia of childhood" they substituted "subcortical syndromes." Finally, for "motor aphasia of childhood" they differentiated the syndromes of "apractognosia of childhood" and "vestibular-proprioceptive disorganization." For each one of these syndromes they tried to define a localization of injury and corresponding language symptoms, which resulted in a classification similar to that of the aphasias in the adult.

Lenneberg (1967) studied sequelae of lesions suffered at different ages and concluded that lateralized brain lesions sustained before the integration of language is accomplished, or in its first stages, do not produce significant language impairment or sequelae, and that only when the injury occurs after age 11 will the aphasic symptoms be irreversible.

Azcoaga, Bello, Citrinovitz, Derman, and Frutos (1981) proposed that language abnormalities of neurologic origin, congenital or acquired before language begins, be called "language retardations." After a profound explanation of the subjacent physiopathological mechanisms, he classified them as "anartric retardation" and "aphasic retardation," since he considered that—even though the child is in the process of acquiring language—the symptoms and pathophysiology found in each syndrome is equivalent to that found in the corresponding syndromes of the adult. He further described specific symptoms depending on whether the physiopathological anomaly is a disequilibrium in the activity of excitatory or inhibitory neuronal circuits. Each syndrome is characterized according to the different stages of development of the infant and child. Azcoaga and his colleagues considered that when the lesion occurs after language development has started, the clinical entity recognizable is no longer a retardation but a syndrome essentially similar to that of the adult, owing to disruption in the activity of the particular analyzer involved. This distinction has important implications for therapy.

As regards childhood aphasia due to brain lesions that occur after language has been organized, Brock and Krieger (1966) recalled 30 cases published by Guttman (1942), including patients with abscess, trauma, tumors, and thrombosis, all between 2 and 14 years of age. In left-hemisphere lesions, aphasia was as frequent as in adults; one case with bilateral lesions also had aphasia, while of 13 patients with right-hemisphere lesions only 1 had aphasia. Temporal lesions produced difficulties in both comprehension and expression; frontal lobe lesions only impaired expression. Guttman considered that children with global aphasia recover slowly and are left with permanent sequelae.

Landau and Kleffner (1957) published the association of acquired aphasia with epilepsy—usually of the partial type (or in some patients only with the EEG expression). This syndrome has since been extensively studied (Billard et al., 1981; Bishop, 1985; Brissaud & Richardet, 1974; Deonna, Beaumanoir, Gaillard, & Assal, 1977; Duloc, Billard, & Arthuis, 1983); language symptoms have been found to be extremely variable, which has induced some to consider it a heterogenous syndrome.

ORGANIC AND FUNCTIONAL SYNDROMES

The foregoing review of the literature presents us with, among other things, an important confusion in terms and concepts. But it could be no other way if we remember that we are but heirs of a dualistic conception that up until today dominates our literature with the distinction between the "organic" and the "functional" (psychogenic, mental) (Eccles, 1970). We have advanced to an understanding (or at least an intuition) that the "functional" demands an "organic housing" (Popper, 1977), but not far enough to accept that neuronal tissue and environment form one complex and inseparable unit when the explanation of psychism is attempted. Thus, neural structure in any given moment—understood in its full morphological, chemical, and electrical aspects—is the sole determinant of the different "constituents" of psychism, language included. But at the same time, the afferent bioelectric input imposed on us by environmental signals—among them those that as feedback come back from the same neuropsychologic expression—are fundamental influences for the modification of that same structure (Horwitz, 1981; McLennan & Hendry, 1981; Meisami & Mousavi, 1982; Mower, Burchfield, & Duffy, 1981). This is so because embryologic development of the human brain is not independent of environmental influences (Cowan, 1979). Right from its very beginnings in the induction of the differentiation of a neural plaque on the ectoderm of the embryo (through the influence of substances that probably originate in the subjacent mesoderm) through well into adult life when myelination is completed, many of the processes involved are under the influence of signals that arise from the environment—inside or outside the body.

We consider the structure as the neural elements (macroscopic, cellular, subcellular, and chemical) and their interrelationships whose functional expressions are the different constituents of psychism. At the same time, we consider that structure as the result—always in a dynamic changing process—of the embryologic development of the nervous system, which depends on individual genetic conditioning as much as on environmental influences.

Health can be understood as the "relatively stable state" in the course of neural processes that results from the presence of "usual" structural elements and also "usual" interrelationships between them (physiologic stable state). Sickness (or disability) instead is the "relatively stable state" in which structural elements or their interrelationships are "erroneous" (pathologic stable state) (Bejtereva, 1984).

We shall therefore discuss initially the embryologic development of the nervous system and then consider (only in reference to language) the physiologic stable state in its evolution (language development in healthy children). Finally, we will proceed to a discussion of the pathologic stable states (language retardations and involution), including the acquisition of reading and writing skills and their abnormalities, also from the perspective of stable states.

BASIC EMBRYOLOGIC CONSIDERATIONS

Volpe (1977) has made an excellent summary of neural embryogenesis. Dorsal induction spans from 3 to 4 gestational weeks; then comes ventral induction from 5 to 6 weeks, followed by neuronal proliferation from 2 to 4 months, then migration from 3 to 5 months, organization from 6 months to "years" postnatal, and, finally, myelination, which prolongs itself at least until the third decade of extrauterine life.

The events described are not exactly limited to that timetable, and not infrequently some overlapping is observed; nevertheless, it is valid as well as convenient to consider the general process of maturation in terms of a sequence of individual events. It should be clearly noted that birth is not shown as a critical borderline because, in the process of neural embryogenesis, birth is but an accident whose only significance is that it influences the characteristics of environmental information.

Around the third gestational week a specialized tissue differentiates on the ectoderm (the neural plaque), which then folds back until a neural tube is formed. This is the origin of the whole nervous system from telencephalon to spinal level L1. This process—the first in neural embryogenesis—is called dorsal induction. Abnormalities in this stage give rise to neural tube closure defects.

Two to 3 weeks later, the rostral portion of this neural tube establishes close interrelationships with the subjacent ecto- and mesoderm, giving rise to craniofacial architecture in the process known as ventral induction. Cerebral hemispheres, diencephalon, thalami, olfactory bulbs and tracts, eyes and optic nerves, and some structures of the posterior fossa are thus formed. It must be remembered that the architectonic elements with which these structures are formed are neural tissue; for this reason, abnormalities in this stage will carry varying degrees of neurologic sequelae (DeMyer, Zeman, & Palmer, 1964), ranging from severe malformations that invariably lead to death (e.g., alobar holoprosencephaly with cyclopia) to subtle neuropsychologic defects in some minor fasciotelencephalic malformations.

In the third stage of embryogenesis—proliferation—the primitive periependymal neuroblasts must multiply themselves to the definite number of neurons that the individual will have for the rest of his life, which Eccles has calculated as approximately 10,000 million. Nevertheless, a considerable individual variability exists which has been difficult to evaluate clinically in its full physiologic or pathologic significance due to the impossibility of quantitating neuronal populations. Thus, in megalencephalies (DeMyer, 1972) descriptions range from profound mental retardation to the genius of Lord Byron (whose brain weighed 1800 gr).

The fourth event—migration—refers to the extraordinarily complex phenomenon whereby thousands of millions of nerve cells move from their sites of origin in the ventricular and subventricular zones to the loci within the central nervous system where they will reside for life (Sidman & Rakic, 1973). According to Volpe, this remarkable phenomenon is bound to suffer some imperfections in every human being. In consequence, minor alterations called neuronal heterotopias are probably present to some degree in all of us. On the other hand, neuropsychological defects have been attributed to these same migration "imperfections" (Galaburda & Kemper, 1979). Abnormalities of the migration process can therefore be understood as a continuum ranging from the most severe forms (schizencephaly, lissencephaly) to subtle defects that produce discrete neuropsychological deficits that impair learning or that may even pass undetected in "normal" subjects, perhaps contributing in all of us to our peculiar "neuropsychological imperfections."

The fifth event in neural embryogenesis is neural organization. Its main developmental features include proper alignment, orientation and layering of cortical neurons, elaboration of dendritic and axonal ramifications, establishment of synaptic contacts, and proliferation and differentiation of glia. Quite evidently, the proliferation of synaptic contacts sets the morphologic substrate for the future enrichment of neuronal circuits (Purpura, 1976), which in turn will be the physiologic substrate of the different "analyzers" (Azcoaga et al., 1983). This stage is highly dependent on environmental stimulation (Chang & Greenough, 1982; Kaye, Mitchell, & Cynader, 1982) in such a way that intensely stimulated neuronal circuits will enrich the number, volume, and electric functional status (Horwitz, 1981) of their synapses, while those poorly stimulated will suffer atrophy (Meisami & Mousavi, 1982), maybe even to the point of functional disappearance of that circuit.

The last stage is myelination. In it, nude axons—both intra- and extraaxial—gradually cover themselves with a myelin sheath that hastens and improves the efficiency of transmission of membrane potentials, with the consequent enhancement of the richness and harmony of the functional expression of the activity of neuronal circuits. Myelination starts in the motor roots of the peripheral nervous system, then proceeds with intra- and extraaxial afferent systems, then with efferent intraaxial pathways, and finally—in a process that prolongs itself at least through the third decade—with intra- and interhemispheric association fibers (Yakovlev & Lecours, 1967). No abnormalities have yet been clearly defined in the process of myelination in the human; in contrast, disease entities in which myelin is destroyed or otherwise injured—the leukodystrophies (Swaiman & Wright, 1982)—are characterized by severe progressive derangement of neuropsychologic abilities—language included.

At some as yet ill-defined time in embryogenesis, an apparently important amount of cell death occurs in some neuronal populations (Levi-Montalcini, 1964; Rabinowicz, 1976). The role of this phenomenon has not been clearly established, but it is tempting to speculate that it might contribute to the "minimization of brain areas necessary and sufficient to sustain a well formed and developed function that will not develop further" (Bejtereva, 1984, pp. 66–67). This is how Bejtereva explain the loss of potentiality in a given analyzer that at the same time both stabilizes and makes it an automatic phenomenon with which the "neuronal effort" to sustain a given functional stereotype is minimized.

It is perhaps important to recall at this stage that, as previously mentioned, neural embryogenesis by no means ends with birth. Consequently, language organization and cerebral maturation occur during—and because of—the events previously mentioned. It follows, then, that abnormalities in these stages (whether originally due to biologic or environmental influences) will cause disorders in language organization.

ANALYZERS AND STEREOTYPES

If we attempt a synthesis of the preceding discussion on neural orthogenesis with certain tendencies in child neuropsychology (Azcoaga, 1981)—deeply rooted in Pavlov's theory of analyzers—and with neurophysiology of language as has been explained mainly by Bejtereva (1984), we could consider the central nervous system as an extremely complex structure that conjugates biologic and environmental conditionants. If at the same time we refuse to explain language solely through the study of the "external expressions" of cerebral activity (language stereotypes) and rather prefer to describe the activity of neural circuits responsible for those stereotypes (or, in Pavlov's conception, the analyzers; Azcoaga et al., 1981), we could arrive at a novel conception of health and sickness on the basis of the stable states theory—both physiologic and pathologic (Bejtereva, 1984). We believe this approach, greatly influenced by Azcoaga's and Bejtereva's contributions, will be extremely productive both from the theoretical and the therapeutic perspective.

The whole embryologic process just described is aimed at the formation and then stabilization of neuronal circuits (analyzers) where the experience or the physiologic substrate of the capacity to react to this experience is "impressed" (Barbizet & Duizabo, 1978). Upon this basis, the analyzer must then combine those elements "impressed" on its circuits through the neurophysiologic mechanisms of neural excitation and inhibition (Azcoaga et al., 1983). "It is known that the phenomenon of language (whose basics can be traced to the close interaction between two signal systems: direct and verbal) obeys the same rules of excitation and inhibition, irradiation and concentration as any other form of cortical activity. The difference lies only in the fact that verbal processes, which reflect reality through relations fixed in language, are accomplished through a process of much greater complexity" (Luria, 1974, pp. 27). The resulting "external expression" of activity of that analyzer—available to the external observer—is the stereotype (Azcoaga et al., 1983).

Environmental signals influencing CNS maturation allow the organization of analyzers that will sustain language and which, under normal conditions, are formed along genetically predetermined pathways. Repetition and coincidence over time of certain stimuli gradually stabilize stereotypes that can be actualized at the "right" time for a "correct language expression" (Azcoaga, 1977). If, as a consequence of structural derangement or "mistaken" relationships between neural elements, these "correct" stereotypes cannot be formed, those same environmental stimuli will influence the CNS, forcing the "impression" of different neuronal circuits. As a consequence, analyzers will then have a different organization, and stereotypes (their functional expression) will thus be abnormal. These abnormal stereotypes can, of course, also be stabilized, and the final consequence of this sequence of events is an abnormal language evolution.

NORMAL LANGUAGE ORGANIZATION: PHYSIOLOGIC STABLE STATES

Reflex or innate orofacial behaviors gradually acquire a communicative function, not yet linguistic, since they are not then symbols or signs. In time they will be, signaling the initiation of language.

We shall describe the stages of development of communicative behavior in man according to Azcoaga's proposal as "first stage in communication (prelinguistic level)," "second stage in communication (first linguistic level)," and "third stage in communication (second linguistic level)" (Azcoaga et al., 1981).

At the prelinguistic level, spanning from 0 to 12 (15) months, it can be observed how certain behavior, which originally had merely a survival function such as crying, shouting, or even breathing, gradually puts itself at the service of communication. Other behaviors such as sucking and swallowing progressively refine themselves to allow the establishment of well-coordinated patterns of movement. All these events establish the basis for the fine orofacial movements and phonorespiratory coordination that will be necessary to articulate sounds, syllables, and words. The role of the adult as moderator and model in this process is almost unanimously accepted. The response the infant obtains will reinforce or stimulate their use with a communicative purpose. But the adult plays other roles different from being a simple reinforcer. Bruner, according to Owens, considers language development as "made possible by the presence of an interpreting adult who operates not so much as a corrector or reinforcer but rather as a provider, an expander and idealizer of utterances while interacting with the child" (Owens, 1984).

Siguan-Soler (1978) emphasizes the importance that early accentuation, modulation, and gesture have in the full development of these initial stages. The child is inmersed in a linguistic environment that continually feeds him verbal messages; sensoriperceptive input then starts pairing with verbal input that accompanies that particular situation, gradually substituting the first signal system for the second one—which initiates semantic recognition. This in turn will serve as basis for future verbal comprehension and expression. It can be stated then that the infant recognizes linguistic meanings before he can express himself in the oral code. The sound emissions that start with crying, whimpering, or shouting gradually differentiate toward vocal play, which basically consists in playful repetition of phonation. This vocal play has two well-differentiated stages: (1) "proprioceptive vocal play," in which sounds are emitted

because of the "pleasure" felt in the oropharynx by the child as he produces sounds (Azcoaga *et al.*, 1981); (2) "auditory proprioceptive vocal
play" in which, as the child produces sounds, hearing aggregates intimately to the proprioceptive afferences (Azcoaga *et al.*, 1981). The lack of
auditory reinforcement "forces" the child to discard sounds not belong-
ing to his linguistic environment. On the contrary, the continuous reinforcement of sounds from his linguistic community trains him in the
production of those first babblings. It is this process of differentiation that,
guided by hearing, will allow the progressive recognition of the distinctive features of phonemes. "From then on, the child does not learn
sounds but phonemes; he no longer is guided by his own articulatory
instinct but rather submits to his environment and tries to imitate what he
hears" (Alarcos Llorach, 1976). From the adequate, coordinated synthesis
of auditory and proprioceptive afferences, two fundamental requisites for
language integration will arise: the recognition of acoustic features of the
phonic emissions from his linguistic environment, and the synthesis between the articulatory pattern and the acoustic image of the phonemes
produced by the same subject. These two accomplishments will result in
the phonematic stereotype, the first step in the process of language
organization.

The posterior synthesis of these phonematic stereotypes will result in
longer chains of emissions called motor verbal stereotypes, and these in
turn will eventually organize themselves in a syntactic ordainment. In
close relation to this process, the child recognizes and synthetizes acoustic features of his linguistic environment and ascribes meaning to them
because of the repetitive spatiotemporal coincidence of the emission with
a certain specific object or event. "The child observes that in a certain
situation the adults repeat the same expression and starts pairing them"
(Alarcos Lorach, 1976).

From the complex connections of those analyzers involved in the
reception and analysis of the various signals pertinent to the recognition
of meaning, verbal stereotypes gradually stabilize as functional expressions of the activity of the verbal analyzer. "At present, no one ac-
cepts that the meaning of words can be reduced to simple visual images
associated with their corresponding verbal designations. The meaning of
a word to a child is always coupled to some practical activity, in the
course of which abbreviation and differentiation gradually take place and
lead to that schematized 'concept of the object' that nominates a word"
(Luria, 1974).

As a concluding remark on this prelinguistic level, the importance of
the auditory control for the understanding of other aspects of communication should be emphasized. The auditory analyzer helps the child understand and differentiate prosodic aspects of adult language and the corre-

sponding affective messages it transmits. At the same time he gradually includes prosody as a communicative resource that accompanies gesture, even though it does not yet have a true linguistic character. Even though gesture will gradually be replaced by verbalization, it never will disappear but rather will be used as a reinforcer of oral expression; indeed, in times of great emotional excitement it can even replace language as a more primitive—and occasionally more efficient—means of communication.

With the first verbal stereotypes, the second stage in communication—first linguistic level—starts. The initial event occurs when, through the repetition of sounds that characterize vocal play, a meaningful monosyllable appears. After that, the first words will gradually surge, in close relation to the vital needs of the child, and of course imbued with a great emotional significance. These words evoke something; they are the representation through a differentiated significance (the word) of a significance (the need) and initially have a generalizer role; because of it their meaning is extended to many other objects or events circumstantially related. An example of this situation is the use of the word bread to mean the act of eating, or any food, the dining room, the dishes, the napkin, and similar objects. Gradually, these words act as sentences in the stage known as holosentence or word sentence, which essentially implies the use of a single word with different possible meanings. At this moment the child can randomly use holosentences or juxtaposed words; in the latter, intensely meaningful words are linked together without any respect for grammatical rules but with a strictly nominative sense, independently of whether they are verbs, adjectives, or other parts of speech. Simple sentences will then gradually appear, plagued with grammatical "errors" since the child has not yet interiorized the "rules" that common use of language dictates. Verbs, nouns, and adjectives appear more frequently than prepositions and linkage elements because the latter require the enchainment of the syntactic structure to highlight their full meaning, since their significance is not linked to concrete objects or events. Verbs in this stage do not respect inflections; nouns, adjectives, and adverbs can likewise be misused. The child guides himself by generalizations of what he hears, obviously without respect for the grammatical exceptions of his native language. With the reinforcement and modeling offered by the adult, he will gradually acquire them.

As the first linguistic level starts, the child shows the symbolic behavior inhering to the preoperational stage—preconceptual phase—which denotes the establishment of a semiotic function defined by Piaget as "being able to represent something (a 'significance'—object, event, conceptual scheme, etc.) through a differentiated 'significant' which only serves that representation: language, symbolic gesture, etc." (Piaget & Inhelder, 1981, p. 59). This symbolic behavior will dominate the activity of the child until 4 years of age, when he will initiate intuitive thinking (still in the preoperational stage). In spite of his having organized important linguistic abilities, they are not yet sufficient to decentrate thinking, which must then rely on perceptual clues. Reversibility is still absent, hence preventing the child from understanding the relation of parts to the totality, explaining conservations after a perceptual transformation, or having categorical criteria for classifications.

The coincidence of this first linguistic level with preconceptual thinking is responsible for the enrichment of semantic aspects of language in this child, busy searching for different ways in which to represent the world he is exploring through symbolic play. This latter is accompanied by egocentric language, first expressed as repetition or echolalia, then as monologue, and finally as collective monologue (Piaget & Inhelder, 1981). The importance of this egocentric language cannot be sufficiently empha- sized because it plays the role that interior language accomplishes in the adult. "It not only escorts the activity of the child but serves his mental orientation and conscious comprehension, and helps him in the difficul- ties that continuously surge; it is the language for himself, intimately and fruitfully linked with infantile thinking. . . . At the end it will transform itself into interior language" (Vigotsky, 1962).

It is important to realize that the gradual enrichment of significances contributes directly to syntactic progress. The handling of complex struc- tures will in turn permit the expression of more abstract situations, pro- gressively separated from purely perceptual aspects—as will be seen in the third stage of communication. At the same time, that handling of complex structures reveals to us a greater conceptual enrichment of the individual. From the phonologic perspective, a gradual acquisition of phonemes from his native language can be seen, but some with greater difficulty than others, thus appearing later. While some explain this delay through the need for finer articulatory movements that require greater maturity of muscles involved (for those that appear later), others believe that "the articulatory delay is rather due to an imperfect bond between the acoustic and the motor image" (Alarcos Llorach, 1976)—that is, to an instability of the kinesthetic motor verbal analyzer, whose functional ex- ternal expressions are phonematic stereotypes.

By the end of this first linguistic level the child is in possession of all the sounds of his native language, even though he sometimes fails in their synthesis to form polysyllables with symphones. From the syntactic per- spective he initiates his first complex sentences—basically of the coordi- nated type—and has a verbal repertoire whose richness depends greatly on his own peculiar environment. The connections and relations among those significances from his repertoire that the child progressively makes will allow the appearance of interior language.

At approximately 5 years of age the child initiates the third stage in communication—second linguistic level—which can in turn be divided in two substages: The first one coincides with intuitive thinking and ends at 7 years of age; the second one, spanning from 7 through 12 years of age, coincides with concrete operational thinking and the initiation of schooling.

In the first substage the phonologic aspects are rapidly perfected, sentences gain in complexity, with great creativity in the use of linkage elements and constructions in general, and a great many significances are added; the child additionally finds new similitudes and differences between those significances and classifies them so that they will expand that creative richness. Language is interiorized, monologue disappears as a guider of activity, and this role is taken over by interior language. "Exteriorized decentrated language gradually diminishes, becomes fragmented and appears only in a scattered, reduced, occasional form which sometimes becomes a mere whisper; it gradually passes to interior language. It is an invariable part of the process of thinking" (Luria, 1979, p. 22).

We can now state that the oral code has been dominated; it will further enrich itself with each new experience, a never-ending process that essentially depends on the particular opportunities of each person.

At approximately 7 years of age the second substage of the second linguistic level starts. A noteworthy event is the enrichment of interior language, made possible by the coincident concrete operational structure with the consequent possibility of categorization of significances, logic, judgment, etc. A final consequence of all these phenomena is the perfect mastery of complex subordinated and coordinated sentences, and heightened creativity and structural richness.

Learning of the written code begins. In that process the already interiorized language will be raw material, but it will need the support of gnosis and praxis different from those learned in oral language. Orofacial praxis and auditory-proprioceptive coordination involved in oral expression are replaced by manual praxis and visuomanual coordination. By the same token, temporoauditory gnosis is replaced by visuospatial gnosis in the comprehension process. Phonetic material is replaced by graphic elements, but with the additional difficulty imposed by the fact that graphic symbols are not univocally and universally paired with the same sound, and also by the necessity of substituting trained channels for specific discrimination for other perceptual discriminatory modalities for the same meaning. In learning these abilities the child spends a great part of his time. By the end of this stage, at approximately 12 years of age, the individual will be in possession of the two codes. Language will then be his best tool for learning new skills and facts, communicating his ideas and feelings, or talking with himself in those long monologues that will help him solve problems, be artistically creative, or amuse himself. From then on, he will enrich and specialize his language in direct relationship to the characteristics of his sociocultural environment.

ABNORMAL LANGUAGE ORGANIZATION: PATHOLOGIC STABLE STATES

Language derangement syndromes of children cannot be classified in the same way as those of adults. Even though certain symptoms are equivalent, it is well known how parenchymal lesions do not produce in the child the clinical manifestations observable in the adult. Descriptions of children severely affected initially but who gradually compensate for those difficulties or (on the opposite) who apparently worsen progressively in their linguistic abilities also abound.

As a general "rule of thumb," parents describe their children's difficulties in two different ways: (1) The child understands and talks poorly. (2) The child understands well but talks poorly or not at all. These descriptions coincide well with what has been a constant in the historical revision: difficulties in comprehension or expression of language. In agreement with the preceding discussion, we consider that these children suffer derangements of their verbal analyzer (semantic code) or their kinesthetic motor verbal analyzer (phonologic-syntactic code).

Abnormalities of language analyzer in children can be grouped basically under three different conditions: (1) retarded organization due to delay in neurophysiologic mechanisms or poor environmental stimulation, which results in the late initiation of the first linguistic level without pathologic symptoms; (2) inadequate organization due to "abnormal analyzer architecture" because of neurologic derangements that occur before the first linguistic level is under way; this will produce a delay in language evolution which will progressively incorporate pathologic symptoms equivalent to those of the adult; and (3) disorganization of analyzers because of neurologic lesions that occur after linguistic levels are well under way, which will determine involution of language milestones already acquired and symptoms similar to those of the adult. We shall attempt a discussion of these abnormalities through the separate study of the verbal and kinesthetic motor verbal analyzers. Nevertheless, it should be borne in mind that in certain conditions (e.g., mental retardation) both analyzers are affected. Hearing impairment will not be discussed.

Kinesthetic Motor Verbal Analyzer

Derangements of the kinesthetic motor verbal analyzer produce difficulties in language expression. A frequent condition is "simple language retardation" characterized by a delay in verbal expression and prolonged persistence of infantile talk without other symptoms, and adequate comprehension. In these children, expression milestones occur in their correct order, but slowly. By the end of the first linguistic level the delay is compensated, and the child continues a normal evolution.

Multiple etiologies have been proposed. Ajuriaguerra and Marcelli (1982) believe it is due to "cerebral inmaturity" or lack of verbal stimulation, or both. Azcoaga et al. (1981) propose chronologic, psychologic, familial, and sociocultural factors. Inadequate or insufficient stimulation in the prelinguistic level could delay connections between the analyzer processing proprioceptive information from orofacial structures and hearing, thereby impeding syntheses necessary for language expression, with the consequent "simple retardation." Nevertheless, if this environmental anomaly prolongs itself into the critical stages, poorly organized kinesthetic motor verbal analyzers may consolidate engrams thus stabilizing abnormal phonematic and motor verbal stereotypes in a pathologic stable state. Otherwise, the almost mandatory enrichment of stimuli that occurs in the first linguistic level corrects this retardation before this second stage ends.

A familial history is frequently encountered. Nevertheless, this history must only be one of simple retardation in acquiring milestones but devoid of pathologic symptoms (Azcoaga et al., 1981); otherwise the retardation will most probably not be a "simple" one.

Quite different is the situation where anomalies in this analyzer are due to neurologic derangements occurring before the first linguistic level is under way. These children likewise suffer a lag in their language milestones, but their expression is also plagued with pathologic symptoms in both phonologic and syntactic aspects. Occasionally the delay in acquiring milestones is not initially evident, but only the pathologic symptoms such as multiple dyslalias and poor syntactic organization appear; with time, the retardation gradually makes itself evident. In these children the kinesthetic motor verbal analyzer must search for new ways of organization, establishing and consolidating different connections that will result in normal or pathologic stable stereotypes, depending on the characteristics of environmental stimuli, and degree and magnitude of neurologic derangement.

Lenneberg (1967) maintains that lateralized lesions suffered between birth and 20 months of age do not interfere with normal language milestones in half the cases, while in the other half, language is retarded but otherwise normal; he likewise feels that prognosis and symptoms are independent of which hemisphere is affected. In this case, the situation would usually pass undetected or, at most, be considered a "simple retardation." Only those with bilateral lesions would be clearly symptomatic. If subtle aspects of linguistic abilities are considered, we believe most

children with early lesions will show language difficulties (Eslava-Cobos
& Mejia, 1985).

A clear genetic factor is advocated by many authors (Gutzmann, 1916;
Orton, 1930; Pfaendler, 1960). Brewer's statement is endorsed by Lenneberg (1967): "Congenital linguistic ability is probably a dominant feature, influenced by sex and with at least a regular penetrance" (p. 283).

When these children are left untreated, their symptoms progressively
worsen. What initially was only multiple dyslalia gradually evolves into a
poor syntactic structure by the end of the first linguistic level: Complex
sentences are impossible because of the difficulties in the syntheses
among different motor verbal stereotypes, dyslalias become fixed, and
abnormal phonematic stereotypes stabilize, hence stabilizing also aberrant motor verbal stereotypes (Azcoaga et al., 1981, p. 85). "[T]he evolutive clinical characteristics of anarthric retardation show well the de-
pendency of the grammatical system on the phonologic in the linguistic
level. . . . By the same token, from the neurophysiologic perspective, the
inadequate organization of the analytic-synthetic activity at different levels starts hampering phonematic stereotypes and ends jeopardizing the
whole syntactic grammatical organization" states Azcoaga, who refers to
this derangement of the kinesthetic motor verbal analyzer as "anarthric
retardation."

The great influence of this deficient organization of the kinesthetic
motor verbal analyzer on the process of learning of the written code must
be emphasized. Azcoaga, Derman, and Iglesias (1979), Launay (1979), and
Quiros and Della Cella (1971), among others, have elaborated on the great
relationship that exists between learning disabilities and language expression retardations. Quite obviously, when the graphic element has to
be paired with the phoneme, this abnormal phonematic stereotype leads
the child to confusion with the written material as it is presented to him;
what he sees and hears does not match with what he has fixed as the
activity of the kinesthetic motor verbal analyzer.

Finally, in conditions that produce disorganization of this analyzer
because of neurologic lesions that occur after linguistic levels are well
under way, symptoms will be more similar to those of adults, the older the
child is by the time he suffers the lesion. Some children can lose expression altogether. The process may then reinitiate, fulfilling all its
stages in an abbreviated form with an almost total compensation. For
others, especially when the child has already attained the second linguistic level, sequelae are usual, with important difficulties in articulation and agrammatism, in spite of vigorous therapy.

Verbal Analyzer

"Simple" retardations, equivalent to the one previously described for
the kinesthetic motor verbal analyzer, are infrequent in verbal analyzer

derangements. Nevertheless, occasionally a child can be seen who starts comprehension of oral language at older stages than what is accepted as normal, not in the general framework of mental deficiency, and devoid of pathologic symptoms. If this delay for verbal stereotypes is due to severe environmental deficiencies, as for example in forlornness that prolongs itself beyond 3 or 4 years of age, it usually is not compensated, especially because other affective factors are also hindered. Not only language, but the totality of communication is then jeopardized.

When the inadequate organization is due to "abnormal analyzer architecture" because of neurologic derangements that occur before the first linguistic level is under way, a delay in the acquisition of guidelines related to language comprehension is seen. As the child progresses in the first linguistic level, symptoms equivalent to those of the adult also appear: verbal paraphasias, anomias, agrammatism, defective articulation.

The greatest problem occurs when the primary level of analysis of nonlinguistic characteristics of phonic material is hampered, since this hinders not only connections essential for other levels involved in decodification but also the coordination of proprioceptive feedback of phonic emissions with recognition of characteristic features of one's own sounds. In this case, both the verbal and the kinesthetic motor verbal analyzer are poorly organized, leading to a mixed language retardation syndrome of poor prognosis. These children cannot perform an adequate analysis and integration of sounds, in spite of normal hearing, a situation referred to as "hearing agnosia" (Launay, 1979) or "congenital auditory imperception" (Worster-Drought & Allen, 1929). A severe lack of comprehension of language occurs; the expression is confined to idioglossia accompanied by gestures. These children are usually misdiagnosed as deaf or—if a profound audiological evaluation rules out deafness—as "dysphasic" at best. The resulting treatment consequently will emphasize verbal symbolism without great concern for discriminatory training of phonic material, a strategy doomed to failure.

In the more frequent, true aphasic retardation (Azcoaga et al., 1981), the verbal analysis is the only one involved without derangement of the acoustic analysis. It is thus named by Azcoaga as he insists that the physiopathologic phenomena are equivalent of those in the aphasias of the adult (differentiating expressive aphasias as "anarthria"). Symptoms are consequently equivalent to those of the adult, although they gradually change and evolve as the child's development progresses. In addition, environmental pressure progressively highlights difficulties that might have gone undetected in previous stages.

Derangements of the verbal analyzer eventually produce impairment of expression. Not infrequently the child is brought for treatment because of those expressive difficulties and not because of miscomprehension. This situation is fostered by the relatively simple communicative environment the young child is exposed to, which allows nonlinguistic comprehension and therefore leaves the expression difficulties as the sole apparent reason for concern. In the clinical setting, these children show difficulty in understanding orders and complex verbalizations, with a contextual—rather than verbal—comprehension. Multiple paraphasias, latencies, and anomias are found, and occasionally language is even restricted to idioglossia. Slight derangements of this analyzer may pass undetected until the child enters school, when he will suffer learning disabilities—not only reading and writing clumsiness, but difficulties in other subjects as well, when they demand abstraction abilities that pull him away from concrete references (Azcoaga et al., 1979).

The disorganization of the activity of the verbal analyzer because of neurologic lesions that occur after linguistic levels are well under way leads to disintegration of language in syndromes gradually more akin to those of the adult, the older the child is when he suffers the lesion. Even when posttraumatic aphasias occur in the first linguistic level, where language apparently fully recovers, academic learning processes are hindered and children require therapeutic support, especially because of difficulties in abstraction (Kiessling, Denckla, & Carlton, 1983).

CONCLUSIONS

The study of disorders in language acquisition in children is hindered by the changes that maturation imposes on the clinical manifestations, thereby forcing their interpretation within a dynamic frame. They must then be considered from the perspective of functional states—either physiologic or pathologic—that progressively stabilize until a stable state is reached. This evolution has its origins in neural embryogenesis, a complex phenomenon, determined by both biologic and environmental factors, which probably extends itself at least until the third decade of life.

Language derangements can be grouped in two large categories: difficulties in the phonologic-syntactic code or in the semantic code, depending on whether the kinesthetic motor verbal or the verbal analyzer is involved. Conditions characterized by difficulties in the organization of analyzers must be differentiated from those where involution is the basic phenomenon, even though the process of stabilization of their stereotypes is still in its initial stages. Derangements of both analyzers or associations with difficulties in other cerebral functions can be frequently seen, leading to more complex pathologic conditions.

REFERENCES

Ajuriaguerra, J., Guignard, F., Jaeggi, A., Kocher, F., Maquard, M., Paunier, A., Quinodoz, D., & Siotis, E. (1969). Organizacion psicologica y perturbaciones del desarrollo del lenguaje. In J. Piaget, J. Ajuriaguerra, F. Bresson, P. Fraisse, B. Inhelder, & P. Oleron *Introduccion a la psicolinguistica* (pp. 119–146). Buenos Aires: Proteo.

Ajuriaguerra, J., & Marcelli, D. (1982). *Manual de psicopatologia del nino*. Barcelona: Toray Mason.

Alarcos Llorach, E. (1976). La adquisicion del Lenguaje por el nino. In A. Martinet, E. Alarcos Llorach, S. Borel-Maisonny, H. Hecaen, D. Mandin, & P. Guiraud *TLE*. (pp. 7–42). Buenos Aires: Nueva Vision.

Azcoaga, J. (1977). *Trastornos del lenguaje*. Buenos Aires: Ateneo.

Azcoaga, J. (1981). *Del lenguaje al pensamiento verbal*. Mexico: Ateneo.

Azcoaga, J., Bello, J., Citrinovitz, J., Derman, B., & Frutos, W. (1981). *Los retardos del lenguaje en el nino*. Barcelona: Paidos.

Azcoaga, J., Derman, B., & Iglesias, P. (1979). *Alteraciones del aprendizaje escolar*. Buenos Aires: Paidos.

Azcoaga, J., Fainstein, J., Ferreres, A., Gonorasky, S., Kochen, S., Krynveniuk, M., & Podliszewski, A. (1983). *Las funciones cerebrales superiores y sus alteraciones en el nino y en el adulto*. Buenos Aires: Paidos.

Barbizet, J., & Duizabo, P. (1978). *Manual de neuropsicologia*. Barcelona: Toray Mason.

Bejtereva, N. (1984). *El cerebro humano sano y enfermo*. Buenos Aires: Paidos.

Billard, C., Autret, A., Laffont, F., Degiovanni, E., Lucas, B., Santini, J., Duloc, O., Ploin, P. (1981). Aphasie acquise de l'enfant avec epilepsie. *Revue Electroencephalographie et Neurophysiologie Clinic, 11*, 457–467.

Bishop, D. (1985). Age of onset and outcome in acquired aphasia with convulsive disorder (Landau–Kleffner syndrome). *Developmental Medicine and Child Neurology, 27*, 705–712.

Brissaud, E., & Richardet, J. (1974). Le syndrome desintégration du langage et comitialité. *Journal Parisien du Paediatrie*, 441–445.

Broadbent, W. (1872). On the cerebral mechanisms of speech and thought. *Med. Chir. Trans. 15*, 155.

Brock, S., & Krieger, H. (1966). *Fundamentos de neurologia clinica*. Barcelona: Jims.

Chang, F., & Greenough, W. (1982). Lateralized effects of monocular training on dendritic branching in adult split-brain rats. *Brain Research, 232*, 283–292.

Coën, R. (1880). *Pathologie und Therapie der Sprachanomalien*. Viena: Urban und Schwarzenberg.

Cowan, W. (1979). The development of the brain. *Scientific American, September*, 112–133.

DeMyer, W. (1972). Megalencephaly in children: Clinical syndromes, genetic patterns and differential diagnosis from other causes of megalocephaly. *Neurology, 22*, 634.

DeMyer, W., Zeman, W., & Palmer, C. (1964). The face predicts the brain: Diagnostic significance of median facial anomalies for holoprosencephaly (arrinencephaly). *Pediatrics, 34*, 256.

Deonna, T., Beamanoir, A., Gaillard, F., & Assal, G. (1977). Acquired aphasia in childhood with seizure disorders: A heterogeneous syndrome. *Neuropaediatrie, 8*, 263–273.

Duloc, O., Billard, C., & Arthuis, M. (1983). Aspects électro-cliniques et évolutifs de l'épilepsia dans le syndrome aphasie-épilepsie. *Archives Francaises du Paediatrie, 40*, 299–308.

Eccles, J. (1970). *Observando la realidad*. Berlin: Springer-Verlag.

Eslava-Cobos, J., & Mejia, L. (1985). Los trastornos de aprendizaje y la organizacion cerebral de funciones. In P. Montanes (Ed.), *Asimetria funcional cerebral* (pp. 133–145). Bogota: As. Col. Neuropsicologia.

Galaburda, A., & Kemper, T. (1979). Cytoarchitectonic abnormalities in developmental dislexia: A case study. *Annals of Neurology, 6*, 94–100.

Guttman, E. (1942). Aphasia in children. *Brain, 65*, 205–219.

Gutzmann, H. (1916). *Die Vererbung der Sprachstoerungen*. Leipzig: Thieme.

Hadden, W. (1891). On certain defects of articulation with cases ilustrating the results of education on the oral system. *Journal of Mental Sciences, 37*, 96.

Horwitz, B. (1981). Neuronal plasticity: How changes in dendritic architecture can affect the spread of postsynaptic potentials. *Brain Rsearch, 224*, 412–418.

Kaye, M., Mitchell, D., & Cynader, M. (1982). Depth perception, eye alignment and cortical ocular dominance of dark reared cats. *Developmental Brain Research, 2*, 37–53.

Kerr, J. (1897). School hygiene in its mental, moral and physical aspects. *Journal of the Royal Statistics Society, 60*, 613.

Kiessling, L., Denckla, M., & Carlton, M. (1983). Evidence for differential hemispheric function in children with hemiplegic cerebral palsy. *Developmental Medicine and Child Neurology, 25*, 727–734.

Landau, W., Goldstein, R., & Kleffner, F. (1954). Congenital aphasia: A clinic pathologic study. *Neurology, 10*, 915–921.

Landau, W., & Kleffner, F. (1957). Syndrome of acquired aphasia with convulsive disorder in children. *Neurology, 7*, 523–530.

Launay, C. L. (1979). Graves en la adquisicion de lenguaje. In C. Launay & S. Burel-Maisonny, *Trastornes del lenguaje la palabre y la voz en el nino* (pp. 128–129). Barcelona: Toray Masson.

Lenneberg, E. (1967). *Biological foundations of language.* New York: Wiley.

Levi-Montalcini, R. (1964). Events in the developing nervous system. *Progress in Brain Research, 4*, 1–29.

Ley, J. (1930). Les troubles du développement du langage. *Journal du Neurologie et Psychiatrie, 30*, 78–90.

Luria, A. (1974). *Cerebro y lenguaje.* Barcelona: Fontanella.

Luria, A. (1979). *El papel del lenguaje en el desarrollo de la conducta.* Buenos Aires: Cartago.

McLennan, I., & Hendry, I. (1981). Effects of peripheral deprivation on mammalian motoneurone development. *Developmental Brain Research, 1*, 440–443.

Meisami, E., & Mousavi, R. (1982). Lasting effects of early olfactory deprivation on the growth, DNA, RNA, and protein content, and Na- K-ATPase and ache activity of the rat olfactory bulb. *Developmental Brain Research, 2*, 217–229.

Morley, M. (1957). *The development and disorders of speech in childhood.* Edinburgh: Livingstone.

Mower, G., Burchfield, J., & Duffy, F. (1981). The effects of dark-rearing on the development and plasticity of the lateral geniculate nucleus. *Developmental Brain Research, 1*, 418–424.

Orton, S. (1930). Familial occurrence of disorders in acquisition of language. *Eugenics, 3*, 140–147.

Owens, R. (1984). *Language development.* Columbus: Merrill.

Pfaendler, V. (1960). Les vices de la parole dans l'optique du geneticien. *Akt Problem der Phoniatriks und Logopaedie, 1*, 35–40.

Piaget, J., & Inhelder, B. (1981). *Psicologia del nino.* Madrid: Morata.

Popper, K. (1977). *Busqueda sin termino: Una autobiografia intelectual.* Madrid: Tecnos.

Purpura, D. (1976). Structure dysfunction relations in the visual cortex of preterm infants. In C. Brazier, (Ed.), *Brain dysfunction in infantile febrile convulsions* (pp. 223–240). New York: Raven Press.

Quiros, J., D'Elia, N., Feldman, J., Galian, M., Lira, E., Lujan Marelli, L., Mercado, M., Pericoli, B., Rincon, M., Rosental, C., Schrager, O., Soto, R., & Tormakh, E. (1971). *Las llamadas afasias infantiles.* Buenos Aires: C.E.M.I.F.A.

Quiros, J., & Della Cella, M. (1971). *La dislexia en la ninez.* Buenos Aires: Paidos.

Rabinowicz, T. (1976). Morphological features of the developing brain. In C. Brazier (Ed.), *Brain dysfunction in infantile febrile convulsions* (pp. 1–23). New York: Raven Press.

Sidman, R., & Rakic, P. (1973). Neuronal migration with special reference to developing human brain: A review. *Brain Research, 62,* 1.

Siguan Soler, M. (1978). De la comunicacion gestual al lenguaje verbal. In J. Bronckart, P. Malrieu, M. Siguan Soler, H. Sinclair, T. Slama-Cazacu, & A. Tabouret *La genesis del lenguaje* (pp. 23–50). Madrid: Pablo del Rio.

Swaimann, D., & Wright, F. (1982). *The practice of pediatric neurology.* St. Louis: C. V. Mosby.

Ucherman, V. (1891). The case of dumbness (aphasia) without deafness, paralysis or mental debility. *Archives of Otolaringology, 20,* 321.

Vigotsky, L. S. (1962). *Thought and language.* Cambridge, MA: M.I.T. Press.

Volpe, J. (1977). Neurologia neonatal. *Clinicas de Perinatologia, 4,* 3–30.

Worster-Drought, C. (1943). Congenital auditory imperception (congenital word deafness) and its relation to idioglossia and allied speech defects. *Medical Press and Circular, 210,* 5460.

Worster-Drought, C. (1968). Speech disorders in children. *Developmental Medicine and Child Neurology, 10,* 427–440.

Worster-Drought, C., & Allen, I. (1929). Congenital auditory imperception. *Journal of Neurology and Psycopathology, 10,* 193.

Wyllie, J. (1894). *The disorders of speech.* Edinburgh: Oliver & Boyd.

Yakovlev, P., & Lecours, A. (1967). The myelogenetic cycles of regional maturation of the brain. In Minkowski, A. (Ed.) *Regional development of the brain in early life* (pp. 3–70). Philadelphia: F. A. Davis.

6

Speech and Language Alterations in Dementia Syndromes

JEFFREY L. CUMMINGS and D. FRANK BENSON

Dementia is an etiologically nonspecific syndrome characterized by acquired persistent disturbance of several areas of neuropsychological function. Once regarded as a syndrome of global intellectual loss, dementia is increasingly approached as a group of disorders with distinct neuropsychological patterns of preserved and impaired abilities reflecting disease-related regional brain involvement. The topography of histologic, biochemical, and metabolic alterations associated with individual central nervous system (CNS) disorders can be correlated with disease-related behavioral profiles. Conversely, behavioral observations are utilized to infer the geography of brain dysfunction and the etiology of the neurologic condition. Such brain–behavior correlations have reached an acceptable degree of reliability with regard to monosymptomatic deficit syndromes such as the aphasias (Benson & Geschwind, 1985) and amnesias (Benson, 1978; Damasio, Graff-Redford, Eslinger, Damasio, & Kassell, 1985) but are in a relatively primitive state of development in polysymptomatic disorders such as the dementias. A crude distinction has been drawn between dementias associated primarily with cortical dysfunction and those occurring with subcortical disturbances (Cummings & Benson, 1983, 1984), but more refined distinctions are necessary both to improve clinical diagnosis and management and to enhance understanding of brain–behavior relationships in the dementia syndromes.

Memory dysfunction has received the most intensive study within the dementias. In the *Diagnostic and Statistical Manual of Mental Disor-*

JEFFREY L. CUMMINGS and D. FRANK BENSON • The Neurobehavior Unit, West Los Angeles Veterans Administration Medical Center, Departments of Neurology and Psychiatry and Behavioral Sciences, UCLA School of Medicine, Los Angeles, California 90024.

ders *(DSM-III)* (American Psychiatric Association, 1980) memory loss is a mandatory criterion for the diagnosis of dementia. The pan-biographic memory loss of the dementias has been contrasted with the temporal gradient present in isolated amnesia syndromes (Freedman, Rivoira, Butters, Sax, & Feldman, 1984; Wilson, Kaszniak, & Fox, 1981), and the learning deficit of the cortical dementias has been contrasted with the recall disturbance of subcortical dementias (Caine, Ebert, & Weingartner, 1977; Cummings, 1986; Cummings & Benson, 1984).

Abnormalities of speech and language occur in nearly all demented patients, but these disturbances are less well recognized as providing criteria for distinguishing between different dementia syndromes. Aphasia as a manifestation of focal left-hemisphere injury following stroke, trauma, neoplastic involvement, or infection has been investigated and categorized (Benson, 1979), and the language disturbance of dementia of the Alzheimer type (DAT) has also been described (Appell, Kertesz, & Fisman, 1982; Cummings, Benson, Hill, & Read, 1985). The value of language profiles in differentiating among the various dementing disorders remains to be determined. Likewise, dysarthria is well recognized as a manifestation of motor system dysfunction, but the usefulness of motor speech abnormalities in dementia diagnosis has not been established. In this chapter, the application of a battery of speech and language tests to normal control subjects and to patients with three varieties of dementia is described. The usefulness of speech and language alterations in distinguishing dementing conditions is investigated and discussed. The dementia syndromes are DAT, Parkinson's disease (PD) with overt dementia, and multi-infarct dementia (MID).

METHODOLOGY

Assessment

The battery of speech and language tests used in these studies was derived from the Boston Diagnostic Aphasia Examination (Goodglass & Kaplan, 1976) and the Western Aphasia Battery (Kertesz, 1979). The battery included 37 operationalized subtests and assessed elements of spontaneous speech, auditory comprehension, repetition, naming, paraphasia, reading aloud, reading comprehension, automatic speech, sentence completion, word list generation (number of animals named in 1 minute), writing, dysarthria, and reiterative speech disturbances. Each subtest received a scale score of 0 (normal) to 6 (most abnormal) based on responses to six (or a multiple of six) scorable questions (e.g., "Is your name Green?") or graded by operationalized anchor points. Table 1 lists the elements of the battery. The Mini-Mental State Examination (MMSE; Folstein, Folstein, & McHugh, 1975) was used to determine the severity of the dementia syn-

TABLE 1. Elements of Speech and Language
Assessed with the Dementia Speech
and Language Instrument

Spontaneous speech	Reading comprehension
Information content	Words
Melodic line	Sentences
Phrase length	Commands
Grammatical complexity	Writing
Auditory comprehension	Mechanics
Word discrimination	Dictation
Yes/no	Narrative
Sequential commands	Automatic speech
Complex commands	Alphabet recitation
Repetition	Counting (1–20)
Words	Completion
Numbers	Sentences
Phrases	Nursery rhymes
Naming	Dysarthria
Paraphasia	Loudness
Literal	Pitch
Verbal	Articulation
Neologistic	Rate
Reading aloud	Intelligibility
Words	Reiteration
Sentences	Stuttering
Commands	Echolalia
	Palilalia
	Logoclonia

dromes. BMDP statistical software (Dixon, Brown, Engleman, & Hill, 1985) was used for all statistical analyses; the Bonferroni adjustment for multiple testing has been applied to all results reported as significant.

Participants

All participants had at least an eighth-grade education and spoke English as their native language. Seventy normal control subjects were tested and all had MMSE scores in the normal range.

All dementia patients were thoroughly evaluated to establish an accurate clinical diagnosis. Each had a thorough historical review, physical examination, neurologic examination, and mental status testing. Standard laboratory studies, including complete blood count, erythrocyte sedimentation rate, serum electrolytes, serum calcium and phosphorus, serum vitamin B_{12} and folate levels, thyroid and liver function tests, and a serological test for syphilis, were obtained and determined to be normal. An electroencephalogram and computerized tomographic (CT) scan of the head excluded hydrocephalus, subdural hematomas, abscesses, neo-plasms, and other occult causes of mental impairment.

DAT subjects met DSM-III criteria for primary degenerative dementia and the NINCDS-ADRDA criteria (McKhann et al., 1984) for probable Alzheimer's disease. In addition, all had an Ischemia Scale score (Hachin-ski et al., 1975) of 4 or less, supportive of a diagnosis of a degenerative disorder. Seventeen men and 13 women were considered to have DAT—15 patients with onset before age 65 and 15 with onset after that age. Patients with stroke-related dementias met DSM-III criteria for MID and had Ischemia Scale scores of 7 or higher. PD patients had bradykinetic-rigid extrapyramidal syndromes consistent with idiopathic PD (Adams & Victor, 1977; Cummings & Benson, 1983). Historical and clinical features were used to exclude patients with progressive supranuclear palsy, post-encephalitic PD, drug-induced PD, and atypical extrapyramidal syn-dromes from the PD group. A total of 21 patients with MID and 52 with PD (18 with overt dementia and 34 without overt dementia) were studied. All comparisons between dementia syndromes are based on patient groups with equally severe dementia syndromes as reflected in their mean MMSE scores (the number of participants in each comparison is shown in the tables).

RESULTS

Normal Control Subjects

Control subjects ranged in age from 20 to 75 years and had a mean age of 42.4 years. Twenty members of the control group were between the ages of 50 and 75, the age range of the patient group. The mean MMSE score for controls was 29.50. There was no significant difference between the MMSE scores of young and old control subjects.

Individuals in the control group performed almost perfectly on the speech and language tests. At least one of the 70 controls made errors on the following subtests: yes/no questions, complex commands, complex comprehension, alphabet recitation, nursery rhyme completion. Using a one-sample t test, however, the means for the performance of the controls did not differ significantly from zero (normal). Young and old controls performed similarly, and the entire group was used for comparison with the patient groups.

Dementia of the Alzheimer Type

Results of DAT patients have been reported previously (Cummings et al., 1985). The mean age of the DAT patients was 71.34 and their mean MMSE score was 10.50.

Mean DAT patient scores on all subtests were abnormal and dis-

TABLE 2. Characteristics of Verbal Output
of Patients with Dementia of the Alzheimer Type

Sample characteristics	
Age (mean with SEM)	71.33 (1.64)
MMSE	10.50 (1.3)
N	30
	Score
Most impaired features (scale score > 3/6)	
Narrative writing	4.63 (0.39)
Information content of speech	3.83 (0.29)
Word list generation (animals/min)	3.37 (0.59)
Nursery rhyme completion	3.17 (0.42)
Comprehension of complex commands	3.09 (0.43)
Naming	3.03 (0.34)
Least impaired abilities (scale score < 2/6)	
Reading sentences aloud	1.97 (0.47)
Phrase repetition	1.87 (0.40)
Sentence completion	1.83 (0.46)
Phrase length	1.80 (0.38)
Grammatical complexity	1.53 (0.38)
Reading words aloud	1.47 (0.45)
Melodic line	1.43 (0.34)
Verbal paraphasia	1.43 (0.32)
Neologistic paraphasia	1.40 (4.40)
Echolalia	1.33 (0.25)
Loudness	1.28 (0.29)
Intelligibility	1.17 (0.27)
Literal paraphasia	1.10 (0.26)
Counting	1.07 (0.38)
Articulation	1.07 (0.24)
Pitch	1.00 (0.23)
Number repetition	0.97 (0.38)
Rate	0.90 (0.24)
Word repetition	0.80 (0.32)
Palilalia	0.70 (0.27)
Logoclonia	0.70 (0.31)
Stuttering	0.33 (0.14)

tinguished the patient from the control population. After Bonferroni adjustment for multiple testing, six subtests no longer differed from the control group: word and number repetition, reading words aloud, stuttering, palilalia, and logoclonia. The most marked disturbances (scale scores > 3/6) involved information content of spontaneous speech, comprehension of complex commands, naming, word list generation, writing to dictation, narrative writing, and completion of nursery rhymes (Table 2). Relatively preserved abilities (scale scores of < 2/6) included counting, sentence completion, phrase length, grammatical complexity, melodic line, paraphasias, oral reading, repetition, dysarthria measures, and reiterative disturbances. The DAT patients exhibited a characteristic pattern comprising a fluent verbal output, impaired auditory comprehension, anomia, and aphasic agraphia, with relative preservation of repetition, oral reading, and motor speech. The language profile resembles that of transcortical sensory aphasia (Benson, 1979).

Analyses revealed that only one subtest had a significant gender effect: Female DAT patients had better performance on the narrative writing portion of the examination. There was a consistent trend for patients whose disease began before age 65 to exhibit more severe deficits in the middle years of the disease course (4 to 9 years' duration), suggesting that an early onset of DAT was associated with more rapid decline of language function. This trend was most obvious for information content of spontaneous speech, auditory comprehension, and writing to dictation. Increasing length of illness was reflected in decreasing phrase length, loss of melody, impaired repetition, declining comprehension, abnormal counting, disturbed speech pitch, and decreased intelligibility. Thus, as the disease progressed, the verbal output acquired some of the characteristics of Wernicke's aphasia along with loss of some aspects of fluency and increasing dysarthria.

There was a consistent correlation between severity of dementia as reflected in MMSE scores and loss of linguistic function. Stepwise multiple regression analyses revealed that three subtests—comprehension, narrative writing, writing to dictation—accounted for 70% of the MMSE score variation. Correlation between disease duration and language alteration was less robust, reflecting the wide range of reported disease durations.

Six patients had family histories suggesting an inherited form of DAT. Those with familial DAT tended to perform better on the speech and language subtests, with significantly better scores on sentence repetition, alphabet recitation, and oral reading, and they had fewer neologisms.

With a separate series of tests, the oral reading and reading comprehension abilities of 13 DAT patients were investigated (Cummings, Houlihan, & Hill, 1986). Patients with a wide range of disease severity (MMSE scores from 19 to 1) were studied. Oral word and letter reading was preserved throughout the entire range of intellectual deterioration even when incomplete or partially obscured letters were presented. Reading comprehension, on the other hand, deteriorated progressively as dementia severity increased. Reading aloud of irregular words was largely preserved, and DAT patients did not recapitulate the errors typical of children first acquiring reading skills.

Parkinson's Disease

There was no difference between the DAT and PD patient groups in age or dementia severity (Table 3). DAT and PD could be distinguished by

TABLE 3. Demographic Features and Significant Speech and Language
Differences between Patients with Dementia of the Alzheimer Type (DAT)
and Parkinson's Disease (PD) with Overt Dementia

	PD score (SEM)	DAT score (SEM)	Bonferroni significance level
Sample characteristics			
N	16	10	
Age	71.81 (0.96)	73.20 (3.30)	n.s.
MMSE	20.25 (0.78)	17.90 (0.84)	n.s.
Distinguishing features			
Phrase length	2.31 (0.31)	0.40 (0.10)	.001
Information content	1.18 (0.24)	2.80 (0.24)	.001
Melody	2.56 (0.15)	0.40 (0.16)	.001
Writing mechanics	3.62 (0.37)	0.60 (0.40)	.001
Naming	0.43 (0.20)	2.10 (0.54)	.05
Grammatical complexity	1.06 (0.28)	0.20 (0.13)	.05
Animal naming (total/min)	10.02 (0.91)	5.50 (1.19)	.01
Loudness	3.81 (0.29)	0.50 (0.22)	.001
Pitch	2.18 (0.31)	0.20 (0.13)	.001
Articulation	2.75 (0.32)	0.50 (0.22)	.001
Rate	2.81 (0.27)	0.30 (0.15)	.001
Intelligibility	2.62 (0.28)	0.30 (0.15)	.001

both speech and language parameters. All five dysarthria measures, writing mechanics, and speech melody were all significantly more abnormal in PD. Phrase length and grammatical complexity were also more disturbed in PD than in DAT. Linguistic compromise, on the other hand, was more evident in DAT patients, who had significantly poorer scores on information content of spontaneous speech, confrontation naming, and word list generation.

Multi-Infarct Dementia

MID and DAT patient groups did not differ significantly in age or dementia severity (Table 4). Two language and four speech parameters were significantly different in the two groups. Information content of spontaneous speech and confrontation naming were more abnormal in DAT, whereas speech pitch, melody, articulation, and rate were more disturbed in MID.

The most abnormal language parameters in MID (scale score > 1.5/6) were narrative writing, writing to dictation, writing mechanics, completion of nursery rhymes, and comprehension of complex auditory commands.

MID patients were also compared with PD patients with overt dementia. The two groups were not significantly different in age or MMSE scores

TABLE 4. Demographic Features and Distinguishing Speech
and Language Characteristics of Multi-Infarct Dementia (MID) and Dementia
of the Alzheimer Type (DAT)

	MID score (SEM)	DAT score (SEM)	Bonferroni significance level
Patient characteristics			
N	18	14	
Age	67.38 (2.45)	73.14 (2.61)	n.s.
MMSE	15.71 (1.31)	18.77 (0.95)	n.s.
Distinguishing features			
Information content	0.72 (0.25)	2.92 (0.24)	.001
Naming	0.77 (0.27)	2.28 (0.45)	.05
Pitch	1.83 (0.39)	0.35 (0.16)	.01
Melody	2.67 (0.45)	0.57 (0.17)	.05
Articulation	1.88 (0.40)	0.50 (0.17)	.05
Rate	1.72 (0.27)	0.28 (0.12)	.05

(Table 5). PD patients exhibited significantly more severe motor disturbances, including speech volume, speech rate, and writing mechanics. In
addition, their spontaneous speech had shorter phrase lengths and they
stuttered more. MID patients had more difficulty completing nursery
rhymes. Classical language functions such as naming, comprehension,
repetition, and reading did not distinguish these two disorders and were
relatively preserved in both conditions.

TABLE 5. Demographic Features and Distinguishing Speech
and Language Characteristics of Multi-Infarct Dementia (MID)
and Parkinson's Disease (PD) with Overt Dementia

	MID score (SEM)	PD score (SEM)	Bonferroni significance level
Patient characteristics			
N	18	17	
Age	67.38 (2.95)	71.94 (0.91)	n.s.
MMSE	18.77 (0.95)	19.70 (0.91)	n.s.
Distinguishing features			
Phrase length	1.05 (0.36)	2.29 (0.29)	.05
Nursery rhyme completion	2.44 (0.47)	0.81 (0.39)	.05
Loudness	1.77 (0.47)	3.64 (0.32)	.01
Rate	1.22 (0.23)	2.76 (0.26)	.001
Stuttering	0.00 (0.00)	0.70 (0.25)	.05
Writing mechanics	1.83 (0.44)	3.70 (0.36)	.01

DISCUSSION

These investigations demonstrate that speech and language observations can distinguish between dementia syndromes even when the patient groups have dementia of equivalent severity. In addition, DAT patients show significantly more disturbed language functions than either MID or PD-dementia patients.

All DAT patients could be distinguished from normal control subjects by their performance on the language tasks utilized in the study. The language abnormalities of DAT resembled transcortical sensory aphasia (Benson, 1979; Cummings et al., 1985): fluent verbal output (impoverished information content of spontaneous speech but preserved phrase length, grammatical complexity, and melodic line), poor auditory comprehension, and relative preservation of repetition abilities. Like transcortical sensory aphasia, DAT also produced impairment of reading comprehension, while reading aloud was strikingly resistant to the effects of declining intellectual function. DAT patients differed from the classical transcortical sensory aphasics in their lack of completion abilities (e.g., completing the final line of familiar nursery rhymes read by the examiner), relative absence of paraphasia and echolalia, and more impaired automatic speech (e.g., alphabet recitation). Similar observations have been made by others studying the verbal output of DAT, including Appell et al. (1982), Bayles and Tomoeda (1983), and Martin and Fedio (1983).

Further progression of DAT is marked by evolution from the transcortical sensory aphasia pattern to a more global linguistic impairment. Comprehension and repetition abilities are increasingly disturbed, as in Wernicke's aphasia, but elements of fluency such as phrase length and speech melody become impaired and elements of motor speech disorder appear. Such alterations may reflect extension of the disease beyond its initial focus to involve other brain regions (Cummings & Benson, 1983).

The pattern of verbal output in DAT indicates that the disease process does not produce a global language loss. Syntactical and phonological aspects of verbalization are preserved until the terminal phases, whereas the semantic and pragmatic aspects of language are disturbed early and are progressively more compromised as the disease progresses. Semantic abilities appear most dependent on posterior cortical structures where DAT has its greatest biochemical, histopathologic, and metabolic impact (Brun & Gustafson, 1978; Cummings & Benson, 1983). In contrast, syntactical elements of language may be mediated by subcortical-frontal systems less affected in DAT.

Observations on reading also contribute to understanding DAT. Although agnosia is frequently described as an early consequence of DAT, the preservation of oral reading skills indicates that competency in grapheme-morpheme translation is spared until late in the disease course. Moreover, the oral reading of DAT patients is not foiled by presenting incomplete letters or partially obscured letters and words—techniques that impair the reading of patients with visual agnosia (Cummings & Benson, 1986; Landis, Graves, Benson, & Hebben, 1982). At most, agnosia is confined to the late stages of DAT.

Two principal explanations have been proposed for the intellectual loss of DAT: (1) that DAT produces instrumental deficits similar to those observed in patients with structural damage underlying vascular aphasia, and (2) that DAT patients undergo a progressive dedifferentiation (regression) of intellectual abilities to the preliterate stages of childhood and infancy (Emery & Emery, 1983). The intact oral reading of irregular words on the New Adult Reading Test (Nelson & O'Connell, 1978) by DAT patients until severe dementia supervenes and the relative rarity of phonetic errors of the type noted during the acquisition of reading skills is more consistent with an instrumental deficit than a dedifferentiation model of DAT (Cummings & Benson, 1986).

The relationship between DAT and the dementia of PD is controversial, and language studies of the type reported may have an impact on this question. The observation that some PD patients with dementia have neuritic plaques and neurofibrillary tangles in the cerebral cortex suggested that DAT and the dementia of PD may represent the same process (Boller, Mizutani, Roessmann, & Gambetti, 1980; Gaspar & Gray, 1984, Hakim & Mathieson, 1979). In addition to histopathologic similarities, some patients with PD also have atrophy of the nucleus basalis of Meynert similar to that found in DAT patients (Arendt, Bigl, Arendt, & Tennstedt, 1983; Whitehouse, Hedreen, White, & Price, 1983). However, distinct neuropsychologic deficits have been associated with subcortical dysfunction, and the dementia of PD may be associated with the subcortical alterations classically occurring in PD (Albert, 1978; Cummings & Benson, 1984; Huber, Shuttleworth, & Paulson, 1986). Language alterations are prominent in DAT, and if the dementia of PD is a product of DAT, similar language defects should be present in PD-dementia. The findings described here demonstrate that the two disorders produce different speech and language changes; in fact, language skills are comparatively spared in the dementia of PD. DAT patients had significantly less information content in their conversational speech ("empty speech"), showed more anomia, and had greater difficulty with word list generation. They also tended to have more problems with auditory comprehension, although the differences did not reach statistical significance. PD patients with equally severe dementia, on the other hand, had more profound dysarthria and disturbances of phrase length, melody, and grammatical complexity. PD patients with dementia did not manifest an aphasic syndrome but suffered severe motor speech disorders. These observations indicate that PD-dementia and DAT have distinguishable speech and language profiles, and, on a clinical basis, it is unlikely that the two dementias represent the same disease process.

Naming and comprehension disturbances were present in some individuals with PD-dementia, and those patients with naming errors accounted for most of the comprehension errors. It could be conjectured that the subset of patients with PD-dementia and language errors may be suffering from an additional disorder, such as DAT. Alternatively, severe disturbances of subcortical processes may be sufficient to interfere with naming and comprehension (Alexander & LoVerme, 1980; Brunner, Kornhuber, Seemuller, Sugar, & Wellesch, 1982; Damasio, Damasio, Rizzo, Varney, & Gersh, 1982).

PD-dementia patients had elements of a nonfluent verbal output, including shortened phrase length, loss of speech melody, and diminished grammatical complexity of spontaneous verbalizations. Thus, PD-dementia patients had more syntactic than semantic abnormalities, a pattern opposite that of DAT. These syntactic disturbances may be a product of the motor abnormalities of PD, but it is also possible that subcortical nuclei and projections have an important role in mediating syntactic functions.

MID could be distinguished from both DAT and PD on the basis of its speech and language profile. Compared with MID patients, those with DAT were more anomic and had significantly less information content of spontaneous speech. MID, on the other hand, caused more motor speech abnormalities than DAT. These distinguishing features resemble the characteristics that distinguished DAT from PD-dementia. In general, MID patients had near-normal performances on the language subtests and did not manifest identifiable aphasic syndromes. They tended to produce grammatically simple and short phrases, the "Brocoid" output described by Hier, Hagenlocker, and Schindler (1985) in patients with stroke-related dementia. These investigators observed that, compared with DAT, MID patients exhibited decreased syntactic complexity, shortened utterance length, diminished total and unique words, and increased sentence fragmentation. They also noted that empty speech and anomia were more prominent in DAT. Together, these observations suggest that aspects of naming, characteristics of spontaneous speech, and dysarthria are important features that distinguish MID from DAT.

MID is a clinically heterogeneous disorder with different syndromes dependent upon the different brain regions involved by infarction. Among the patients studied here, a wide range of deficit severity was present on speech and language subtests. Most MID patients also manifested elements of dysarthria; motor speech abnormalities appear common to MID patients regardless of the linguistic and neuropsychological diversity within the syndrome. The prevalence of motor deficits may reflect the high frequency of subcortical lacunar infarctions involving descending motor tracts (Hachinski, Lassen, & Marshall, 1974; Hughes, Dodgson, & MacLennan, 1954; Roman, 1985).

PD-dementia and MID could be differentiated primarily by the considerably greater motor disability of the former. PD-dementia patients had shorter phrase lengths, lower voice volume, slower speech, more stuttering, and poorer writing mechanics than MID patients. PD-dementia patients, however, were better able to complete partially presented nursery rhymes. Language functions such as naming, comprehension, reading, narrative writing, word list generation, and repetition did not distinguish the two disorders since they were relatively spared in both conditions within the range of dementia severity studied. The similarity of the speech and language profiles of these two conditions supports the suggestion that both involve dysfunction of common subcortical sites.

CONCLUSIONS

Systematic assessment of speech and language abilities reveals different profiles of preserved and impaired functions in each dementia syndrome investigated. Differences in the patterns cannot be attributed to dementia severity since patients with equivalent degrees of intellectual deterioration were studied. DAT patients manifested significantly more language and significantly less motor speech impairment than patients with PD-dementia or MID. DAT and PD-dementia patients had different patterns of linguistic compromise, suggesting that DAT is not the cause of all PD-dementia. MID patients had motor speech abnormalities in common despite the heterogeneity of their disorder. DAT had its greatest impact on the semantic aspects of language; PD-dementia and MID had more effect on syntactic and phonologic functions. Thus, speech and language assessment provides valuable information for the differentiation of dementia syndromes, reveals different patterns of abnormalities in different dementing conditions, and contributes to the understanding of brain–behavior relationships within the dementias.

ACKNOWLEDGMENTS

This project was supported by the Veterans Administration, the John Douglas French Foundation, and the Los Angeles Chapter of the Alzheimer's Disease and Related Disorders Association. The authors are indebted to the following Neurobehavior Fellows who contributed to data collection: Sandra Horowitz, Michael Frankel, Stephen Read, Mario Mendez, Adam Darkins, and Artiss Powell. They also thank Mary Ann Hill,

Ph.D., for her aid with the statistical analyses, and Bonita Porch and Wendy Kashitani for preparing the manuscript.

REFERENCES

Adams, R. D., & Victor, M. (1977). *Principles of neurology.* New York: McGraw-Hill.

Albert, M. L. (1978). Subcortical dementia. In R. Katzman, R. D. Terry, & K. L. Bick (Eds.), *Alzheimer's disease: Senile dementia and related disorders* (pp. 173–180). New York: Raven Press.

Alexander, M. P., LoVerme, & S. R., Jr. (1980). Aphasia after left hemisphere intracerebral hemorrhage. *Neurology, 35,* 1193–1202.

American Psychiatric Association. (1980). *Diagnostic and statistical manual of mental disorders* (3rd ed.). Washington, DC: Author.

Appell, J., Kertesz, A., & Fisman, M. (1982). A study of language functioning in Alzheimer patients. *Brain and Language, 17,* 73–91.

Arendt, T., Bigl, V., Arendt, A., & Tennstedt, A. (1983). Loss of neurons in the nucleus basalis of Meynert in Alzheimer's disease, paralysis agitans, and Korsakoff's disease. *Acta Neuropathologica, 61,* 101–108.

Bayles, K. A., & Tomoeda, C. K. (1983). Confrontation naming impairment in dementia. *Brain and Language, 19,* 98–114.

Benson, D. F. (1978). Amnesia. *Southern Medical Journal, 71,* 1221–1228.

Benson, D. F. (1979). *Aphasia, alexia, and agraphia.* New York: Churchill Livingstone.

Benson, D. F., & Geschwind, N. (1985). The aphasias and related disturbances. In A. B. Baker & R. J. Joynt (Eds.), *Clinical neurology* (Vol. 1). Philadelphia: Harper & Row.

Boller, F., Mizutani, T., Roessmann, U., & Gambetti, P. (1980). Parkinson disease, dementia, and Alzheimer disease: Clinicopathological correlations. *Annals of Neurology, 7,* 329–335.

Brun, A., & Gustafson, L. (1978). Limbic lobe involvement in presenile dementia. *Arch Psychiatr Nervenkr, 226,* 79–93.

Brunner, R. J., Kornhuber, H. H., Seemuller, E., Sugar, G., & Wellesch, C. W. (1982). Basal ganglia participation in language pathology. *Brain and Language, 16,* 281–299.

Caine, E. D., Ebert, M. H., & Weingartner, H. (1977). An outline for the analysis of dementia. The memory disorder of Huntington's disease. *Neurology, 27,* 1087–1092.

Cummings, J. L. (1986). Subcortical dementia: Neuropsychology, neuropsychiatry, and pathophysiology. *British Journal of Psychiatry, 149,* 682–697.

Cummings, J. L., & Benson, D. F. (1983). *Dementia: A clinical approach.* Boston: Butterworths.

Cummings, J. L., & Benson, D. F. (1986). Dementia of the Alzheimer type. An inventory of diagnostic clinical features. *Journal of the American Geriatrics Society, 34,* 12–19.

Cummings, J. L., & Benson, D. F. (1984). Subcortical dementia: Review of an emerging concept. *Archives of Neurology, 41,* 874–879.

Cummings, J. L., Benson, D. F., Hill, M. A., & Read, S. (1985). Aphasia in dementia of the Alzheimer type. *Neurology, 35,* 394–397.

Cummings, J. L., Houlihan, J. P., & Hill, M. A. (1986). The pattern of reading deterioration in dementia of the Alzheimer type: Observation and implications. *Brain and Language, 19,* 315–323.

Damasio, A. R., Damasio, H., Rizzo, M., Varney, M., & Gersh, F. (1982). Aphasia with nonhemorrhagic lesions of the basal ganglia and internal capsule. *Archives of Neurology, 39,* 15–20.

Damasio, A. R., Graff-Radford, N. R., Eslinger, P. J., Damasio, H., & Kassell, N. (1985). Amnesia following basal forebrain lesions. *Archives of Neurology, 42*, 263–271.

Dixon, W. J., Brown, M. B., Engleman, L., & Hill, M. A. (1985). *BMDP statistical software* (2nd ed.). Los Angeles: University of California Press.

Emery, O. B., & Emery, P. E. (1983). Language in senile dementia of the Alzheimer type. *Psychiatry Journal of the University of Ottawa, 8*, 169–178.

Folstein, M. F., Folstein, S. E., & McHugh, P. R. (1975). Mini-mental state. *Journal of Psychiatric Research, 12*, 189–198.

Freedman, M., Rivoira, P., Butters, N., Sax, D. S., & Feldman, R. G. (1984). Retrograde amnesia in Parkinson's disease. *Canadian Journal of Neurological Science, 11*, 297–301.

Gaspar, P., & Gray, F. (1984). Dementia in idiopathic Parkinson's disease. *Acta Neuropathologica, 64*, 43–52.

Goodglass, H., & Kaplan, E. (1976). *The assessment of aphasia and related disorders.* Philadelphia: Lea and Febiger.

Hachinski, V. C., Iliff, L. D., Zilkha, E., Du Boulay, G. H., McAllister, V. L., Marshall, J., Russell, R. W. R., & Symon, L. (1975). Cerebral blood flow in dementia. *Archives of Neurology, 32*, 632–637.

Hachinski, V. C., Lassen, N. A., & Marshall, J. (1974). Multi-infarct dementia. *Lancet, 2*, 207–210.

Hakim, A. M., & Mathieson, G. (1979). Dementia in Parkinson disease: A neuropathologic study. *Neurology, 29*, 1209–1214.

Hier, D. B., Hagenlocker, K., & Shindler, A. G. (1985). Language disintegration in dementia: Effects of etiology and severity. *Brain and Language, 25*, 117–133.

Huber, S. J., Shuttleworth, E. C., & Paulson, G. W. (1986). Dementia in Parkinson's disease. *Archives of Neurology, 43*, 987–990.

Hughes, W., Dodgson, M. C. H., & MacLennan, D. C. (1954). Chronic cerebral hypertensive disease. *Lancet, 2*, 770–774.

Kertesz, A. (1979). *Aphasia and associated disorders: Taxonomy, localization, and recovery.* New York: Grune & Stratton.

Landis, T., Graves, R., Benson, D. F., & Hebben, N. (1982). Visual recognition through kinaesthetic mediation. *Psychological Medicine, 12*, 4515–531.

Martin, A., & Fedio, P. (1983). Word production and comprehension in Alzheimer's disease: The breakdown of semantic knowledge. *Brain and Language, 19*, 124–141.

McKhann, G., Drachman, D., Folstein, M., Katzman, R., Price, D., & Stadlan, E. M. (1984). Clinical diagnosis of Alzheimer's disease: Report of the NINCDS-ADRDA Work Group under the auspices of Department of Health and Human Services Task Force on Alzheimer's Disease. *Neurology, 34*, 939–944.

Nelson, H. E., O'Connell, A. (1978). Dementia: The estimation of premorbid intelligence using the new Adult Reading Test. *Cortex, 14*, 234–244.

Roman, G. C. (1985). Lacunar dementia. In J. T. Hutton & A. D. Kenny (Eds.), *Senile dementia of the Alzheimer type* (pp. 131–151). New York: Alan R. Liss.

Whitehouse, P. J., Hedreen, J. C., White, C. L., III, & Price, D. L. (1983). Basal forebrain neurons in the dementia of Parkinson disease. *Annals of Neurology, 13*, 243–248.

Wilson, R. S., Kaszniak, A. W., & Fox, J. H. (1981). Remote memory in senile dementia. *Cortex, 17*, 41–48.

III

Oral and Written Language Disorders

7

Mechanisms Underlying Aphasic Transformations

HUGH W. BUCKINGHAM

This chapter treats the various "mechanisms" that may be said to underlie aphasic transformations. I have quoted the word *mechanisms* for a reason, since that term implies some sort of device (actually, another metaphor) or internal agent that does things. Whatever these mechanisms are in their neurophysiological instantiations, they must be understood psychologically as manipulating some types of elements in some domain of operation. Without first attempting to characterize what the mechanisms might be at a psycholinguistic level of explanation and what they might do, we will not be in any position to begin to characterize aphasic transformations. That is, in order to start I must lay out a production model of some sort that can justifiably be said to form part of the cognitive system for language—a model constructed from evidence external to the data from aphasia.

The justification for the type of model I intend to use comes from modern studies in the philosophy of psychology (e.g., Fodor, 1983), where the claim (p. 29) is made that "contemporary cognitive theory takes it for granted that the paradigmatic psychological process is a sequence of transformations of mental representations and that the paradigmatic cognitive system is one which effects such transformations." Like Fodor, I will assume for the purposes of the present chapter that if I am going to speak of psychological mechanisms, then I must assume that these mechanisms will be computational systems of one sort or another. Concurring further with Fodor (1982, p. 279), I will assume that these computational processes are both *symbolic* and *formal*. The processes are termed sym-

HUGH W. BUCKINGHAM • Program in Linguistics and Communication Disorders, Louisiana State University, Baton Rouge, Louisiana 70803.

bolic because they are defined over (operate upon) representations that consist of symbolic elements. The processes are termed formal because they apply to the various representations in virtue of the configuration or syntax of those representations. The formal operations apply, as it were, to various types of symbols without "understanding" anything about what those symbols may or may not mean. Or, to put it another way, the operations manipulate the symbols in terms of their shapes, not their meanings.

Once we spell out the levels of representation and the various types of computations that map one level onto another, we will be in a position to consider what types of derailments of the computations could occur to account for the production of aphasic transformations.

THE GARRETT MODEL

Over the past 10 years or so, Merrill Garrett (1975, 1976, 1980) has been developing a model for sentence production based on data he and others have collected from the slips of the tongue of normal, non-brain-damaged subjects. More recently Garrett (1982, 1984) has shown how his model may be used to characterize aphasic syndromes. Schwartz (1987) and Buckingham (1980, 1985, 1986, 1987) have incorporated and extended Garrett's model in explaining their aphasic data. Garrett's publications (1982, 1984), however, have ensured that his model will play a major role in psycholinguistic accounts of the aphasias for some time to come. That there is, indeed, a clear relation between slips of the tongue and many types of aphasic errors has been indicated in Cutler and Fay's (1978) introduction to the reissue of the landmark study of Meringer and Mayer (1895) and in Buckingham (1980). It is therefore not without precedent that I utilize a model such as Garrett's to characterize the computational and representational breakdowns seen in aphasic language.

The overall model of Garrett (Garrett, 1984, p. 174) consists of inferential processes that map conceptual structures onto a message level representation, which is viewed by Garrett as a real-time construct that determines all subsequent sentence level production. It is in this sense that all subsequent mental processes are "executive driven" (Fodor, 1986, p. 81). At these higher levels, which, parenthetically, have not been arrived at through data from slips of the tongue but rather through philosophical argument (e.g., Searle, 1983), intentionality is the key, and since "executive control" is established at the message level, it may be said that "intentionality is the key to the mental" (Fodor, 1986, p. 81). Again, the message level is based upon the speaker's current perceptual and affective states of mind and on his general knowledge of how the world is. So-called scripts and plans as well as other schemata are crucial in the memorial structures pertaining to knowledge of the world, and are the *sine qua non* for characterizing message level representations. In addition, representations of the message level must be composed of a basic symbology of simple concepts and some sort of syntax. That the representations are composed of symbols in an arrangement follows from the requirement that computational processes be both symbolic and formal. It is also important to emphasize that there is a syntax at every level of representation.

Mapping from the message level to the functional level in Garrett's model (e.g., Garrett, 1984, p. 176) is realized through what he calls logical and syntactic processes. There are three principal computations here. First, there is a determination of functional level structures. Although they are not the same, as Garrett points out, these functional level structures are strikingly similar to the "deep case" structures of Fillmore (1968), and they are couched in $f(x)$ notation consisting of atomic predicates and arguments. The second computation is that of a meaning-based lexical identification. The computations that operate here access the lexicon solely in terms of meaning,[1] but a "linking address is set up here that establishes an association with the shape of the word in question. The shape here, however, may be very abstract (see Caplan, 1987, pp. 246–247). Moreover, it should be pointed out that these computations are very fast and may initially access *all* the meanings of some word or perhaps initially *all* meaning-related words. The meaning "sphere" or semantic field may be what is pointed to, and initially the linking addresses of all members of the sphere apparently present themselves in a rapid, and almost reflexlike, fashion (e.g., Swinney, 1982). Derailments here would ultimately cause incorrect selections of the shapes of words that were nevertheless in the semantic sphere of the target, and consequently it is within these computations that one would locate the mechanism of semantic paraphasia. Meaning-related, lexical slips of the tongue are located precisely here by Garrett. The third computation in the message to functional mapping is the assignment of the semantically selected lexical items to functional structures. The Functional Level structure is thereby computed and the representation is a syntactic one but, again, a very

---

[1]Given Fodor's stipulation that computations manipulate symbols only in terms of their shapes, we may question the status of the operations involved in the first, or meaning-based, lexical lookup at the functional level. Is there any essential computational difference between "appreciating" the meaning of a word and "selecting" that word from the mental lexicon on the basis of its phonological shape? It is certainly logical that a word can be "selected" on the basis of its meaning, but how is this carried off as a computation if that selection does not involve symbol manipulation. "Symbol" implies form as well as meaning. So, it would appear that even at the functional level where the selection processes do not have access to the phonological shape of a word, those processes do have access to the word in terms of its semantic symbolic form. Phonological form is connected to the first lexical lookup computations through the "linking address."

abstract syntax cast in the atomic predicate-argument form of deep case structure. It still must be viewed, however, as a real-time construct, rendering it quite unlike the deep case structural level in Fillmore's theory.

Syntactic and phonological processes then work off of the functional level representation and map it onto Garrett's positional level representation (e.g., Garrett, 1984, p. 178). These processes are exceedingly important, since evidence to date indicates that many aphasic transformations are the result of derailments that would appear to involve them. According to Garrett, there are four processes here. Later on I will augment the list of computations in this domain, bringing to bear mechanisms proposed by Butterworth (1979) and by Shattuck-Hufnagel (1979, 1983).

The first of the positional level computations[2] construct phrasal frames or matrices, which carry superficial constituent structure information, markings for functor morphemes, and grammatically positioned empty slots for the contentives (nouns, verbs, adjectives, and adverbs). Phrasal intonational contours are also coded with the frames.

The second computation feeding into the positional level is extremely important and involves the retrieval of lexical items in terms of the form or shape of those items. Thus, retrieval here is distinguished from functional level retrieval, which, as we saw, involved selection exclusively on the basis of meaning. The "linking address," recall, will have previously been established at the functional level retrieval in order to assure that in the normal situation, the form-based retrieval will match the meaning-based retrieval. That is, if book has been retrieved initially in terms of its meaning, we want to ensure that that item's formal counterpart will subsequently be accessed in terms of its phonological shape. Ultimately, both retrieval computations must operate correctly to produce the proper target. Data from slips of the tongue and aphasia demonstrate that these two retrieval processes may be dissociated—one operating, the other failing. Words may be appreciated in terms of their meaning, while their forms are completely inaccessible. Forms of words may be accessed at times when there is absolutely no appreciation of their meaning.

The third computation is the actual assignment of the form-retrieved lexical items to their respective frame slots. It is important to point out that the computations here are also manipulating the segmental units of the words as well and are readying them for utterance order. That is, at some point, the representative shapes of words as they exist in the lexicon must be, in a sense, reordered for real-time production. I view this reordering as taking place in parallel with the assignment of the whole word to its phrasal frame slot; however, in order to discuss these additional

---

[2]We call them positional level computations, but in a strict sense only representations are understood to exist at the levels in Garrett's model. Computational processes map levels onto levels and they exist between the levels, not at them. Often in the wording of the operations in this model, by x level processes we mean that map onto level x.

computations, I will borrow from Shattuck-Hufnagel, since Garrett in his original work did not consider segmental ordering manipulation in any detail. Later on, I will further augment the computational structure at this location by adding a mechanism that will supply phonological syllabic forms when no regular target forms can be accessed, and subsequently these "de novo" forms will be assigned to the empty contentive slots. The notion of a separate segmental "generator" comes from Butterworth (1979).

The fourth computation leading to the positional level of representation is one that assigns the frame elements (the functors, both bound and free) to their respective positions in the lexically interpreted phrasal frames. These computations place items such as affixal morphemes, determiners, and the like onto their positions. Again, data from slips of the tongue as well as aphasia demonstrate that the processes that assign contentives to their slots and the processes that assign functor morphemes to their slots can be separately disrupted, and thus those computations are functionally dissociated.

After these computations have operated, we arrive at the positional level of representation, where the utterance order is more directly reflected. The representation here is phonological, and, although it is a level in a real-time model of sentence production, it closely parallels the "systematic phonetic" level in the sense of Chomsky and Halle (1968).

The basic computations that map from the positional level to the phonetic level are akin to the so-called regular phonological processes, and these essentially establish the allophonic and allomorphic manifestations of the phonemic and morphemic units as they are represented at the positional level. The computations that map the positional onto the phonetic are clearly dissociated from the positional level process just discussed. There is a wealth of data from slips of the tongue and from aphasia that demonstrates derailments with the later and none with the former. That is, the literature on aphasia or slips of the tongue is replete with examples of errors where, despite what has occurred above, all the allophonics and allomorphics are computed correctly. If, for example, a /p/ slips out of a nonaspirated position into a syllable initial position in a stressed syllable, its allophonic realization will be aspirated. In the error *papple,* the unaspirated /p/ in the target, will pick up its aspirated allophone in the initial position of the error. If the past-tense morpheme moves to a new slot, such as in *he added ten* spoken as *he add tened,* the past-tense allomorph will be /-d/, instead of the /-əd/ after *add.*

A lower set of computations will then map the phonetic level of representation onto the articulatory level, off of which are computed the motor commands to the articulators. The phonetic-to-articulatory processes compute ever finer phonetic detail (below that of the allophones and allomorphs) and construct units that will more naturally feed into

actual motor commands. The computations that run off of the phonetic
level take into consideration all other nonlinguistic contextual factors of
articulation that exist in each speaking situation, factors such as temporary obstructions in speech cavities (such as bite blocks and chewing
gum), attentional states, and other factors that do not play a role in the
underlying linguistic system but which must be accounted for on each
speaking occasion, since the information is nevertheless relevant for
motor production.

For the purposes of this chapter, however, we need only focus upon
the functional and positional levels of representations and the computations that construct them. I will now turn to the various additions to the
Garrett model that I feel are necessary for a more complete picture of the
computations between the functional and positional levels of that model.

THE AUGMENTATIONS OF THE GARRETT MODEL

As additions to the syntactic and phonological processes that map
onto the positional level, I will propose two mechanisms and a buffer
from the world of Stephanie Shattuck-Hufnagel (1979, 1983). On Shattuck-Hufnagel's view, phonological *forms* are retrieved from the lexicon
and placed into a buffer that can hold up to a clause. There is some sort of
interlocking between this buffer and the initially constructed phrasal
frames of Garrett, since the content words operated upon segmentally are
destined for the empty slots designated by the frames. The words are
placed in the buffer in their representative shapes, whereupon a device
termed the *scan copier* scans the segments by syllable position and copies
those segments into their productive orders. In the normal case, the productive order will be quite similar to the order of the lexical segments as
they are stored in their representative shapes. Obviously, a somewhat less
abstract phonology will work better here, but where the dictates from
underlying systems force a more abstract analysis, production models
such as Garrett's will have to settle for more recondite representative
forms and proceed accordingly.

Once a segment is copied onto its productive order position, it must
be eliminated from the buffer in order to avoid repetitive copying, which
would lead to copious reiteration (or perseveration). Accordingly, Shattuck-Hufnagel has suggested a mechanism she calls the "checkoff
monitor." Once the segment is copied, the monitor "checks it off." The
scan copier operates in accordance with the syntax of the phonological
material, which means that it operates over the syllabic structure of representative forms, and it copies segments onto a syllabically coded productive order structure.

To fully understand this, we must take a closer look at the constituent structure of the syllable. The model I incorporate goes back to the work of Pike and Pike (1947) and is further discussed in Bell and Hooper (1978). To begin with, the syllable bifurcates into an "onset" and a "core," as illustrated in Figure 1. The onset consists of any initial consonants of the syllable. The core bifurcates into a "peak" and a "coda." The peak is the syllabic element that may carry stress, and is thus usually the slot for the vowels, although certain of the sonorant consonants in English may function as syllabics. The core consists of any terminal consonants assigned to the syllable. Like the onset, the core may be empty. The only unit of the syllable that must be filled is, of course, the peak. On this view, the syntax of syllables is essentially binary. Coda consonants are more strongly glued to the peak than are onset consonants, and there is much data to support this (e.g., Shattuck-Hufnagel, 1987). We can now return to the scan copier.

It scans the segmental elements of the phonological forms in the buffer by syllable position. That is, it scans onsets and cores, but within the core there is some evidence that the scanner is sensitive to whether it is manipulating a peak item or a coda. Slips of the tongue have instructed us here. The literature on them is replete with examples where the slip involves the movement of a segment to some other location in another syllable. However, it has been noted that in practically every case, the segment that switches syllables ends up in the same position as it occupied in its original syllable. That is, onsets move to onset positions,

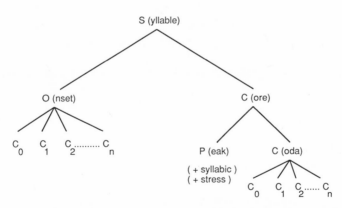

FIGURE 1. A hierarchical representation of the major syllable constituents. This is essentially a binary view of the structure of the syllable. Onsets and codas may be empty or may consist of one or more consonants, depending upon the language. The specific arrangements of the consonants that make up the onsets and codas are first conditioned by the universal principle of sonority. Language-specific phonotactic constraints then account for slightly different possibilities for consonantal sequences in the onsets and codas for different languages. The range of phonotactic differences among languages is, however, highly constrained by the overriding universal principle of sonority.

peaks go only to positions for peaks, and codas move to coda positions. The only recent finding is that ambisyllabic consonants have a greater range of choice as to where they may end up, since by their very nature they are ambivalent as to whether they are the coda of one syllable or the onset of another (Buckingham, 1980; Stemberger, 1982). Consonants that are unambiguously assigned to a syllable are called "tautosyllabic." The scanner, then, scans and copies segments by syllable position. If it mis-scans, then some onset that occurs later on in the form will be copied in an earlier onset position. At times there will be an exchange of segments, and at other times either the original segment will be deleted by the checkoff monitor or it will remain in its original position—the checkoff monitor failing to check the misscanned segment off from its original slot. In this latter case, the so-called doublet error will be the result (see Lecours & Lhermitte, 1969). In the end, all of the processes suggested by Shattuck-Hufnagel will have to interact with the computations suggested by Garrett at the positional level, since phonological shape and utterance order are crucial at this point in the production process.

The next augmentation to the positional level processes in the Garrett model is the so-called random generator suggested by Butterworth (1979). Butterworth suggested this device on the basis of data from neologistic jargonaphasia. That is, there appeared to be a need for getting some sort of phonological material into the buffer in those cases where it seemed that the speaker could not retrieve target words on the basis of their form. The neologisms Butterworth analyzed consisted of phoneme aggregates that did not follow the normal distributional characteristics of words in English. In fact, his statistical analysis showed them to be randomly distributed, not in terms of phonotactic arrangement but in terms of expectancy. He therefore posited a "random generator" that would go into operation at the point of blocked access to phonological shapes. Again, by "random" Butterworth did not mean haphazard ordering of phonemes but rather that the frequency-based expectancies for phoneme use were not followed in the construction of the neologisms. The ability assumed by this random generator is not so strange and should not be taken to be some recondite capacity that results from brain damage (Buckingham, 1987). Merrill Garrett (1982, p. 46) discusses Butterworth's proposal in the following manner: "Butterworth hypothesizes that the neologistic forms are generated by jargon aphasics in response to a word retrieval difficulty—rather than halt, the speaker generates a phonetically acceptable slot filler using the phonological and morphological structure building systems normally at one's disposal."

In a footnote supporting the assumption that this random generator is not some de novo creation by the brain lesion but rather part of the normal cognitive system, Garrett (1982, p. 72) writes: "Any speaker can generate nonsense forms on request, and everyone on occasion produces nonce forms. . . . investigations of voluntary glossolalia are convincing in the former regard."

Butterworth suggested that this device was a segment generator, but it is more reasonable to suppose that it produces syllable-sized chunks of phonological material. It is also likely that the syllable stock that this device has recourse to abides by the phonotactic patterns of the language, since, no matter how bizarre they are, neologisms do not in general disobey the constraints that condition permissible syllable patterns of the aphasic's language. Figure 2 illustrates how the scan copier, the checkoff monitor, and the random generator fit in with Garrett's positional level processes.

Having now characterized a model for normal sentence production, we are in a position of analyzing the computational derailments that produce aphasic transformations. I will begin with lexical phenomena.

LEXICAL SUBSTITUTIONS

Full lexical substitutions are triggered either on a meaning-similarity base or on a form-similarity base. The point of the present chapter is not to present a wealth of new data for these kinds of paraphasias but rather to suggest the type of computational breakdown involved and the location of the breakdown. As should be obvious by now, meaning-based lexical errors and form-based lexical errors would take place at different points in

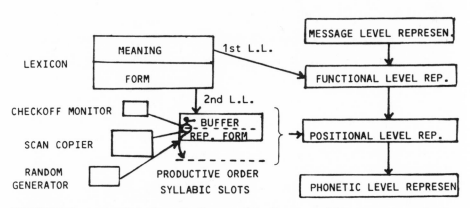

FIGURE 2. An augmented schematic diagram of the Garrett model for sentence production demonstrating the additions of the scan copier, the checkoff monitor, the random generator, the working memory buffer for the serial ordering of segments, and the productive-order syllabic slots. The diagram highlights the fact that these processes enter into the computations that operate between the functional level and the positional level, and as such they feed into the positional level. (From Buckingham, 1987, p. 382.)

the production process, which is to say that they occur in different computational domains in a model such as Garrett's.

Meaning-based lexical errors take place owing to derailments of the functional level computations of meaning-based selection (or appreciation). These so-called semantic paraphasias have been catalogued and described in numerous publications, such as Buckingham (1981), Buckingham and Rekart (1979), and Rinnert and Whitaker (1973). Recently, disturbances of lexical semantic representations have been summarized in Caplan (1987, chap. 12). The semantically related substitutive errors all indicate that the subject nevertheless correctly arrives at the semantic sphere of the word sought, so, in a sense, there really is no semantic field disturbance—at the level of the sphere itself. These spheres are many and are discussed fully in Buckingham and Rekart (1979), in Rinnert and Whitaker (1973), and in the references found in those works. For these kinds of lexical substitutions, the linking address serves only to hold onto the semantic field of the target word, to ensure that at the point of form-based retrieval, the phonological shape found will be from the necessary semantic area. Form-based retrieval need not be disrupted, and in fact cannot be, if there is to be a semantic substitute for the target, since in an obvious sense the error must nevertheless be accessed in terms of its shape. Consequently, there may be a disruption with the linking address. Anomias that are characterized by numerous semantic substitutions are quite different in nature from anomias where no forms are accessed whatsoever. In addition, the semantic paraphasia does not necessarily take into account phonological structure, since a typical error would be to substitute *Thanksgiving* for *Easter*, the two forms having little in common in terms of their shapes. Caplan (1987, p. 212), however, observes that there is often formal similarity between target words and their semantically related substitutes. This need not be the case, however.

The network of connections in the lexicon is a web-shaped structure that stretches in the horizontal as well as in the vertical plane. There are vertical (paradigmatic, hyponymic relations as well as horizontal (syntagmatic) modificational/attributive relations. These are semantic relations; but there are form relations as well, since in some obvious sense words with similar phonological makeup must be linked (see Fay & Cutler, 1977). And this in turn allows for the form-based selection errors. Form-based selection derailments, in the Garrett scheme, take place at the positional level, well after meaning-based selection has been computed. This does not mean, of course, that it would not be possible in some instances to claim that some failure to appreciate semantic connectiveness could give rise to form-based selection difficulties. It only means that form-based selection disturbances can be dissociated from meaning-based appreciation of words. There is ample evidence of this type of dissociation (e.g., Buckingham, 1985).

The so-called malapropism is indicative of a form-based lexical substitution, but at least two types of malapropism must be distinguished. The "classical" malapropism is a product of learning and is not considered to be an "on-line" slip or an aphasic derailment (Zwicky, 1982). The sociolinguistically relevant malapropism is the classical one described in Sheridan's novel *The Rivals*, where through lack of familiarity and use, some word is misperceived (a sort of slip of the ear) and initially stored in memory incorrectly. For example, the word *discretion* may be misperceived (or perceived, but subsequently misanalyzed) and stored in the lexicon as *discrepancy*. As a result, the speaker may on some occasion say of a boss that he often leaves decisions up to the *discrepancy* of his employees. The classical malapropism is an *advertent* error. The "on-line" malapropism, however (Fay & Cutler, 1977) is of a very different nature and truly represents a selection error based upon shape similarity; it is *inadvertent*. The phonologically based errors, therefore, will not be meaning-related, and those who commit them will quite often catch themselves in the act and correct the error. Aphasics tend to produce fewer on-line malapropisms than semantic paraphasias.

LEXICAL BLENDS

It can occur that two lexical items will be selected simultaneously, the result being a blended form. Blends can take place both at the lexical and at the phrasal level (Fay, 1981). In fact, slips of the tongue that had been classified as derailed transformational processing turned out, upon close inspection, to look more like the simultaneous blending of two— semantically related—phrases. Lexical blends also involve two words that are related semantically. For example, a blend of *slightest* and *least* would result in the error form *sleast* (Ellis, 1980). Most often, the blended error is not a word in the language, but interestingly enough it will conform to the phonotactics. Another example would be the blend of *gripping* and *grasping* to yield *grisping* (Fay & Cutler, 1977). In some rare cases, the error will match a word in the dictionary, but that word will not bear the meaning relation that the two input items shared. Fay and Cutler (1977) provide an example where the semantically related words *heritage* and *legacy* blend to form *heresy*, most certainly unrelated to the semantics of the blended items.

Phrasal blends would be characterized according to the Garrett model as an example of a derailed positional level computation of phrasal frame construction with concurrent lexical selections. For example, the error *when you boil down to it*, would come from the blend of *when you come down to it* and *what it boils down to* (Fay, 1981). Note that the two blended phrases share very similar semantic properties. However, since meaning is crucially involved, the similarity in meaning between the blended forms must implicate the functional level as well. Many of the fluent aphasics exhibit blended forms of this nature (Buckingham & Kertesz, 1976, pp. 60–61).

Pure lexical blends most certainly argue for a functional level derailment because those forms must share meaning, but the blending itself involves the simultaneous form-based selection of two words. Blended errors clearly argue for a more parallel processing view of the functional and positional levels, which of course does not mean that the computations themselves are not encapsulated and cognitively impenetrable in the sense of Fodor (1983). As indicated above, the linking addresses serve as crucial mediating processes between functional and positional lexical manipulation. Consequently, the lexical blend may be viewed as some sort of coalescence of different linking addresses eminating from the same semantic domain. In other words, there is very close interaction between these two levels in the production of blends. They are coalescences of shapes that share meaning.

Before leaving blends, I should point out that there are other sorts of blends that have been discussed in the aphasia literature, but these result from the perseveration of one of the forms to be blended. For example, Buckingham, Whitaker, and Whitaker (1978) describe many instances where some perseverated form will carry over into the production of some subsequent response, blending in with that response. For example, as discussed in that paper, a patient who was perseverating on the word *drink* would contaminate other forms, such as *cross* and *crack*, such that they were produced as *dross* and *drack*. In these cases, of course, the blended forms will not share meaning. Perseverated blends, therefore, are more likely to be derailments at the positional level and to involve items that somehow get "stuck" in the buffer through computational derailments of the checkoff monitor, thereby interfering with newly selected items. So much for the whole-word derailments. I now turn my attention to the disruption of computations that manipulate the segments of the words.

PHONEMIC SUBSTITUTION

The nature of the phonemic substitution is not transparent, although at the outset it would appear to be. The important question to ask is from where does the substituting phoneme originate? For there to be a strict phonemic substitution, some phoneme must be substituted for some other phoneme—or so it would seem. However, even this apparently obvious point is deceiving, since the substitution may not be of one phonemic unit for another but rather simply a switch of one distinctive feature of some phonemic unit, the result being the appearance of some other phonemic unit that differs from the original by that one feature. In that event, the substitution is really simply the reversal of some feature + or − marking. Shattuck-Hufnagel and Klatt (1979) have argued that, at least for slips of the tongue, accounting for phonemic substitutions in terms of distinctive feature switches buys one very little, and that the proper way of viewing these kinds of transformations is in terms of whole phonemic units substituting for whole phonemic units. In any event, usually only phonemes that are similar in terms of their distinctive feature makeup substitute for one another. Practically every investigator of phonemic substitutions has pointed this out (e.g., Blumstein, 1973). The ambiguity in analysis (feature vs. whole phoneme unit) is still a serious problem for the substitution of phonemes that differ minimally in their feature array; however, it represents less of a problem for the substitution where the two phonemes involved differ in several features, which is apparently the case for many of the so-called conduction aphasics (see Caplan, 1987, p. 220). For substitutions involving two or three features, it would seem more likely that the transformation involves whole phonemic units. The issue, however, is still unresolved, and in many instances we simply cannot be sure whether the substitution involves whole segments or switches in feature markings.

We now ask ourselves where in the production process could phonemic substitutions take place. In terms of the combined model presented in this chapter, errors in the selection of unit phonemes would appear minimally to occur somewhere during the manipulation of the phonological structure of words and the copying of representative forms onto levels more in line with articulatory production. It must be admitted, however, that the investigator who proposed the scan-copier model of phonological production (i.e., Shattuck-Hufnagel) did not observe many exclusively paradigmatic phonemic substitutions in her slip of the tongue data and, accordingly, did not set up her model to readily account for them. In fact, Shattuck-Hufnagel's findings lead her to the conclusion that few if any strict phonemic substitutions occur—that is, phonemic substitutions that do not implicate linear ordering disruptions. Be that as it may, the scanner could on occasion somehow select a closely related segment (or perhaps not so closely related) and copy it onto the productive level. Just how this may come about is not well defined from the analyses provided by Shattuck-Hufnagel, since, again, she does not think that pure phonemic substitutions account for much of her error data. This finding from slip data is rather puzzling, given the fact that one of the most detailed studies of phonemic paraphasias to date (Blumstein, 1973) assumed that most of the phonemic paraphasias across syndromes (Broca, Conduction, and Wernicke) were, in fact, phonemic substitutions.

To get around the puzzling "no-source" (purely paradigmatic) phonemic substitution, Shattuck-Hufnagel (1979, pp. 317–318) offers several suggestions. First, it may be the case that the source of the substituting phoneme was in part of the utterance not recorded or written down by the investigator. Here we must recall that Shattuck-Hufnagel is talking about data collection for slips of the tongue, not aphasia. Consequently, this suggestion is bound to the research methodology. Most investigators, given the very nature of the data they are collecting, do not accumulate slip of the tongue samples through lengthy tape recordings, but rather in one setting or another they overhear a slip and quickly try to write it down with paper and pencil. They may, of course, fail to write down enough of the utterance that surrounded the slip to spot a possible linear source of a slip recorded as a pure phonemic substitution originally. For this reason, Shattuck-Hufnagel's first alternative is a real possibility for slips of the tongue. The aphasia researcher, on the other hand, is more likely to at least audiotape-record the speech output of the patient. That being the case, a fairly distant linear source for a phonemic substitution may be somewhat easier to ascertain.

Second, it may happen that the information specifying a target segment is incompletely or incorrectly copied onto its syllabic slot by the scanning mechanism. How this might occur is left undescribed by Shattuck-Hufnagel. This account may simply reduce to the claim that the phonemic units that get to the buffer are underspecified in their featural makeup, and the error occurs during the computations that fill in the rest of the feature matrix, as suggested by Beland and Nespoulous (1985).

A third possibility suggested by Shattuck-Hufnagel is that some component of a segment (i.e., a feature) in an analogous syllable slot down line interferes with (contaminates) the segmental array currently being copied. Admittedly, though, Shattuck-Hufnagel pays little attention to the feature level of explanation for her error corpus.

A fourth alternative account considered by Shattuck-Hufnagel is a more intriguing one. It is that the substituting segment's source is in a *word* that somehow mistakenly presents itself as a competing or alternative element into the set of ongoing planning units. Competing plan errors are discussed in detail in Baars (1980). This type of lexical account for phonemic substitution errors is also considered by MacNeilage, Hutchinson, and Lasater (1981).

Although I cannot go into much detail in this chapter, an additional possible confounding factor involved in the observation of so many supposedly nonsource phonemic substitutions could be that subtle articulatory asynchronies, which are not generally perceived without technical measurement, give rise to shifts in the acoustic spectrum. These acoustic shifts may in some cases be affecting crucial perceptual cues for the hearers. The altered acoustic cue may be such that the perceiver "hears" another phonological unit. In that case, the hearer would make the claim that the speaker *substituted* the phonemic unit that was actually constructed in the perceiver's own mind. This process has been referred to as "phonemic false evaluation," and the clinical and theoretical repercussions of it have been discussed in Buckingham and Yule (1987). Suffice it to say that, consequently, in many cases, what have been tagged as phonemic substitutions may in reality be substitutions in the minds of hearers only—the speaker having selected the correct target phoneme only to produce it with some sort of articulatory aberration, thereby shifting the acoustic quality such that the hearer constructs another phoneme. In this case, it would be incorrect to claim that the speaker selected the wrong segment, and thus it would not be a case of phonemic substitution. To the extent that Shattuck-Hufnagel's alternative accounts have some feasibility and in fact could represent what is actually going on, then those processes, together with presumed instances of phonemic false evaluation, may be robust enough to rule out pure phonemic substitutions altogether, for aphasia and for slips of the tongue.

PHONEMIC TRANSPOSITION

Phonemic transpositions, on the other hand, constitute a majority of phonological errors in aphasia, and they may or may not condition phoneme substitutions. Transpositions of this sort involve linear ordering derailments and are seen in great quantities in both slips of the tongue and aphasia. Fromkin (1971), Garrett (1980), and Shattuck-Hufnagel (1979) provide ample cases of linear segmental slips of the tongue, while Blumstein (1973), Buckingham and Kertesz (1976), Buckingham et al. (1978), Kohn (1984, 1985), and Lecours and Lhermitte (1969) are but a few of the many studies that have documented linear switches in aphasic patients.

Transpositional errors among segments are either anticipatory or perseverative, or in some cases there may be complete exchanges, although the latter type are seen much more in slips of the tongue than in aphasia. Anticipatory errors may result in the addition of the anticipated segment to the total stock of segments in the original word. For example, the error *papple* for the word *apple* creates an additional /p/ to the total word string. In other words, a doublet is created. The error *nondon* for the word *London* does not create an additional segment, but rather the anticipated /n/ substitutes for the /l/ of the target. Note that in both these cases the anticipated segment remains in its original slot. Not all anticipated segments will necessarily remain in their original positions. Whether they will or will not remain in their original positions is usually conditioned by syllable structure constraints. That is, if by its not appearing in its original slot an unpermissible sequence of two segments would result, the anticipated segment will most often remain in that position. If upon its disappearing from that slot a permissible sequence still obtains, the antic-ipated segment may delete from its original position in a word. Buck-ingham (1987, 1989) details the constraints involved in whether doublets are produced or not. We will briefly consider the nature of these con-straints later on in this chapter.

Now it should be clear that the above transformations would most likely occur as derailments with the scan copier and checkoff mecha-nisms postulated earlier in this chapter. The scanner would erroneously scan ahead a syllable or two down line and copy, for example, some syllable onset too early. That onset could then be added to the stock of segments of the word by filling an empty slot (see Beland & Nespoulous, 1985) or it could substitute for the original consonant onset. Moreover, the anticipating segment may or may not be deleted from its original position by the checkoff monitor. That is, if there is a disruption of the checkoff monitor, it will fail and the anticipated item will not be checked off. So, in a sense, the checkoff monitor's operation appears to be constrained by principles of syllable structure (again, see Buckingham, 1987, 1989, for more details).

Virtually everything that has been said about anticipatory transposi-tions can be said of perserverative transpositions, except in this case the process works from left to right, whereas the anticipatory shifts went from right to left. Perseverated segments may be added to the total stock of segments of some word or they may substitute for some segment that is down line. Furthermore, the perseverated segment may or may not delete from its original slot, again depending upon the sequence that would remain. Here again, the scan copier would copy, for instance, an initial onset consonant onto an onset position somewhere down line in the word, or phrase, either adding another segment by filling an empty slot (see Beland & Nespoulous, 1985) or by substituting for some other conso-nant originally in that position. Once again, it appears that the derail-ments that result in perseverative phonemic transpositions take place during the operation of the scan copier mechanism.

Since practically all of the phonemic transpositions take place in the segmental structuring of content words, it would appear that these errors occur during the manipulation of the contentives. Furthermore, the ma-nipulation must involve the form of the content words, since form is crucially involved with phonemic errors. The forms of content words are being uniquely manipulated as they are inserted into the phrasal frame slots at the positional level in the Garrett model. It may very well be during this phrasal frame placement that the scan copier operates as well (perhaps in parallel) on the segments of the contentives. Consequently, I would assign the location of phonemic paraphasia to the stage at which lexical phonological representations of individual content words are in-serted into the developing phrasal matrices at the positional level.

CONSTRAINTS ON ERRORS CONDITIONED BY
REPRESENTATIVE/COMPUTATIONAL KNOWLEDGE

Up to this point, we have characterized a model of normal language production, specified representative levels and computational mappings between the levels, considered different types of aphasic transformations, and located those transformations in terms of breakdowns in the computations at certain points in the production process according to the model. In this final section, we must consider some overriding constraints that are built into the structure of the model and which serve to ensure that, although errors are produced, they practically always abide by general structural principles of the language in question—in our case, English. Or, if the constraints are universal, they will work to condition the error typology regardless of which language is being spoken.

If we consider, first, lexical substitutions, we first note that they involve content words almost exclusively. Lexical substitutions based on meaning similarity most likely take place prior to the establishment of phrasal frames. Accordingly, they would occur at the functional level, where the sentential arguments (together with their predicates) are established on a meaning base. Derailments here will predictably involve semantic associates, as opposed to phonological associates, and the semantic paraphasia is simply placed into the functional level structure. Its phonological form is normally retrieved at the positional level, and it is produced in normal fashion and in the phrasal slot specified for the target word. This picture explains why semantic paraphasias always agree in grammatical category with the target. Not only are the phrasal frames evoked normally in the production of semantic paraphasias, but the allophonic and allomorphic computations are produced in normal fashion through the processes that map the positional level onto the phonetic level. This predicts that phonetic processes will await the production of the semantic error in order to ensure that phonetic realization rules will apply to the error and not to the target. Further, since the evocation of phrasal frame matrices is not involved in these errors, the syntax of the speech output containing semantic paraphasias will remain in the normal confines of English word order.

Phonemic substitutions and transpositions are highly constrained by the general patterns of segmental and syllabic structure in the language in question. Three patterns must be considered here: syllable position, syllable phonotactics, and syllable sonority. All phonemic paraphasias seem to abide by these conditions, no matter how severe the aphasic transformations seem to be.

We have indicated that phonemic substitutions and transpositions in aphasia are constrained by the syllable slots from which the original target segments come in their representative forms. In substitutions of phonemes, the resulting error must be allowed to occur in the position it occupies. For example, the bilabial nasal /m/ may substitute for the /n/ in a word like nut, since /m/ may occur in syllable onset position. However, the velar nasal may never substitute for some other initial nasal (or any other consonant for that matter) onset in English, since English does not permit velar nasals in onset position.

Phonemic transposition paraphasias always respect syllable position. That is, onset segments move only to other onset positions of other syllables, peaks move only to other peak positions, while codas move to other coda positions. This has been observed quite often in slips of the tongue and has been recently observed to operate in paraphasia (e.g., Buckingham, 1980). This constraint holds for all tautosyllabic elements. Ambisyllabic consonants, however, appear to have freer mobility, which makes sense since, phonologically, they may be viewed as either onsets or codas. By the same token, any tautosyllabic consonant may move to an ambisyllabic position. Obviously, what we are considering here are constraints under which mechanisms like the scan copier operate. That is, scan copier errors are very highly constrained by language-specific syllable structure patterns.

Language-specific phonotactic patterns are also observed by phonemic substitutions and transpositions. For example, /t/ may substitute for /s/ in a word like sip, since /t/ is a permissible singleton onset consonant in English. However, /t/ may not substitute for /s/ in a word such as slip, since English-based phonotactic constraints rule out onset clusters */tl-/. Similarly, no segment can move to a position whereby a nonpermissible sequence would be set up. For example, the /l/ in slip of the tongue cannot move to the second position of the onset in tongue, since, again, */tl-/ is not permitted.

The so-called sonority principle of syllable structure (Buckingham, 1987, 1989) also appears to be an overriding constraint in the production of many phonemic transposition errors. One very apparent type of error that seems to be conditioned by this principle is the so-called doublet creating error, to which I alluded above. First, let me briefly describe the sonority hierarchy. This universal phonetic principle extends over the domain of the syllable and involves a continual increase (crescendo) in vocal apperture and degree of relative prominence through spontaneous voicing from the initiation of the onset to the syllable peak (the initial demisyllable). From the peak, there is a gradual decrease (decrescendo) in sonority out to the last segment of the coda (the final demisyllable). The order of phonetic segments from least sonorous to most sonorous is obstruents, nasals, liquids, glides, and vowels. Within the obstruents are the oral stops, the affricates, and the fricatives, the oral stops being the least sonorous. The only problem here is that it is often the case that /s/ will appear before oral stops in onset clusters; /s/ seems to be the only recalcitrant segment on the sonority scale. The liquids /r/ and /l/ are between the nasals and glides in terms of sonority. The glides /y/ and /w/ are quite close to the vowels in sonority, but note that glides may never be the peaks since they are never stressed. The liquids, on the other hand, may serve as syllabic elements in English. A typically acceptable syllable on this scale would be the word *gland*, where the outermost elements are oral stops /g/ and /d/ (the least sonorous), the internal consonants /l/ and /n/ being more sonorous, and the peak *a* being the most sonorous. Consequently, a syllable is composed of an increasing degree of sonority inward toward the stressed elements and from there a decreasing degree of sonority to the final item of the coda. A syllable such as *put* would consist of a steep incline and decline in terms of sonority, whereas a syllable such as *ground* would have a more gradual incline and decline: oral stop, liquid, vowel, glide, nasal, oral stop. It is a universal fact of syllable structure (Clements, 1988) that the most preferred, least complex, least marked, or simplest type of CVC syllable involves sharp inclines and gradual declines in sonority (very sharp crescendos and less sharp decrescendos). Syllables such as /ba/ are simpler or more preferred than syllables such as /wa/. The unmarked final VC syllable has a more gradual decrescendo. In this way, we can set up a complexity metric for syllable types and in a sense for sequences of two segments. Simple, two-segment sequences are those pairs where the segments involved are far apart on sonority hierarchy. Accordingly, there would be an enhancement of a contrast in prominence, or what Donnegan and Stampe (1978) refer to as an "attraction of opposites." This is why geminate consonant clusters and sequences of two vowels are so rare in languages. It also explains why children's earliest syllables involve segments far apart on the sonority scale (i.e., CVs, where the Cs are oral stops). Onset consonant clusters composed of two oral stops are rare as well, as are onset clusters with sequences of segments that are adjacent on the sonority hierarchy (e.g., Harris, 1983, p. 21, for Spanish). Again, the attraction of opposites holds more strongly in initial demisyllables, where sharp crescendos are preferred.

If we turn our attention back to doublet creating phonemic paraphasias, we note that in order to produce the doublet, the checkoff monitor must not work, leaving the moved segment (having been either anticipated or perseverated) in its original position as well. In Buckingham (1989), several examples are cited that demonstrate the operation of the sonority principle. When some segment is erroneously transposed by the scan copier, it is generally the case that it will not be checked off from its original position, if by so doing a highly marked sequence of segments would be set up. I should note that, heretofore, doublets have been *described* but not explained. The sonority principle attempts to offer an explanation of why we get doublets in some instances and not in others. Take the doublet creation of two /p/'s in the paraphasia *papple* for the word *apple*. If the doublet had not been created—that is, if the antici-pated /p/ had been correctly checked off by the monitor—that would have left a highly marked cross-syllabic sequence of two vowels: /æ/ and /ə/. Most linear transpositions of the doublet-creating sort come from syllable peripheries and cross syllable boundaries. Consequently, the so-called "syllable contact law," which follows from sonority principles (Clements, 1988), provides a partial account here. In the syllable contact sequence X$Y (where $ indicates a syllable boundary), X is usually more sonorous than Y. Therefore, a situation in which X and Y are both vowels would be highly undesirable. It turns out that on close inspection, doublet errors are most often created when the misscanned consonant that crosses syllable boundaries comes from an intervocalic position. The principle of sonority and the syllable contact law neatly explain why this should be the case. Again, the computations carried out by the scan copier and by the check-off monitor must be sensitive to the syllabic structure.

SUMMARY

The mechanisms underlying aphasic transformations have distinct characteristics and are located at different junctures in the overall produc-tion of sentences. In this chapter I have outlined a production model set up for normalcy, a model based on errors that all normal speakers make (i.e., slips of the tongue). To that model I added other components sug-gested from related research on language production. The underlying as-sumption of this chapter has been that without some notion of how the normal linguistic productive system operates, we have little hope of fully understanding aphasic errors. Rather than viewing lesions as creating new mechanisms that produce errors, it is the present author's view that aphasic breakdowns arise through derailments of computations that are carried out in normal language production, except, of course, where one commits a slip of the tongue. And for this reason, I am in general agree-ment with Eric Lenneberg (1968, p. 345), who argued that certain aphasic errors are simply augmented and sustained productions, which in more transient conditions are not uncommon in persons without demonstrable pathology. Furthermore, these computations operate at different levels in the overall system, and as a consequence, one can tease out the location of the aphasic error, while at the same time demonstrating which representa-tive levels and which computations remain intact. Overall constraints on the operation of the mechanisms also play an important role, and the intriguing aspect here is that brain damage practically never disrupts these hard-wired structural principles of pattern. In sum, it is my firm conviction that only through psycholinguistically sound models of normal production can we hope to characterize the various mechanisms underlying aphasic transformations. This chapter has been written in such a spirit.

REFERENCES

Baars, B. J. (1980). On eliciting predictable speech errors in the laboratory. In V. A. Fromkin (Ed.), Errors in linguistic performance: Slips of the tongue, ear, pen, and hand. New York: Academic Press.

Beland, R., & Nespoulous, J. L. (1985). Recent phonological models and the study of aphasic errors. Paper presented at the Academy of Aphasia, Pittsburgh.

Bell, A., & Hooper, J. B. (Eds.). (1978). Syllables and segments. Amsterdam: North-Holland.

Blumstein, S. E. (1973). A phonological investigation of aphasic speech. The Hague: Mouton.

Buckingham, H. W. (1980). On correlating aphasic errors with slips-of-the-tongue. Applied Psycholinguistics, 1, 199–220.

Buckingham, H. W. (1981). Lexical and semantic aspects of aphasia. In M. T. Sarno (Ed.), Acquired aphasia. New York: Academic Press.

Buckingham, H. W. (1985). Perseveration in aphasia. In S. Newman & R. Epstein (Eds.), Current perspectives in dysphasia. Edinburgh: Churchill Livingstone.

Buckingham, H. W. (1986). The scan-copier mechanism and the positional level of language production: Evidence from aphasia. Cognitive Science, 10, 195–217.

Buckingham, H. W. (1987). Phonemic paraphasias and psycholinguistic production models for neologistic jargon. Aphasiology, 1, 381–400.

Buckingham, H. W. (1989). The principle of sonority, doublet creation, and the checkoff monitor. In J. L. Nespoulous & P. Villiard (Eds.), Morphology, phonology and aphasia. New York: Springer-Verlag. (in press).

Buckingham, H. W., & Kertesz, A. (1976). Neologistic jargon aphasia. Amsterdam: Swets & Zeitlinger.

Buckingham, H. W., & Rekart, D. M. (1979). Semantic paraphasia. Journal of Communication Disorders, 12, 197–209.

Buckingham, H. W., Whitaker, H., & Whitaker, H. A. (1978). Alliteration and assonance in neologistic jargon aphasia. Cortex, 14, 365–380.

Buckingham, H. W., & Yule, G. (1987). Phonemic false evaluation: Theoretical and clinical aspects. Clinical Linguistics and Phonetics, 1, 113–125.

Butterworth, B. (1979). Hesitation and the production of verbal paraphasias and neologisms in jargon aphasia. Brain and Language, 18, 133–161.

Caplan, D. (1987). Neurolinguistics and linguistic aphasiology: An introduction. Cambridge: Cambridge University Press.

Chomsky, N., & Halle, M. (1968). The sound pattern of English. New York: Harper & Row.

Clements, G. N. (1988). The role of the sonority cycle in core syllabification. Working Papers of the Cornell Phonetics Laboratory, No. 2, April.

Cutler, A., & Fay, D. (1978). Introduction. In R. Meringer & C. Mayer (Eds.), Versprechen und Verlesen. Amsterdam: John Benjamins.

Donegan, P. J., & Stampe, D. (1978). The syllable in phonological and prosodic structure. In A. Bell & J. B. Hooper (Eds.), Syllables and segments. Amsterdam: North-Holland.

Ellis, A. W. (1980). On the Freudian theory of speech errors. In V. A. Fromkin (Ed.), Errors in linguistic performance: Slips of the tongue, ear, pen, and hand. New York: Academic Press.

Fay, D. (1981). Substitutions and splices: A study of sentence blends. In A. Cutler (Ed.), *Slips of the tongue and language production*. Amsterdam: Mouton.

Fay, D., & Cutler, A. (1977). Malapropisms and the structure of the mental lexicon. *Linguistic Inquiry, 8,* 505–520.

Fillmore, C. J. (1968). The case for case. In E. Bach & R. T. Harms (Eds.), *Universals in linguistic theory*. New York: Holt, Rinehart & Winston.

Fodor, J. A. (1982). Methodological solipsism considered as a research strategy in cognitive psychology. In H. L. Dreyfus (Ed., with H. Hall), *Husserl, intentionality, and cognitive science* (a Bradford book). Cambridge, MA: M.I.T. Press.

Fodor, J. A. (1983). *The modularity of mind: An essay on faculty psychology* (a Bradford book). Cambridge, MA: M.I.T. Press.

Fodor, J. A. (1986). Information and association. In M. Brand & R. M. Harnish (Eds.), *The representation of knowledge and belief*. Tucson: University of Arizona Press.

Fromkin, V. A. (1971). The non-anomalous nature of anomalous utterances. *Language, 47,* 27–52.

Garrett, M. F. (1975). The analysis of sentence production. In B. Gordon (Ed.), *The psychology of learning and motivation: Advances in research and theory*. New York: Academic Press.

Garrett, M. F. (1976). Syntactic processes in sentence production. In R. J. Wales & E. Walker (Eds.), *New approaches to language mechanisms*. Amsterdam: North-Holland.

Garrett, M. F. (1980). Levels of processing in sentence production. In B. Butterworth (Ed.), *Sentence production 1: Speech and talk*. London: Academic Press.

Garrett, M. F. (1982). Production of speech: Observations from normal and pathological language use. In A. W. Ellis (Ed.), *Normality and pathology in cognitive function*. London: Academic Press.

Garrett, M. F. (1984). The organization of processing structure for language production: Applications to aphasic speech. In D. Caplan, A. R. Lecours, & A. Smith (Eds.), *Biological perspectives on language*. Cambridge, MA: M.I.T. Press.

Harris, J. W. (1983). *Syllable structure and stress in Spanish: A nonlinear analysis*. Cambridge, MA: M.I.T. Press.

Kohn, S. E. (1984). The nature of the phonological disorder in conduction aphasia. *Brain and Language, 23,* 97–115.

Kohn, S. E. (1985). *Phonological breakdown in aphasia*. Unpublished doctoral dissertation. Boston: Tufts University.

Lecours, A. R., & Lhermitte, F. (1969). Phonemic paraphasias: Linguistic structures and tentative hypotheses. *Cortex, 5,* 193–228.

Lenneberg, E. H. (1968). Review of *Speech and brain mechanisms* by W. Penfield & L. Roberts. In R. C. Oldfield & J. C. Marshall (Eds.), *Language*. Middlesex, England: Penguin.

MacNeilage, P. F., Hutchinson, J. A., & Lasater, S. A. (1981). The production of speech: Development and dissolution of motoric and premotoric processes. In J. Long & A. Baddeley (Eds.), *Attention and performance* (Vol. 9). Hillsdale, NJ: Erlbaum.

Meringer, R., & Mayer, C. (1895). *Versprechen und verlesen, Eine psychologisch-linguistische Studie*. Stuttgart: Goschense Verlagsbuchhandlung.

Pike, K. L., & Pike, E. (1947). Immediate constituents of Mazateco syllables. *International Journal of American Linguistics, 13,* 78–91.

Rinnert, C., & Whitaker, H. A. (1973). Semantic confusions by aphasic patients. *Cortex, 9,* 56–81.

Schwartz, M. F. (1987). Patterns of speech production deficit within and across aphasia syndromes: Application of a psycholinguistic model. In M. Coltheart, G. Sartori, & R. Job (Eds.), *The cognitive neuropsychology of language*. London: Erlbaum.

Searle, J. (1983). *Intentionality: An essay in the philosophy of mind*. Cambridge: Cambridge University Press.

Shattuck-Hufnagel, S. (1979). Speech errors as evidence for a serial ordering mechanism in speech production. In W. E. Cooper & E. C. T. Walker (Eds.), *Sentence processing: Psycholinguistic studies presented to Merrill Garrett*. Hillsdale, NJ: Erlbaum.

Shattuck-Hufnagel, S. (1983). Sublexical units and suprasegmental structure in speech production planning. In P. F. MacNeilage (Ed.), *The production of speech*. New York: Springer-Verlag.

Shattuck-Hufnagel, S. (1987). The role of word-onset consonants in speech production planning: New evidence from speech error patterns. In E. Keller & M. Gopnik (Eds.), *Motor and sensory processes of language*. Hillsdale, NJ: Erlbaum.

Shattuck-Hufnagel, S., & Klatt, D. (1979). Minimal use of features and markedness in speech production. *Journal of Verbal Learning and Verbal Behavior, 18*, 41–55.

Stemberger, J. P. (1982). The nature of segments in the lexicon: Evidence from speech errors. *Lingua, 56*, 235–259.

Swinney, D. (1982). The structure and time-course of information interaction during speech comprehension: Lexical segmentation, access, and interpretation. In J. Mehler, E. C. T. Walker, & M. F. Garrett (Eds.), *Perspectives on mental representation: Experimental and theoretical studies of cognitive processes and capacities*. Hillsdale, NJ: Erlbaum.

Zwicky, A. (1982). Classical malapropisms and the creation of a mental lexicon. In L. K. Obler & L. Menn (Eds.), *Exceptional language and linguistics*. New York: Academic Press.

8

Alexia and Agraphia in Spanish Speakers

CAT Correlations and Interlinguistic Analysis

ALFREDO ARDILA, MONICA ROSSELLI, and
OSCAR PINZON

Interest in reading alterations arose toward of the last century when Dejerine described two types of alexia: alexia with agraphia and alexia without agraphia. The first type was correlated with a lesion in the angular region and the second with a lesion of the occipital lobe in which the corpus callosum was involved. The relationship between the angular region and alterations in both reading and writing has been repeatedly confirmed in the literature (e.g., Benson, 1979; Geschwind, 1965; Hecaen, 1962). The topography of alexia without agraphia has, however, been debated by several authors (Damasio & Damasio, 1983; Greenblatt, 1983), and the presence of this reading disturbance has been accepted in cases of exclusive occipital lesions (Damasio & Damasio, 1983).

Almost a century after Dejerine described the two cases of alexia classically known in the literature, Benson in 1977 proposed the term *frontal alexia* to describe the reading alterations observed in patients with Broca's aphasia.

Although reading seems to be a strongly lateralized function, since alterations are usually a product of left-hemisphere lesions, right-hemi-

ALFREDO ARDILA and MONICA ROSSELLI • Konrad Lorenz Foundation University, Bogotá, Colombia, and Miami Institute of Psychology, Miami, Florida 33166-6612. OSCAR PINZON • San Juan de Dios Hospital, National University of Colombia, Bogotá, Colombia.

sphere lesions can produce reading alterations that cannot be correlated with the ability to code or decode written language, but rather with spatial organization abilities (Ardila & Ostrosky, 1984; Hecaen & Albert, 1978). Patients with right-hemisphere lesions can present what is known as spatial alexia, but very little is known about its anatomical correlates.

In an attempt to find reading models that comply with the knowledge we have about cerebral organization, Marshall and Newcombe (1973) developed a classification system for alexias depending on the type of paralexias presented by the patient: visual, semantic, or phonemic. The differential presence of these types of paralexias corresponds to a particular type of alexic disturbance: phonological dyslexia, deep dyslexia, and surface dyslexia (Marshall & Newcombe, 1980). A very important limitation to this classification of alexias is that in the case of paralexias the description has been made in languages, such as English, whose writing system is not strictly phonological. In English, the phoneme–grapheme conversion system plays an indirect role, while the semantic channel (understanding of the read word) and recall of orthographic rules play a principal role (Miceli, Silveri, & Caramazza, 1985). In languages such as Spanish and Italian, there is an almost one-to-one relationship between pronunciation and orthography; the letters are pronounced in almost always the same way independently of the word they are found in. In spite of some exceptions, shown in Table 1, a person with phonological knowledge of the graphemes can read and write in Spanish even though he may not know the meaning of the words.

These considerations would therefore suggest that the use of a phonological and/or semantic system will depend on the particular linguistic system and will not be an intrinsic part of the cognitive system. The characteristics of reading alterations observed in patients with cerebral lesions have not yet been determined in languages such as Spanish.

Errors in writing can become apparent at different levels: (1) in graphic quality (calligraphy), (2) in letter sequence (orthography), (3) in the correct choice of words, lexical and syntactic organization, and morphological composition, and (4) in spatial organization (e.g., distribution of spaces, direction of the line). However, with regard to writing alterations, no classification exists that has been completely accepted by aphasiologists. Many authors use the term *agraphia* for all types and degrees of writing alterations, and *agraphia* has thus become a confused term that has not been sufficiently studied. Different attempts at classification have been made (e.g., Benson & Cummings, 1985; Hecaen & Albert, 1978; Luria, 1977). Most authors agree that agraphias can be divided into two large groups: agraphias that accompany aphasic language disturbances and agraphias that do not. The first group comprises those aphasic agraphias that include fluent and nonfluent agraphias and agraphia with alexia. The second group includes agraphias such as motor, apraxic, visuospatial, and hemiagraphic agraphias.

TABLE 1. Phoneme and Grapheme Correspondence
in Spanish

Phoneme	Grapheme
/b/	b, v
/s/	c (before e, i), s, z
/tʃ/	ch
/d/	d
/f/	f
/g/	g (before a, o, u) and gu (before e, i)
/i/	i, y (as a conjunction and in diphthongs)
/h/	j, g (before e, i)
/k/	c (before a, o, u) and qu (before e, i)
/l/	l
/λ/ or /j/	ll
/m/	m
/n/	n
/ɲ/	ñ
/p/	p
/r/	r
/ɾ/	rr, r (at the beginning of a word)
/t/	t
/k/ + /s/	x
/j/	y
—	h
/a/	a
/e/	e
/o/	o
/u/	u

In 1982 Bub and Kertesz suggested the term *deep dysgraphia* to describe the profile characterized by the semantic substitutions in writing
that one of their patients presented. Similarly, Roeltgen, Sevush, and
Heilman (1983) gave the name *phonological agraphia* to the inability
another patient presented to write nonsense words to dictation in spite of
a good ability to write known words. Roeltgen, Rothi-Gonzalez, and
Heilman (1986) have proposed the existence of a *semantic agraphia* in
five patients who could spell irregular words but had difficulties in giving
them their meaning.

Little is known about the relationship between writing alterations
and cerebral damage in reading-writing systems like the one used in
Spanish. The classifications used are very vague and do not sufficiently
satisfy observations made in clinical practice. Furthermore, no studies
have been carried out to correlate reading-writing alterations in Spanish-
speaking patients with lesions in particular areas of the brain.

One of the methods that has probably allowed us to advance furthest
in our knowledge about cerebral lesion topography is the brain scan or

computerized axial tomography. By means of this radiological method it has been possible to visualize and exactly determine the location of cerebral pathologies of different etiologies and, as a result, establish correlations between clinical manifestations and structural damage to the brain (Ardila, Montanes, Bernal, & Serpa, 1986; Damasio & Damasio, 1983; Greenblatt, 1983; Kertesz, 1983, Chapter 3 this volume; Naeser, 1983; Novoa & Ardila, 1987; Poeck, Bleser, & Von Keyserlingk, 1984; Rosselli, Rosselli, Vergara, & Ardila, 1985).

In this work, 62 Spanish-speaking patients with cerebral focal lesions were studied and their alterations in reading and writing were correlated with the topography of the damage found by the scanning method.

METHOD

Subjects

Sixty-two patients with cerebral damage were studied (27 women, 35 men; average age = 41.43, SD = 13.92, age range = 16–65). These subjects presented various etiologies (vascular = 44, tumoral = 14, traumatic = 4). Sixty-two normal subjects matched for age, sex, and schooling with the first group were also studied. The cerebral damage had evolved in a period varying from 1 to 4 months. Patients had no background of previous neurological or psychiatric illnesses. Average schooling was 8.14 years (range = 4–19, SD = 4.54). Table 2 shows the general characteristics of the population studied. All lesions were confirmed by means of computerized axial tomography, and the analysis of damage topography was carried out by a neuroradiologist.

Procedure

The patients included in the sample were taken from the neuropsychological services of the San Juan de Dios Hospital and the Colombian Institute of Neurology. Each patient was administered a neuropsychological battery consisting of the following tests: (1) Boston Diagnostic Aphasia Examination (Goodglass & Kaplan, 1979), (2) Token Test (De Renzi & Faglioni, 1978), (3) a reading and writing test specifically designed for Spanish-speaking subjects and standardized in a population of normal subjects (Rosselli & Ardila, 1987), (4) the Rey-Osterrieth Complex Figure (Osterrieth, 1944). The specific language tests (Boston Diagnostic Aphasia Examination and the Token Test) were applied only to patients with left-cerebral damage. Normal subjects were given only the reading and writing test.

Patients with left-hemisphere lesions were divided into seven groups, and the following criteria were jointly considered: results on the Boston Diagnostic Aphasia Examination, topography of the damage as shown on scans, and the general neuropsychological and neurological examination. The following groups were formed: (1) prefrontal (PF—6 patients), (2) Broca's aphasia (BA—5 patients), (3) conduction aphasia (CA—6 patients), (4) Wernicke's aphasia (WA—13 patients), (5) anomic or amnesic aphasia (AA—4 patients), (6) alexia without agraphia (AWA—3 patients), and (7) global aphasia (GA—4 patients). As well as being classified in this way, patients with left-hemisphere lesions were divided into two large groups: prerolandic and retrorolandic, depending on whether the scans revealed their lesions to be in front of or behind the fissure of Rolando.

Patients with right-hemispheric lesions were divided into two groups according to damage topography: (1) prerolandic (6 patients) and (2) retrorolandic (15 patients).

The results obtained by the patients on the reading and writing tests were grouped into tables in order to carry out the pertinent comparisons. Their scores were compared with those obtained by the matched sample from the normal population. Comparisons were also made between the means obtained by patients with right and left lesions. The means obtained by prerolandic patients were compared with those obtained by patients from the retrorolandic group, in the case of patients with right-hemisphere lesions. The means of patients from the different left hemisphere lesion groups were compared one with the other. A t test (Edwards, 1968) was used to carry out the comparisons between means. After carrying out the pertinent comparisons between the means obtained by the different groups in the reading and writing test, an analysis was made of the types of error made for each item. The means of some types of error were subsequently compared for patients with right and left lesions, as were the means of the types of error for the right subgroups and for the left subgroups. The results obtained on the Boston Diagnostic Aphasia Examination and the Token Test were used as classificatory criteria for the patients in the different groups. Similarly, the Rey-Osterrieth Complex Figure test was used to relate spatial alterations in writing with the presence or absence of constructional apraxia. The classification criteria used in the Rey complex figure were taken from Lezak (1983).

In order to transcribe the patients' lesions, a template was designed with 10 standard scanner cuts from the base of the brain to the highest region. Each lesion identified by the scan was transcribed to the standard template. The lesions corresponding to the different patients in the same category or group were then superimposed onto one template, following the method described by Kertesz (1983) and Naeser (1983) in order to identify the critical compromised zone in the appearance of the deficit analyzed.

TABLE 2. General Characteristics of the Sample

	Sex	Age	Educational level	Topography	Hemisphere	Etiology	Token	Category
Pat. 1	F	34	5	Frontal	Right	Tumor	—	Prerolandic (1)
Pat. 2	F	53	5	Frontal	Right	Vascular	—	Prerolandic (2)
Pat. 3	M	19	8	Frontal	Right	Trauma	—	Prerolandic (3)
Pat. 4	M	39	5	Frontal	Right	Vascular	—	Prerolandic (4)
Pat. 5	M	63	10	Frontal	Right	Tumor	—	Prerolandic (5)
Pat. 6	M	32	15	Frontal	Right	Tumor	—	Prerolandic (6)
Pat. 7	M	50	11	Occipital	Right	Vascular	—	Retrorolandic (1)
Pat. 8	F	44	4	Par-occ	Right	Vascular	—	Retrorolandic (2)
Pat. 9	F	65	11	Par-occ	Right	Vascular	—	Retrorolandic (3)
Pat. 10	F	33	5	Par-tem	Right	Vascular	—	Retrorolandic (4)
Pat. 11	M	55	5	Par-occ	Right	Vascular	—	Retrorolandic (5)
Pat. 12	M	26	5	Tem-par	Right	Vascular	—	Retrorolandic (6)
Pat. 13	F	44	11	Tem-par	Right	Tumor	—	Retrorolandic (7)
Pat. 14	F	16	7	Parietal	Right	Vascular	—	Retrorolandic (8)
Pat. 15	M	45	5	Parietal	Right	Vascular	—	Retrorolandic (9)
Pat. 16	F	49	5	Tem-ins	Right	Vascular	—	Retrorolandic (10)
Pat. 17	M	38	5	Temporal	Right	Tumor	—	Retrorolandic (11)
Pat. 18	F	19	11	Tem-par	Right	Vascular	—	Retrorolandic (12)
Pat. 19	M	55	5	Tem-par	Right	Vascular	—	Retrorolandic (13)
Pat. 20	F	29	5	Tem-par	Right	Vascular	—	Retrorolandic (14)
Pat. 21	M	60	5	Tem-par	Right	Vascular	—	Retrorolandic (15)
Pat. 22	M	55	6	Frontal	Left	Vascular	26	Prefrontal (1)
Pat. 23	M	20	11	Frontal	Left	Vascular	33	Prefrontal (2)
Pat. 24	F	47	5	Frontal	Left	Tumor	20	Prefrontal (3)
Pat. 25	F	56	16	Frontal	Left	Tumor	24	Prefrontal (4)
Pat. 26	M	45	4	Frontal	Left	Vascular	26	Prefrontal (5)
Pat. 27	F	23	11	Frontal	Left	Tumor	28	Prefrontal (6)
Pat. 28	F	43	16	Frontal-tem	Left	Vascular	28	Broca (1)
Pat. 29	M	26	16	Frontal	Left	Vascular	31	Broca (2)

Patient	Sex	Age		Location	Side	Etiology		Diagnosis
Pat. 30	F	30	5	Frontal-par	Left	Vascular	18	Broca (3)
Pat. 31	F	64	4	Frontal-par	Left	Vascular	29	Broca (4)
Pat. 32	M	36	16	Frontal-par	Left	Vascular	30	Broca (5)
Pat. 33	M	35	5	Frontal-par	Left	Tumor	26	Conduction (1)
Pat. 34	F	61	8	Parietal	Left	Vascular	22	Conduction (2)
Pat. 35	F	39	5	Insular	Left	Vascular	31	Conduction (3)
Pat. 36	M	33	8	Parietal	Left	Vascular	32	Conduction (4)
Pat. 37	F	43	5	Parietal	Left	Tumor	31	Conduction (5)
Pat. 38	F	26	11	Parietal	Left	Vascular	27	Conduction (6)
Pat. 39	M	63	6	Tem-par	Left	Vascular	17	Wernicke (1)
Pat. 40	M	34	11	Tem-par	Left	Tumor	18	Wernicke (2)
Pat. 41	M	31	8	Temporal	Left	Vascular	14	Wernicke (3)
Pat. 42	F	48	5	Temporal	Left	Vascular	18	Wernicke (4)
Pat. 43	M	18	9	Tem-occ	Left	Trauma	15	Wernicke (5)
Pat. 44	F	53	4	Temporal	Left	Vascular	5	Wernicke (6)
Pat. 45	M	28	5	Temporal	Left	Trauma	22	Wernicke (7)
Pat. 46	M	63	9	Temporal	Left	Vascular	14	Wernicke (8)
Pat. 47	M	60	11	Temporal	Left	Vascular	10	Wernicke (9)
Pat. 48	M	46	16	Tem-par	Left	Tumor	8	Wernicke (10)
Pat. 49	M	28	5	Temporal	Left	Trauma	18	Wernicke (11)
Pat. 50	F	37	16	Tem-par	Left	Vascular	4	Wernicke (12)
Pat. 51	M	46	4	Temporal	Left	Vascular	24	Wernicke (13)
Pat. 52	F	43	7	Temporal	Left	Tumor	30	Amnesic (1)
Pat. 53	M	36	5	Par-occ	Left	Tumor	17	Amnesic (2)
Pat. 54	M	65	11	Angular	Left	Vascular	27	Amnesic (3)
Pat. 55	M	30	11	Tem-par	Left	Vascular	24	Amnesic (4)
Pat. 56	M	54	5	Occipital	Left	Malfor	27	Alexia w/o agraphia (1)
Pat. 57	M	47	5	Occipital	Left	Vascular	30	Alexia w/o agraphia (2)
Pat. 58	M	65	16	Occipital	Left	Vascular	30	Alexia w/o agraphia (3)
Pat. 59	F	25	5	FPT	Left	Vascular	8	Global (1)
Pat. 60	M	31	5	FPT	Left	Vascular	11	Global (2)
Pat. 61	F	46	5	FPT	Left	Vascular	11	Global (3)
Pat. 62	F	22	5	FPT	Left	Vascular	13	Global (4)

Instrument

A reading and writing test designed for Spanish-speaking subjects was used (Rosselli & Ardila, 1987). The test consisted of the following subtests:

Reading

Reading of letters (20; 15 consonants, 5 vowels)
Reading of syllables (12; e.g., *pa, li, clus, trans*)
Reading of logotomes (11; e.g., *talo, fasaja*)
Reading of words (13; e.g., *casa, libro, ventana, bicicleta*)
Reading of sentences (5; e.g., *La cantina es de Juan*)
Understanding orders (9; e.g., close your eyes)
Reading and comprehension of texts (9; 108-word text, 4 questions; and 185-word text, 5 comprehension questions)
Ideographic reading (7; e.g., Coca-Cola)

Writing

Writing of letters (dictation and copy) (14; 9 consonants, 5 vowels)
Writing of syllables (dictation and copy) (10; e.g., *pa, cla*)
Writing of words (dictation and copy) (6; e.g., *casa, caballo*)
Writing of sentences (dictation and copy) (4; e.g., *La gente se reune*)
Written description of a picture (cookie theft)

The test uses a scoring system based on the number of errors; the possible number of errors is indicated in brackets. The written description of a picture was taken from the Boston Diagnostic Aphasia Examination (Goodglass & Kaplan, 1979) and the proposed scoring method was used.

RESULTS

Seven patients of the 62 with cerebral damage were excluded from the statistical analysis (patients 11, 12, 21, 59, 60, 61, and 62 in Table 2) because their lesions were considered to be too extensive, and for that reason, the very large number of errors they made on all the subtests could have contaminated the results. Of these 7 patients, 4 had an infarct of the whole left-middle cerebral artery and presented global aphasia, and 3 had widespread lesions of the right hemisphere as a result of an extensive infarct of the right-middle cerebral artery. The results obtained by the patients with global aphasia were analyzed separately.

Population with Cerebral Damage and Normal Population

On comparing the means of the scores obtained by patients with left-hemisphere lesions with those obtained by the matched normal controls, a significantly greater number of errors were observed in the patients in all the subtests of the reading and writing sections.

Significant differences were observed in the results produced by the t test when comparing the means of the scores obtained in the reading and writing subtests in patients with right-hemisphere lesions with those obtained by the matched normal subjects only in the reading of syllables, logotomes, words, sentences, and understanding-of-orders subtests. In the writing subtests the average number of errors was significantly higher in patients with right-hemisphere lesions than in normal subjects.

Patients with Right-Hemisphere Lesions and Patients with Left-Hemisphere Lesions

The results obtained on comparing the means corresponding to the reading subtests of patients with right-hemisphere lesions and those with left-hemisphere lesions are shown in Table 3. The average number of errors (scores) obtained by patients with left lesions were significantly greater in all the subtests except for the reading of sentences, in which the difference in scores did not reach significance level.

The results of the t test used to compare the performance of patients with right- and left-hemisphere lesions on the writing subtests showed significant differences for the writing of syllables and sentences subtests but not for the writing of letters and words (Table 4). The average number of total errors obtained by the two groups of patients (with right and left lesions) show that the patients with left-hemisphere lesions presented a greater number of errors in both reading and writing.

Intrahemispheric Comparisons

After comparing the results obtained by patients with right and left lesions, intrahemispheric comparisons were then carried out. For this purpose, the patients in each group were divided into two subgroups: prerolandic and retrorolandic, depending on whether the scanner image was found in front of or behind the central fissure.

The left retrorolandic group showed a significantly greater number of errors in reading [$\bar{X}$ = 41.65 (43% errors)], and in writing [$\bar{X}$ = 15.81 (47%)], than the prerolandic group [reading: $\bar{X}$ = 23.55 (25%); writing: $\bar{X}$ = 9.18 (27%)]. The group of patients with right retrorolandic lesions presented an almost equivalent number of errors to the right prerolandic

TABLE 3. t Test of Means Obtained by Patients with Right and Left Cerebral Lesions in the Reading Subtests[a]

Subtest group	LTR[b]	SLB	LGT	WOR	SEN	ORD	TXT	IDG
Right hemisphere n = 18	$\bar{X}$ = 0.5 2.5%	$\bar{X}$ = 1.00 8%	$\bar{X}$ = 2.72 25%	$\bar{X}$ = 2.00 15%	$\bar{X}$ = 1.44 29%	$\bar{X}$ = 1.21 13%	$\bar{X}$ = 3.05 34%	$\bar{X}$ = 0.22 3%
Left hemisphere n = 37	$\bar{X}$ = 2.8 14%	$\bar{X}$ = 3.64 30%	$\bar{X}$ = 5.89 54%	$\bar{X}$ = 5.10 39%	$\bar{X}$ = 2.24 45%	$\bar{X}$ = 3.91 43%	$\bar{X}$ = 5.78 64%	$\bar{X}$ = 1.29 18%
df	53	53	53	53	53	53	53	53
t	2.27	2.11	2.006	2.15	1.08	2.33	1.71	2.18
p	.02	.02	.05	.02	.15	.02	.05	.02

[a]Percentage of errors of each group is shown in relation to the total possible.
[b]Reading of letters (LTR), reading of syllables (SLB), reading of logotomes (LGT), reading of words (WOR), reading of sentences (SEN), comprehension of written orders (ORD), comprehension of text (TXT), ideographic reading (IDG).

TABLE 4. t Test of Means Obtained by Patients with Right and Left Cerebral Lesions on the Writing Subtests[a]

Subtests groups	Letters	Syllables	Words	Sentences
Right hemisphere $n = 18$	$\bar{X} = 1.44$ 10%	$\bar{X} = 1.72$ 17%	$\bar{X} = 1.44$ 24%	$\bar{X} = 1.83$ 46%
Left hemisphere $n = 37$	$\bar{X} = 3.08$ 22%	$\bar{X} = 4.56$ 46%	$\bar{X} = 2.81$ 47%	$\bar{X} = 3.10$ 78%
df	53	53	53	53
t	1.44	2.11	1.61	1.73
p	.10	.02	.10	.05

[a]Percentage of errors of each group is shown in relation to the total possible.

group in both reading [retrorolandic: $\bar{X} = 18.67$ (19%); prerolandic: $\bar{X} = 10.67$ (11%)], and in writing [retrorolandic: $\bar{X} = 7.17$ (21%); prerolandic: $\bar{X} = 5.00$ (15%)].

On comparing the means of each subtest for the left prerolandic group with those of the left retrorolandic group, the latter group was found to present a significantly greater average number of errors on all the subtests with the exception of the ideographic reading subtest. In the writing section, the left retrorolandic group obtained significantly greater means than the left prerolandic group on the writing of letters and words subtests.

The statistical differences between the means of the right pre- and postrolandic groups can be seen in the reading section, in which differences were observed in the means obtained on the reading of logotomes, words, and text comprehension subtests. In these subtests, the retrorolandic group had a greater number of errors. In the writing section, no differences in the performance by the two groups could be appreciated.

As explained in the procedure, the patients with left-hemisphere lesions were also divided into six groups according to lesion site and to the neuropsychological alterations presented in the Token Test and the Boston Diagnostic Aphasia Examination. The means and standard deviations obtained by each group on the two sections of the reading and writing test were compared. Maximum number of errors in reading was found in AWA group; minimum number of errors in reading and writing tasks was found in PF patients.

Table 5 shows the percentage of errors obtained by each of the subgroups with cerebral lesions (excluding the global aphasics) on each of the

TABLE 5. Percentage of Errors Obtained by Patients from Different Groups
in the Reading Subtests

	LTR[a]	SYL	LGT	WOR	SEN	ORD	TXT	IDE
Prefrontal								
n = 6	0	7	15	14	2	8	4	0
Broca								
n = 5	15	38	49	29	60	47	47	37
Conduction								
n = 6	29	28	64	48	40	42	48	14
Wernicke								
n = 13	17	28	55	42	48	57	84	14
Anomic								
n = 4	13	25	73	42	50	50	89	16
Alexia without agraphia								
n = 3	30	50	82	69	86	100	100	51
Right prerolandic								
n = 6	7	4	11	6	6	11	12	3
Right retrorolandic								
n = 12	25	18	36	25	43	22	50	6

[a]Reading of letters (LTR), reading of syllables (SYL), reading of logotomes (LGT), reading of words (WOR), reading of sentences (SEN), comprehension of written orders (ORD), comprehension of a text (TXT), ideographic reading (IDE).

reading subtests. The greatest number of errors was made in the reading of letters and words by the CA and AWA groups. The AWA, AA, and CA group showed the greatest number of errors in the reading of logotomes; in reading comprehension AWA, AA, and WA were most impaired. In the case of ideographic reading, the greatest numbers of errors was observed in patients with AWA. Patients with PF presented the lowest mean for errors. Table 6 shows the percentage of patients presenting errors in each reading subtest.

In Table 7, we can appreciate the percentage of errors obtained by each subgroup of patients in each subtest of the writing section. After the GA group (79% errors), the patients in the WA (36%), CA (30%), and AWA (30%) groups presented the largest number of errors in the writing of letters. In the writing of syllables, the greatest number of errors was made by groups AA, AWA, CA, and WA, and in the writing of words, the groups AWA, WA, and CA presented a higher average number of errors in relation to the other groups. The AA and AWA groups presented the greatest number of errors in the writing of sentences in spite of the fact that the number of errors was very similar in all groups except for the groups with right lesions and the PF left group, for which the average of errors was lower. Table 8 shows the percentage of patients presenting errors in each writing subtest.

TABLE 6. Percentage of Patients Presenting Errors in Each Reading Subtest

	LTR[a]	SYL	LGT	WOR	SEN	ORD	TXT	IDE
Prefrontal	17	33	83	67	17	33	67	0
Broca	80	80	100	100	80	100	80	60
Conduction	50	83	100	100	83	100	83	67
Wernicke	69	69	100	92	62	100	100	38
Anomic	75	75	100	100	100	75	100	75
Alexia without agraphia	100	100	100	100	100	100	100	100
Right prerolandic	17	33	50	50	33	66	33	17
Right retrorolandic	33	41	83	91	66	83	100	25

[a]Letters (LTR), syllables (SYL), logotomes (LGT), words (WOR), sentences (SEN), comprehension of orders (ORD), comprehension of a text (TXT), ideographic reading (IDE).

TABLE 7. Percentage of Errors in Different Groups for Writing Subtests

	Letters	Syllables	Words	Sentences
Prefrontal	4	26	22	58
Broca	20	42	43	75
Conduction	30	48	55	83
Wernicke	36	48	55	75
Anomic	18	57	33	88
Alexia without agraphia	30	53	60	100
Right prerolandic	7	13	18	38
Right retrorolandic	14	24	27	55

TABLE 8. Percentage of Patients Presenting Errors in Each Writing Subtest

	Letters	Syllables	Words	Sentences
Prefrontal	33	50	66	83
Broca	40	80	60	100
Conduction	83	83	83	100
Wernicke	77	92	100	100
Anomic	75	75	50	100
Alexia without agraphia	100	100	100	100
Right prerolandic	33	50	50	50
Right retrorolandic	75	75	41	75

Quantification of the Type of Errors

Table 9 shows different types of errors in some reading subtests. Literal substitutions on reading letters, syllables, logotomes, words, and sentences were more evident in the AWA, CA, and WA groups. Of these literal substitutions, changes in consonants were more frequent than changes in vowels. Neologisms were observed in some patients with WA, AA, and AWA. Morphological substitutions were recorded in the group of patients with AWA. A tendency to literal reading was apparent in the AWA group, and defects in naming a letter by means of words (e.g., for the letter *D*, the patient would say "that's the one for donkey") that would give the desired letter were observed only in the AA group. Anticipations were found in patients with BA and CA. Omissions of letters within words were principally observed in the BA group. In the AWA and CA groups, a tendency was observed to present fewer of errors in the left portion of the syllables or words read. The left PF group showed the smallest number of errors.

Patients with right-hemisphere retrorolandic lesions mainly presented errors due to left hemi-inattention, with a tendency to confabulate the left half of the word. In some patients with left lesions, particularly in the AWA and WA groups, a phenomenon similar to invention was observed, which consisted in meaningfully reading syllables and logotomes—e.g., instead of reading *sligo* (nonsense), they read *le digo* ("I tell him"). Finally, patients with right retrorolandic lesions had difficulty in following the lines of the text on reading, and this prevented them from following the content of the text. Patients with right prerolandic lesions presented minimal errors as a result of neglect in the reading of logotomes; in the other subtests they presented no errors.

Analysis of the types of error in the writing subtests showed the presence of literal paragraphias in all the subgroups with left lesions; the greatest number, however, were made by patients with WA. Perseverations were registered in the groups with left PF, BA, WA, and AWA. Omissions were frequent errors in the CA, WA, and AWA groups. Errors due to anticipation were more evident in the BA group and neologisms were observed in the groups with AA, WA, and CA. Paragrammatism in spontaneous writing was observed in WA. The group with CA was the only one to show evident self-correction. Errors due to agrammatism were found in the writing of sentences in the CA and BA groups. In the writing of sentences a tendency was observed to present fewer of errors on the left side of the sentence in groups AWA, WA, and left PF. The AWA subgroup increased the number of errors when copying (Table 10).

In patients with right-hemisphere lesions (in particular in the retrorolandic group), omissions of letters and omissions of the strokes of a letter were observed. Similarly, a tendency was observed to fragment

TABLE 9. Type of Errors in Five Reading Subtests (Letters, Syllables, Logotomes, Words, Sentences)[a]

	LSU	NEO	VMS	ANT	PER	ANO	LRE	SLM	LOM	NOM	LAD	NEG	CON
Prefrontal	1.0	0.0	0.0	0.0	0.0	0.0	0.0	4.0	2.0	0.0	0.5	0.0	0.0
Broca	5.0	0.0	0.0	5.0	6.5	0.0	0.0	0.5	8.0	0.0	2.0	0.0	0.0
Conduction	11.5	1.5	2.0	3.5	1.5	0.0	3.5	3.5	3.5	0.0	3.5	0.0	0.0
Wernicke	11.5	8.0	2.5	1.0	1.0	0.0	2.5	3.0	5.0	2.0	2.0	0.0	0.0
Anomic	9.0	6.0	1.0	0.0	0.5	6.5	6.5	1.5	4.0	10.0	0.0	0.0	0.0
Alexia without agraphia	15.0	5.0	11.0	0.0	9.0	0.0	15.0	2.5	1.5	1.5	4.0	0.0	0.0
Right prerolandic	0.5	0.0	0.0	0.0	0.0	0.0	0.0	1.0	0.0	0.0	0.5	0.5	3.0
Right retrorolandic	1.5	0.0	0.0	0.0	0.0	0.0	0.0	3.0	3.0	0.0	1.5	5.5	8.5

[a]Each cell represents the average number of errors. Literal substitutions (LSU), neologisms (NEO), verbal morphological substitutions (VMS), anticipations (ANT), perseverations (PER), anomic errors (ANO), literal reading (LRE), substitution of logotomes for meaningful words (SLM), letter omissions (LOM), noun omissions (NOM), letter additions (LAD), neglect (NEG), confabulation (CON).

TABLE 10. Type of Errors in Writing Test[a]

	PER	LIT	NEO	LAD	LOM	FAD	FOM	ANT	GEL	COP
Prefrontal	3.2	2.0	0.0	0.0	1.6	0.0	0.0	0.4	0.0	0.0
Broca	3.2	5.6	0.0	1.2	0.8	0.0	0.0	5.2	0.0	8.8
Conduction	1.6	7.2	6.0	1.6	6.4	0.0	0.0	2.0	0.0	4.0
Wernicke	3.2	8.8	9.6	2.8	6.0	0.0	0.0	0.0	0.0	0.4
Anomic	0.0	5.2	12.0	2.0	1.2	0.0	0.0	2.4	0.0	2.0
Alexia without agraphia	3.2	7.6	4.0	3.6	6.4	0.0	0.0	1.2	0.0	37.2
Right prerolandic	0.0	1.2	0.0	2.8	2.4	5.2	0.8	0.0	1.2	0.0
Right retrorolandic	0.0	1.2	0.0	2.4	8.0	3.2	2.4	0.0	12.0	0.0

[a]Each cell represents the average of errors. Perseverations (PER), literal substitutions (LIT), neologisms (NEO), letter additions (LAD), letter omissions (LOM), feature additions (FAD), feature omissions (FOM), anticipations (ANT), grouping of elements (GEL), copying errors (COP).

words by separating the syllables of one word in an inadequate way, and grouping of words was clear. They wrote obliquely at an angle of 13 degrees to the line on average. An increase or decrease of approximately 3 cm of the left-hand margin was observed as the patient wrote words and sentences and in the written description of the picture (spontaneous writing).

Reading was impossible for the patients with global aphasia since they had no language (or their language had been reduced to a verbal stereotype) and identification was purely by chance. Some patients sporadically recognized syllables or words by the number of letters they contained and pointed to a syllable with the equivalent number of elements to those asked for. It was of note, however, that these patients had on average a better performance in ideographic reading than patients from the AWA group. In writing, patients from this group presented a severe impossibility owing to hemiparesis or apraxia. Those who managed to write with the left hand presented stereotype writing in a perseverative way; they were even less able to copy correctly, and none of them could present spontaneous writing.

Scores on the Rey-Osterrieth Complex Figure

The Rey-Osterrieth Complex Figure could be applied only to 19 patients with left-hemisphere lesions (14 with retrorolandic lesions) and to 12 patients with right-hemisphere lesions (1 with prerolandic lesions and 11 with retrorolandic lesions). Scoring criteria for performance on the copy of the Rey-Osterrieth Complex Figure were taken from Lezak (1983). According to this scoring system, 2 points are given for a perfect copy of each of the 18 parts into which the figure is divided; omissions or a performance different from the figure copied score zero, half a point, or 1 point, depending on the severity of the error. The maximum score possible is 36 points.

Patients with left-hemisphere lesions had a mean score of 28.39 and a standard deviation of 6.93, and patients with right hemisphere lesions a mean of 13.09 and a standard deviation of 6.93. The Student t test showed the significance level for this difference in the means to be .005 ($t = 5.83$, $df = 29$).

The errors observed in patients with left-hemisphere lesions were due to their simplifying the figure and omissions of details, particularly those on the right-hand side; disintegration or fragmentation of the figure were never observed. In all cases of left lesion, the drawn figures could be identified by an observer as figures from the Rey. In the performance by patients with right-hemisphere lesions, disintegration of the figure was evident, as were disarticulation of its elements, the tendency to perseveration of the strokes, and the omission of elements in the left part of the figure, and, on occasion, it was impossible to identify the figure drawn as the Rey figure. None of the patients with right lesions showed attempts at self-correction or made comments indicating their concern over their bad performance.

Superimposition of Scans

The scans of the patients from each group were superimposed in accordance with the steps explained in procedure. In this way, templates were obtained corresponding to the groups studied, seven of which are shown in Figures 1 to 7. Owing to the small sample in the AWA and GA groups, the superimposition of their scans did not produce important data. The templates of the figures indicate the areas that had a certain level of superimposition: 20–40%, 50–60%, 70–90%, and 100%.

Figure 1 shows the regions of the left hemisphere that were involved in the PF group ($n = 6$). The anterior prefrontal cortex and the paramedian and parasagittal region of the left frontal lobe are those principally involved. Figure 2 shows how in patients with BA there is an extensive damage of the motor and premotor cortex and also of the anterior portion of the insular cortex. In the CA group ($n = 6$), a damage principally of the anterior portion of the insula appeared, involving a small portion of the sensitive cortex in the middle part and extending to the beginning of the supramarginal region (Fig. 3).

The topographical findings obtained from the superimposition of scans of patients with WA ($n = 13$) are shown in Figure 4. The posterior third of the insular cortex was the site of the lesions in all the patients.

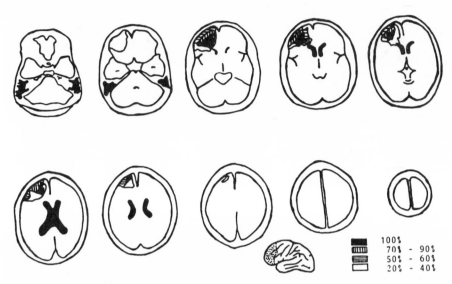

FIGURE 1. Scan superimposition: Left prefrontal (*n* = 6).

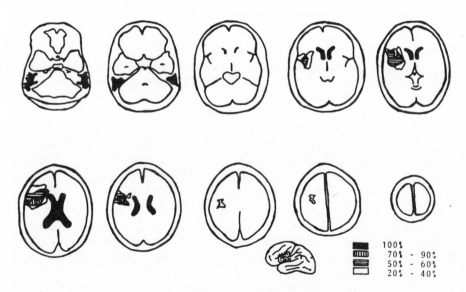

FIGURE 2. Scan superimposition: Broca's aphasia (*n* = 5).

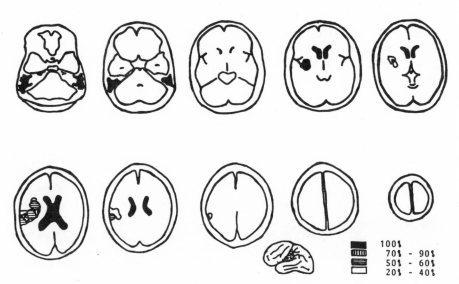

FIGURE 3. Scan superimposition: Conduction aphasia (n = 6).

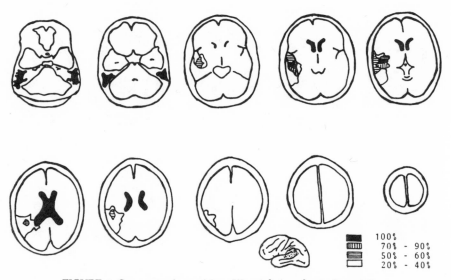

FIGURE 4. Scan superimposition: Wernicke's aphasia (n = 13).

The posterior temporal cortex, particularly the first gyrus, was also observed to be involved and, to a lesser degree, the posterior parietal cortex (angular gyrus). The scanner results of the patients with AA (n = 4) can be seen in Figure 5. Deep involvement of the posterior temporal lobe and angular gyri predominated. There were very few patients with AWA (n = 3), and it was therefore not possible to produce an adequate superimposition of the lesions; the posterior portion of the occipital lobe was observed to be involved in all the patients, and 1 patient also presented a certain posterior parietal damage. The patients with global aphasia (n = 4) presented an extensive cortical and subcortical damage that extended from the premotor regions of the frontal lobe to the parieto-temporo-occipital junction.

The superimposition of scans of the lesions presented by the patients with right-hemisphere lesions is shown in Figures 6 and 7. The patients with prerolandic lesions (n = 6) had involved the superior region of the right prefrontal area, and, on occasions, this damage reached the premotor area. The cerebral compromise observed in the patients from the retro-rolandic group was located principally in the deep cortical portion of the parietal lobe. In some patients, however, a deep posterior temporal and anterior occipital damage was also observed.

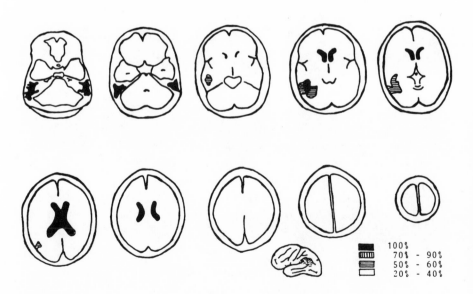

100%
70% - 90%
50% - 60%
20% - 40%

FIGURE 5. Scan superimposition: Amnesic aphasia (n = 4).

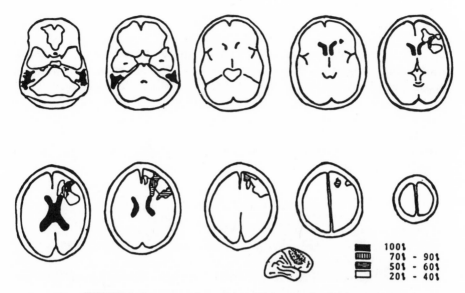

FIGURE 6. Scan superimposition: Right prerolandic (n = 6).

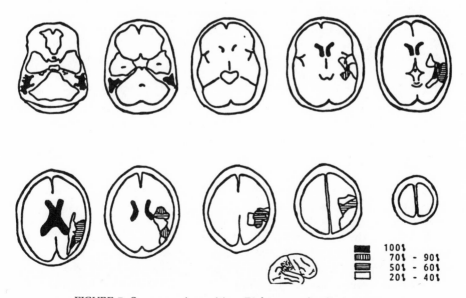

FIGURE 7. Scan superimposition: Right retrorolandic (n = 12).

DISCUSSION

In general, patients with left lesions showed a considerably greater number of errors than those with right lesions. However, the fact that patients with right lesions showed differences between their means and those of normal subjects suggests some type of relation between this hemisphere and written linguistic processes. It is also interesting to observe the similarity between the performance of patients with right lesions and normal subjects on some of the reading subtests (e.g., letters and ideographic reading).

Patients with Right and Left Lesions

The patients with right lesions presented better reading abilities than the left patients with the exception of the reading of sentences, in which the two groups of patients had an equivalent number of errors. These results would suggest that the items used in the reading of sentences could have had an equivalent level of difficulty for the patients because the items had a semantic content.

The results of the writing tests show that the writing of syllables and sentences is more sensitive to left lesions than to right while the writing of letters and words presented a similar level of difficulty for the two groups of patients. However, for both groups of patients, the level of difficulty increased with the number of written elements: Writing letters is easier than writing syllables, but syllables are easier than words, and so on. The patients with left lesions presented defects in verbal memory and therefore had a reduced memory volume. As a consequence, they could more easily retain items with a few elements.

Intrahemispheric Comparisons

If the left prerolandic and retrorolandic groups are compared, a greater number of errors can be observed in the retrorolandic group on both the reading and writing tests, while no important differences were observed in the two groups of patients with right-hemisphere lesions. Several aspects could be related to these findings: (1) The posterior areas of the left cerebral cortex have classically been considered to be principally responsible for the symbolic aspects of reading and writing, while the anterior areas have been related to the motor aspects of the same. (2) Several authors (e.g., Bradshaw & Nettleton, 1981) have spoken of the homogeneousness of the right-hemisphere areas, with a supposedly more diffuse, less localized organization of functions, in contrast to the heterogeneity of the left hemisphere areas, with a supposedly more defined organization of its functions.

In a more specific analysis, by subtests, it was observed that ide-ographic reading was conserved without difficulty in left (except AWA) retrorolandic patients, probably indicating that this type of reading is performed in a gestaltic way, with the right hemisphere playing a very large part. In the writing section, the patients with posterior lesions made a larger number of errors in all subtests, thus showing that these patients were the ones responsible for the low scores the left group had on these subtests in relation to the right group.

On analyzing the means obtained on the reading tests by the groups with left lesions, it was observed that the PF patients who presented no aphasic compromise of language had the smallest number of errors, while the GA patients, whose language involvement was maximum, had the greatest number of errors, showing the close connection between altera-tions in oral language and written language. The other groups each had a similar average number of errors, with the AA group obtaining the lowest mean. The WA, AWA, and CA groups obtained a fairly similar number of errors and shared some types of mistake. However, the types of error could be defined for some groups: The WA group presented literal para-lexias and neologisms, errors very similar to those presented in their oral language; the CA group, as well as presenting literal substitutions, also showed anticipations and self-corrections. Omissions of letters were ob-served in the BA group, but the omission of grammatical connectors de-scribed in these patients by Benson (1977) were not necessarily observed. A tendency to literal reading was observed in the AWA group, as was the tendency to invent the right half of the word, thus producing mor-phological paralexias. These patients usually recognized and read the initial letter in a word adequately but invented the rest of it. This defect, which has already been defined in these patients (Benson, 1979), could be explained by their greater verbal alexia and lesser literal alexia. It was of note that none of the three patients in this group was aware of the alexical defect presented and constantly tried to spell the words they were pre-sented with as if it were the usual reading procedure they used. Naming errors of letters were evident only in the AA group; the circumlocutions these patients used when reading a letter were very similar to those used in spontaneous language. None of the patients presented semantic verbal substitutions, while morphological verbal substitutions were observed in the AWA group.

It is important to emphasize that none of the patients presented se-mantic paralexias. The nearest to semantic paralexias were the mor-phological verbal paralexias principally presented by patients in the AWA group and the tendency in the WA group to make the logotomes meaningful. It would seem that semantic paralexias are not produced in Spanish speakers as a result of cerebral lesions. A further point could be added here: The reading of logotomes is equivalent in Spanish to the reading of low-frequency words. Perhaps the lack of meaning would give the logotomes a greater level of difficulty, but the reading strategies used (grapheme-phoneme decoding) would probably be the same.

Analysis of the results obtained in the writing subtests of each of the left groups showed that the largest number of errors were presented by the WA, CA, and AWA groups and smallest number by the PF group. In spite of the fact that the patients with AWA presented a greater defect in reading than in writing, they made numerous writing errors due to omissions. Moreover, this was the only group whose copy writing showed more errors than writing to dictation. The patients from the WA group presented paragraphias due to literal substitutions, perseverations, omissions, and even neologisms. Paragrammatism in spontaneous writing was observed in this group.

Agrammatism and, to a lesser extent, neologisms and omissions were characteristic of the CA group. Awareness of their errors was evident in this group since they presented numerous attempts at correction; these patients seemed to have forgotten the graphemic representation of phonemes since they repeated the word they wanted to write several times to themselves as if they were trying to recover the written memory trace of the words. Difficulty to write spontaneously was also frequent in these patients, as it was in some patients with BA, and they made comments such as "I can't think how to write." In the BA group anticipations, literal paragraphias, and agrammatism were observed.

Although the patients with right-hemisphere lesions (pre- and postrolandic) showed very similar results in the overall scores on the reading and writing tests, differences were observed on some reading subtests, such as the reading of logotomes and words and the comprehension of texts. These tests were particularly compromised as a result of errors due to the left neglect, which frequently made them invent the omitted half of the word in order to produce a semantic content (e.g., on reading *caballo* ("horse"), the patient initially read *allo* but in order to give it a meaning placed a *t* in front to obtain the word *tallo* ("stem"). As well as this type of error, the retrorolandic patients presented defects in following the lines. Although the patients with right lesions did not present defects in the symbolic recognition of letters, the spatial defects mentioned above together with a complex anosognosia resulted in low scores on some of the subtests and a great difficulty in text comprehension.

In the writing tests, patients with right retrorolandic lesions presented omissions and additions of letters in words, and omissions and additions of strokes in letters. The additions of strokes and letters can be explained in two ways: On the one hand, they could be the result of the tendency to perseverate and not inhibit an initiated movement—this tendency was clearly observed in their copy of the Rey figure. On the other hand, it could be explained also by their left hemi-inattention—the patients forget the letter they have just written since it is in the left visual field, which is neglected, and as a consequence the patient repeats the letter; e.g., on writing the word *libro* ("book"), the patient writes *libbroo*. Other errors observed in this group of patients were related to an inadequate separation of the words, since the patients forgot the spaces between them and sometimes even grouped words together or put in spaces in the middle of a word, thus fragmenting it. Furthermore, the wide left-hand margins due to hemi-inattention were very clear, as was the presence of the "cascade phenomenon"—that is, an increasingly greater increase or decrease of the left-hand margin (Figure 8). The right patients began to write at one point on the page, and as they went on writing, they would begin the following lines at points increasingly apart (or closer), thus forming an oblique line traced with the first letter of each line. Great difficulty in conserving the written line in a horizontal position was also observed. These spatial difficulties in writing were related to the greater or lesser difficulty the patients had in copying the Rey figure. It could then be supposed that spatial agraphia is secondary to constructional apraxia.

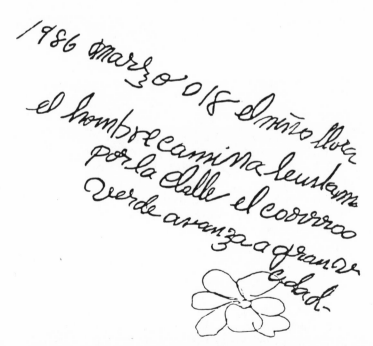

FIGURE 8. Sample of writing of a patient with right hemisphere lesion. "Cascade" phenomenon: Margins increase each time a new line is begun.

Topography of the Clinical Findings

If we correlate the clinical findings with the scans we could conclude the following:

1. Lesions of the insula could alter oral and written language in a differential way. The most anterior portion of the insula associated with left motor lesions (the opercular area) was related to Broca-type aphasias, agrammatism, and substitutions due to anticipations in writing; in reading, omissions of letters were observed. The middle portion of the insula seems to be correlated with conduction aphasias and hence with defects in repetitive language. This insular region with the anterior portion of the parietal lobe was correlated with a certain written agrammatism, phonological paragraphias, and omissions in writing. Finally, lesions of the posterior portion of the insula associated with lesions of the upper temporal cortex (first gyrus) were correlated with Wernicke-type aphasias, with phonological substitutions and neologisms in reading and with phonological paragraphias, perseverations, omissions, neologisms, and paragrammatism in writing. It is important to remember the fact that some patients with WA and AA presented a certain degree of involvement of the angular region, and perhaps for this reason similarities could be observed in the alterations in written language in these two groups.

2. The posterior region of the parietal and temporal lobes (the parieto-temporo-occipital junction) was correlated with defects in the naming of objects (anomic aphasia), with difficulties in naming letters and literal substitutions in writing.

3. Damage of the occipital lobe was correlated with alexia without agraphia. Although there were few cases in this group, it was observed that in all the patients there was a tendency to spell written words, but performance in reading letters was much better than in reading words. Confabulation in the three patients, secondary to their tendency to guess the written word, constituted morphological paralexias. The three patients presented a dissociation between their ability to read and their ability to write. However, they all presented some paragraphias characterized by the omissions and substitutions of letters.

4. The deep cortical parietal region of the right hemisphere on the side of the deep posterior temporal region was associated with left hemi-inattention, a tendency to invent the left side of the words and difficulties in following the line in reading. In writing it was correlated with omissions and additions of strokes, cascade phenomenon, fragmentation, and grouping of elements. These alterations were correlated with constructional apraxia in copying the Rey figure.

5. The prefrontal regions of the two hemispheres were only slightly correlated with alterations in written language.

An Interlinguistic Consideration

Finally, it is worthy to mention that the psycholinguistic models of the alexias and agraphias developed in other languages, particularly in English, do not seem to be applicable to Spanish. In this work (and in *all* the authors' personal experience) no semantic paralexia appears in Spanish-speaking aphasic patients. Morphological verbal paralexias do, however, frequently appear: One part of the word is read correctly (usually the first morpheme) and the rest is deduced (e.g., /konsiderando/ - /konsiderasyon/; "considering", "consideration"). Moreover, given the writing system of Spanish, there are no appreciable differences between the reading of logotomes and the reading of low-frequency words. The writing system of the Spanish allows the correct reading of even completely unknown words. Spelling is a task with a low level of difficulty.

The existence of a double system of reading (phonological and semantic) would not then seem to be acceptable, as has been proposed for English. This seems to be a fundamental point of view: while Spanish presents an almost complete phonological writing system, the English writing system is partially phonological and partially logographic (Sampson, 1985).

For Spanish speakers, the underlying cognitive operation during reading is to convert graphemes into phonemes. This is not totally true in English: Reading is achieved at a more morphological level. For Spanish speakers it is just surprising to approach the English writing system, as it is perhaps for English speakers to approach an ideographic system. A Latin-American woman living in the United States for many years expressed this feeling in a very descriptive way: "The problem with English is that you read one thing, but you have to say another." For her, of course, reading could be thought of only as converting graphemes into phonemes. Our point, simply, is that reading in English and reading in Spanish represent quite different cognitive activities. Consequently, brain representation of written language and models for alexias and agraphias have to be somehow different. Many more studies are needed in this regard.

ACKNOWLEDGMENTS

This research was possible thanks to a grant received from Colciencias (Fondo Colombiano de Investigaciones Cientificas y Proyectos Especiales "Francisco José de Caldas") and the support received from the Faculty of Psychology of the Fundacion Universitaria Konrad Lorenz (Bogotá, Colombia). All the patients were taken from the Departament of Neurology of the Hospital San Juan de Dios (National University of Colombia) and the Neurological Institute of Colombia. Beatriz Penagos, Angela Flores, Catalina Ramirez, and Lissy Sperber helped in the collection of the data. The English version was prepared by Jenny Lewis. To all of them our gratitude.

REFERENCES

Ardila, A., Montanes, P., Bernal, B., & Serpa, A. (1986). Partial psychic seizures and brain organization. *International Journal of Neuroscience, 30*, 23–32.
Ardila, A., & Ostrosky, F. (1984). *The right hemisphere: Neurology and neuropsychology.* London: Gordon and Breach.
Benson, D. F. (1977). The third alexia. *Archives of Neurology, 34*, 327–331.
Benson, D. F. (1979). *Aphasia, alexia and agraphia.* New York: Churchill Livingstone.
Benson, D. F., & Cummings, J. L. (1985). Agraphia. In J. A. M. Frederiks (Ed.), *Handbook of clinical neurology, Vol. 45: Clinical neuropsychology.* Amsterdam: Elsevier.
Bradshaw, J. L., & Nettleton, N. C. (1981). The nature of the hemispheric specialization. *Behavioral and Brain Sciences, 4*, 146–165.
Bub, D., & Kertesz, A. (1982). Deep agraphia. *Brain and Language, 17*, 146–165.
Damasio, A., & Damasio, H. (1983). The anatomical basis of pure alexia. *Neurology, 33*, 1573–1583.
De Renzi, E., & Faglioni, P. (1978). Normative data and screening power of a shortened version of the Token Test. *Cortex, 13*, 424–433.
Edwards, A. L. (1968). *Experimental design in psychological research.* New York: Holt, Rinehart & Winston.
Geschwind, N. (1965). Disconnection syndromes in animals and man. *Brain, 88*, 237–294.
Goodglass, H., & Kaplan, E. (1979). *Evaluacion de las afasias y de transtornos similares.* Buenos Aires: Editorial Medica Panamericana.
Greenblatt, S. H. (1983). Localization of lesions in alexia. In A. Kertesz (Ed.), *Localization in neuropsychology.* New York: Academic Press.
Hecaen, H. (1962). Clinical symptomatology in right and left hemisphere lesions. In V. B. Mountcastle (Ed.), *Interhemispheric relations and cerebral dominance.* Baltimore: Johns Hopkins.
Hecaen, H., & Albert, M. (1978). *Human neuropsychology.* New York: Wiley.
Kertesz, A. (1983). Localization of lesions in Wernicke's aphasia. In A. Kertesz (Ed.), *Localization of neuropsychology.* New York: Academic Press.
Lezak, M. D. (1983). *Neuropsychological assessment.* New York: Oxford University Press.
Luria, A. R. (1977). *Las funciones corticales superiores en el hombre.* La Habana: Editorial Orbe.
Marshall, J. C., & Newcombe, F. (1973). Patterns of paralexia: A psycholinguistic approach. *Journal of Psycholinguistics, 2*, 175–199.
Marshall, J. C., & Newcombe, F. (1980). The conceptual status of deep dyslexia. In M. Colheart, K. Patterson, & J. V. Marshall (Eds.), *Deep dyslexia.* London: Routledge and Kegan Paul.
Miceli, G., Silveri, M. C., & Caramazza, A. (1985). Cognitive analysis of a case of pure dysgraphia. *Brain and Language, 25*, 187–212.
Naeser, M. A. (1983). CT scan lesion size and lesion locus in cortical and subcortical aphasias. In A. Kertesz (Ed.), *Localization in neuropsychology,* New York: Academic Press.
Novoa, O. P., & Ardila, A. (1987). Linguistic abilities in patients with prefrontal damage. *Brain and Language, 30*, 206–225.

Osterrieth, P. A. (1944). Le test de copie d'une figure complexe. *Revue de Psychologie, 30,* 206–256.

Poeck, K., Bleser, R., & Keyserlingk, T. (1984). Computed tomography localization and standard aphasic syndromes. In J. J. C. Rosen (Ed.), *Advances in neurology: Progress in aphasiology* (Vol. 42). New York: Raven Press.

Roeltgen, D. P., Rothi-Gonzalez, E., & Heilman, K. M. (1986). Linguistic semantic agraphia: A dissociation of the lexical spelling system from semantics. *Brain and Language, 27,* 257–280.

Roeltgen, D. P., Sevush, S., & Heilman, K. M. (1983). Phonological agraphia, writing by the lexical-semantic route. *Neurology, 33,* 755–765.

Rosselli, M., & Ardila, A. (1987). Alteraciones de la lectura, la escritura y el calculo. In J. Bustamante & F. Lopera (Eds.), *El lenguaje: Principios de neurolinguistica.* Medellin: Prensa Creativa.

Rosselli, M., Rosselli, A., Vergara, I., & Ardila, A. (1985). Topography of the hemi-inattention syndrome. *International Journal of Neuroscience, 27,* 165–172.

Sampson, G. (1985). *Writing systems.* Stanford, CA: Stanford University Press.

9

Semantic Aphasia Reconsidered

ALFREDO ARDILA, MARIA VICTORIA LOPEZ, and
EUGENIA SOLANO

In 1920 Head described a language alteration that he defined as an inability to recognize simultaneously the elements within a sentence, and he called this *semantic aphasia*. Only a few authors referred to this aphasia during the following years (Conrad, 1932; Goldstein, 1948; Zucker, 1934). Luria (1966, 1970, 1973, 1976) took up the concept again and analyzed it extensively. With the exception of a few references to it in Western literature over the last few years (Ardila, 1981, 1984; Brown, 1972; Kertesz, 1979) and the report of three cases elaborated by Hier, Mogil, Rubin, and Komros in 1980, few authors have shown special interest in studying semantic aphasia. However, an analysis of this aphasia is of great help in the clarification of the organization of spatial concepts, the mechanisms underlying acalculia and certain types of apraxia and agnosia, the understanding of the role of the left posterior parietal region in the organization of cognitive activity and of its interhemispheric asymmetry. Probably the term itself, *semantic aphasia*, is not very appropriate, but neither are other terms such as *transcortical* or *conduction* aphasia, broadly used in aphasiology.

Luria (1970, 1976) considers that difficulties in the following aspects of language appear in semantic aphasia:

1. Sentences that include a complex system of successive subordinate clauses, particularly forms that include the conjunction *kotory* ("which" or "that"), prepositions and conjunctions of the type *nesmatria* ("in spite of"), *vsledstvie chego* ("as a result of").

ALFREDO ARDILA • Konrad Lorenz Foundation University, Bogotá, Colombia, and Miami Institute of Psychology, Miami, Florida 33166-6612.   MARIA VICTORIA LOPEZ • Colombian Association of Neuropsychology, Bogotá, Colombia.   EUGENIA SOLANO • Neurologic Institute of Colombia, Bogotá, Colombia.

2. Reversible constructions, particularly of the temporal and spatial type (*krug pod kvadratom*—"the circle underneath the square").
3. Constructions with a double negative (*Ia ne privyk ne podchiniatsa preavilam*—"I am not used to not obeying the norms").
4. Comparative sentences (*slon volshe muhi*—"the elephant is bigger than the fly").
5. Passive constructions (*zemlia tsvetlaetsa solntsem*—"the earth is illuminated by the sun").
6. Constructions with transitive verbs (*prosit*—"to ask").
7. Constructions with attributive relations (*brat otsa, otets brata*—"the father's brother, the brother's father").

According to Luria (1976), left posterior parietal or parietal-temporal-occipital lesions produce components of spatial apraxia and agnosia, semantic aphasia, and acalculia. Patients do not show alterations in phonemic discrimination or word articulation, nor do they exhibit defects in the comprehension of words and simple sentences. However, these patients do experience difficulty in understanding grammatical structures, especially the relationships between words within a sentence. Therefore, although word comprehension does not suffer, this is not true of comprehension of the sentence structure. The patient is unable to handle prepositions and spatial or quasi-spatial structures (Luria, 1973).

On occasion, it has been shown that patients with difficulties in understanding syntax suffer from spatial disorders characterized by some constructional apraxia and elements of the Gerstmann syndrome. Luria (1973) suggested that these spatial disorders do not just incidentally accompany semantic aphasia, but the semantic aphasia is a defect in the perception of simultaneous spatial structures only transferred to a higher symbolic level. Consistent with Luria's hypothesis, patients with semantic aphasia have difficulty in understanding the meaning of words tinged with spatial or quasi-spatial meaning.

Thus, semantic aphasia is not merely a deterioration in the understanding of words tinged with spatial meaning, but the comprehension of logicogrammatical structures has also deteriorated. These patients have lost their ability to integrate the elements of a sentence into a whole. As a result, they are unable to grasp the meaning of relationships. The patient is aware of the fact that certain words in the sentence should be combined for him to find the meaning he is looking for but is unable to understand the interrelations. In grammatical constructions there is a common factor: All of them in one way or another are a verbal expression of logicogrammatical relations of a quasi-spatial kind that become apparent, for example, in the use of prepositions.

We shall analyze two cases of left posterior parietal damage with semantic aphasia in an attempt to compare its characteristics with those of patients who have been systematically reported in the literature (Figure 1). And we shall analyze the basic cognitive defects underlying the deficits found in these patients.

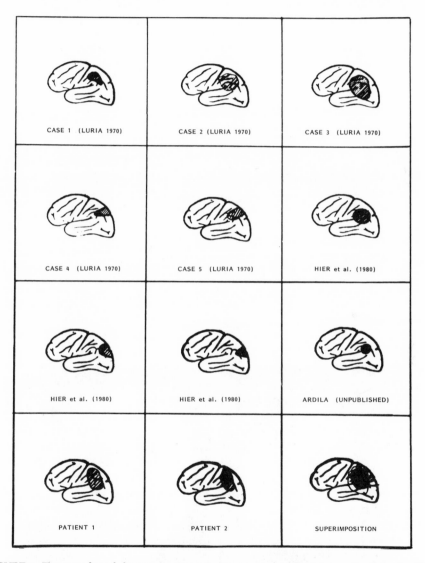

FIGURE 1. Topography of damage in 11 patients reported to have semantic aphasia. The existence of a posterior parietal superimposition can be observed. The last two cases (patient 1 and patient 2) correspond to the two cases analyzed in this chapter.

CASE REPORTS

Patient 1

This is a 21-year-old right-handed woman with 12 years of schooling, monolingual (Spanish), who in November 1983 presented involuntary contraction of her right arm with subsequent loss of consciousness. The only important fact in her history is a bilateral fronto-parieto-temporal pulsatile headache from the age of 13. Her examination on admittance to the Neurological Institute of Colombia proved to be normal except for a discrete hypoesthesia in the right hemibody. As a result of the scans she was taken to the operating room, where a left posterior parietal glioma was removed. She subsequently received cobalt therapy. During the following years, she remained apparently symptom-free, suffering occasionally from paresthesias; on one occasion she had a right hemibody focal seizure. However, she stopped studying and worked sporadically as a manicurist. In June 1986 a control scan was taken (Figure 2) that recorded the presence of a mixed-density lesion. This clearly showed the contrasting medium with well-defined borders and an irregular shape with no great contralateral deviation from the structures of the middle line.

Her neurological examination showed her to be an alert, cooperative patient, with adequate affect, fluent conversational language, and no evidence of agrammatism or dysprosody. She exhibited occasional verbal paraphasias and word-finding difficulties. No comprehension defect was evident in casual conversation. There was extinction in the presence of simultaneous double tactile stimulation, moderate diffi-

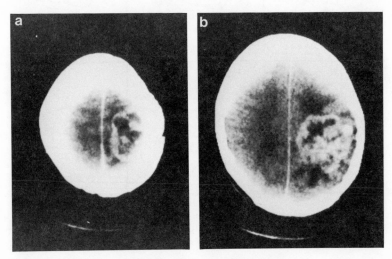

FIGURE 2. Patient 1—brain scan.

culty in the localization of right hemibody stimuli together with agraphesthesia, astereognosis, finger agnosia, strange feelings in her hand, and ideomotor and ideational apraxia. The rest of the neurological examination was found to be within normal limits.

Patient 2

This is a 28-year-old right-handed man with 14 years of schooling, monolingual (Spanish). He was diagnosed as having a left parietal astrocytoma, which was removed in 1981 after an episode of right hemibody partial motor seizure with subsequent generalization. The patient subsequently returned to his work in the government, but only on a part-time basis, owing to what he called his "tiredness and slowness." He still had a four-fifths right hemiparesis and moderate hypoesthesia. Since then he has had frequent partial somatosensory and motor seizures on his right side, some of them with subsequent generalization. In May 1986 a control scan was taken (Figure 3) that showed a zone of lesser density in the operative region, multiple calcifications that do not exert any apparent effect, and dilatation of the left occipital horns.

His neurological examination showed him to be an alert, cooperative patient, depressed in affect, with fluent language, no evidence of agrammatism, dysprosody, or articulatory defects, and with occasional verbal paraphasias and word-finding difficulties. A right hemihypoesthesia and a four-fifths hemiparesis was observed. There was tactile extinction, right agraphesthesia and astereognosia, finger agnosia, and apraxia. The rest of the examination proved to be within normal limits.

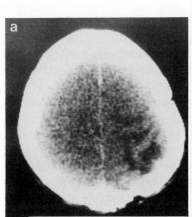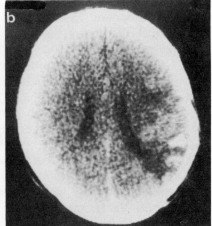

FIGURE 3. Patient 2—brain scan.

Testing Procedure

Each of the patients was given a battery of tests that lasted approximately 10 hours and was divided into 1-hour sessions. The battery included the following:

1. Wechsler Adult Intelligence Scale (WAIS; Wechsler, 1955).

2. Boston Diagnostic Aphasia Examination (BDAE; Goodglass & Kaplan, 1972).

3. Token Test-shortened version (De Renzi & Faglioni, 1978).

4. Rey-Osterrieth Complex Figure.

5. Right-left orientation: The patient indicates on his body and on the examiner's body simple and crossed instructions, recognition of right and left on a drawing, reproduction of the examiner's movements with the appropriate hand (Head's test).

6. Finger gnosis: The patient names/shows the fingers on his and the examiner's hand; shows, on his hand, the finger that corresponds to the one indicated by the examiner; indicates that one or two of his fingers are being touched; says how many fingers there are between the two touched by the examiner.

In addition to these tests, the following were designed for the purpose of this research:

7. Reading: letters, syllables, meaningless sequences, words of different levels of difficulty, sentences, comprehension of written instructions, reading of text aloud, reading of ideograms (e.g., Coca-Cola), recognition of symbols (e.g., danger).

8. Writing: letters, syllables, words with different levels of difficulty, copying words, dictation and copying sentences, changes in the type of writing.

9. Calculation: reading of numerals, writing of numbers, transcription of numbers to letters and vice versa, pointing out the largest number in a pair, arithmetical operations (mental and written), reading of arithmetical signs, successive operations (100 − 13; 1, 4, 7 . . .), counting forward and backward, ordering numbers in columns, arithmetical problems, appreciation of quantities (e.g., how much does an egg weigh?) and of time (e.g., how long does it take a person to walk around a block?).

10. Grammar: conversational language, completion of sentences (verbs, adverbs, prepositions), changing the tense, article—noun agreement (Spanish has masculine/feminine, singular/plural forms of nouns and articles), indicating the verb that corresponds to a noun (e.g., thought—to think) and vice versa, antonyms (with the use of affixes and with a change in the stem), saying what action is being performed in a drawing, ordering the parts of a sentence, understanding of passive sentences, understanding of comparative sentences, understanding of coordination (e.g., the secretary you sent with your cousin is a friend of Peter),

spatial relationships (with reference to a drawing, say yes/no to a series of statements (e.g., the square is above the circle).

RESULTS

Intelligence. Table 1 shows the two patients' scores on the WAIS. Patient 1's IQ was 95 and Patient 2's was 91. In both cases, the lower scores were obtained on the Arithmetic, Digit Span, and Digit Symbol subtests. Both had higher Verbal than Performance IQs.

BDAE. Patient 1 had errors in auditory and reading comprehension. Performance was impaired in naming tasks, especially with regard to body parts. Writing proved to be involved with mistakes due to literal omission and some verbal paragraphias. Praxic mistakes were also observed in tasks such as blowing out a match, greeting someone, lighting a cigarette, putting a piece of paper in an envelope. In Patient 2, greater involvement appeared in the items of auditory and reading comprehension, which became more accentuated with the increase in the volume of verbal material. Performance on naming tasks was deficient especially when they referred to parts of the body. In the case of writing, there were omissions of letters and syllables, and literal paragraphias. Some praxic errors to verbal instructions were also evident in tasks such as greeting someone, teeth cleaning, and using screwdrivers. Figure 4 shows the assessment scale for the language characteristics of both patients. As ex-

TABLE 1. Scaled Scores of the Wechsler Adult
Intelligence Scale

	Patient 1	Patient 2
Full scale IQ	93	91
Verbal IQ	95	93
Performance IQ	91	90
Information	10	10
Comprehension	10	13
Arithmetic	7	4
Similarities	10	9
Vocabulary	10	11
Digit span	7	6
Digit symbol	7	5
Picture completion	10	8
Block design	8	10
Picture arrangement	10	8
Object assembly	8	9

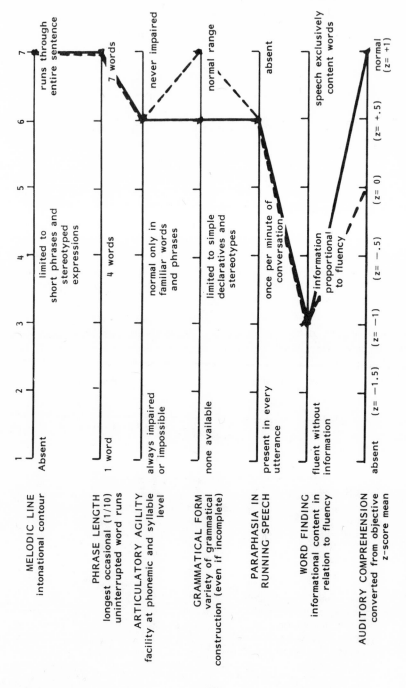

FIGURE 4. Rating scale profile of speech characteristics (continuous line = patient 1, dotted line = patient 2).

pected, the profile is close to that for anomic aphasia (and, indeed, both patients presented associated anomic defects). However, auditory comprehension has been fairly well retained, being almost normal in Patient 1, with a low quantity of paraphasias in discursive speech.

Token Test. The comprehension deficit was slight in Patient 1 (28/36) but greater in Patient 2 (15/36), who found it impossible to carry out instructions in which two tokens were involved simultaneously.

Rey-Osterrieth Complex Figure. For both patients, minor errors appeared in their copies of the figure. In particular, there was confusion of spaces and the omission of details.

Right–Left Orientation. Patient 1 correctly showed right-left on her and the examiner's body and performed crossed instructions. The only mistakes were on Head's test. Patient 2 was unable to perform any of the tasks correctly, and all the answers were at random. He also showed particularly long latencies.

Finger Gnosis: Neither of the patients was able to perform all the tests of recognition and naming of fingers. A certain difference was observed in Patient 1, where performance with the left hand was discretely better.

Reading. In letter reading, both patients revealed spatial confusion (e.g., p - q, b - d). The reading of words, sentences, and texts showed some literal paralexias, but comprehension of written instructions and texts was relatively good. The patient recognized ideographic words and symbols satisfactorily.

Writing. Both patients used their right hand to write. Their writing was slow, hesitant, and poorly legible, with incorrect spacing, distortions of letters, and some literal paragraphias (Figure 5). In the case of the 10-word dictation in the BDAE, correct oral spelling scores were higher than in the written spelling scores, suggesting that the writing defect is apraxic or spatial rather than linguistic. The same difficulties were found in copying.

Calculation. The reading of simple numbers was correct. However, there were confusions in the reading of compound numbers (e.g., 391 instead of 3,091) and in the reading of Roman numerals. The transcription of numbers into letters (e.g., 7–seven) and vice versa was correct. The selection of the larger or smaller of two numbers showed two mistakes (out of six) in Patient 1 and three in Patient 2. Mental arithmetic opera-

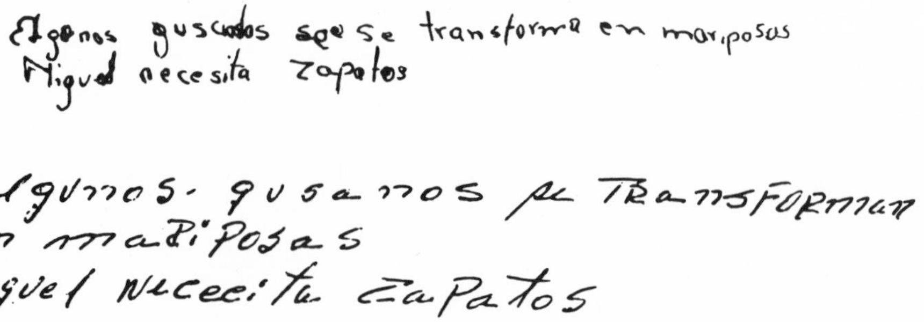

Algonos guscados sqese transforme en mariposas
Miguel necesita zapatos

algunos· gusanos se Transforman
en mariposas
Miguel Necesita Zapatos

FIGURE 5. Samples of writing of patient 1 (above) and patient 2 (below). The two sentences dictated are *Miguel necesita zapatos* ("Miguel needs shoes") and *Algunos gusanos se convierten en mariposas* ("Some worms become butterflies"). Patient 2 needed approximately 5 min to write these two sentences.

tions with just one figure (e.g., 3 + 5) were possible but impossible with two digits (e.g., 93 − 13). The same results were found with written operations. Recognition of arithmetical symbols (+, −, ×, :) was correct. The patients could count adequately forward and backward but could not perform successive calculations (e.g., 1, 4, 7 . . .). The ordering of numbers in columns was adequate. Both made mistakes in solving simple arithmetic problems and in the appreciation of quantities and time.

Grammar. Conversational speech in both patients was grammatically correct, and on answering simple questions they always used grammatical connectors. Table 2 shows their performance on the designed grammar test. No defects were observed in the use of verbs or tenses, the naming of actions, and organizations of the parts of a sentence. Errors (or inability) appeared in the use of adverbs, prepositions, transformations (noun–verb, verb–noun, adjective–verb), antonyms (particularly with prefixes), passive sentences, comparative sentences and coordination, and the handling of spatial relationships.

DISCUSSION

Our two patients and all the other patients reported in the literature presented acalculia in association with the difficulties in the comprehension of different elements within language. Also, to a certain extent, spatial, praxic, and gnosic defects would point to the proposal that they form a unified syndrome (Luria, 1976). According to the results of the BDAE, both patients exhibited mistakes in auditory comprehension (minimal in case 1, moderate in case 2), some naming defects (particularly with regard

TABLE 2. Performance on the Grammar Test

Part	Example	Patient 1	Patient 2
Adverb of place	The dog hid _____ the door.	2/3	2/3
Adverb of manner	Clara took the drug. Now she feels _____	2/5	3/5
Appropriate verb	Yesterday the secretary _____ a letter.	6/6	4/6
Past	Now I'm going to say your name. Yesterday, _____ your name.	3/3	3/3
Future	Today Susana came to say hello to you. Tomorrow _____ to say hello to you.	3/3	3/3
Present	Yesterday I listened to a concert. Now _____ to a concert.	3/3	3/3
Verb to go in its appropriate form	Next week _____ to your house.	5/5	5/5
Prepositions	Most people write _____ their right hands.	22/27	14/27
Change verb into noun	To think: thought	3/5	4/5
Change noun into verb	Entrance: enter	3/5	3/5
Change adjective into verb	Obedient: obey	4/5	3/5
Antonym (with a different stem)	Fat: thin	5/6	5/6
Antonym (prefix)	Real: unreal	0/6	3/6
Naming actions	A picture showing a person eating. Correct answer: "to eat"	5/5	5/5
Organizing the parts of a sentence	in/fishes/the/river/the/boy	5/5	5/5
Passive sentences	A drawing of a doctor examining a patient. Say yes or no: "The doctor is examined by the patient."	1/4	3/4
Comparative sentences	Planes are faster than cars.	9/12	7/12
Coordinations	"The secretary you sent with your cousin is Peter's friend." Who is Peter's friend?	5/10	7/10
Spatial relationships	"The square is above the circle." Say yes or no.	5/10	6/10

to parts of the body), some paraphasias in conversational language, and moderate deficits in reading and writing. The Token Test shows that comprehension of simple orders is adequate, but comprehension of complex orders, particularly if they include elements of a spatial nature, is found to be compromised. The agraphia is more of the apraxic than the

aphasic type, and certain spatial confusions appear in reading. Both patients present finger agnosia—moderate left-right disorientation in Patient 1 and severe disorientation in Patient 2; severe acalculia; and difficulties in the use and comprehension of adverbs, prepositions, passive
sentences, comparative sentences, and verbal elements with a spatial
content.

The similarity between our cases and those reported by Hier et al.
(1980) is striking. The WAIS, for example, shows, in these authors' results
and in our own, a Verbal IQ higher than a Performance IQ, with decreases
in Arithmetic, Digit Span, and Digit Symbol. The associated disorders
(right-left disorientation, finger agnosia, acalculia, and apraxic agraphia)
are the same. However, despite the apparently similar lesion location and
lesion volume in our patients, the performance in our two patients is
somehow different in some tasks. For example, Patient 1 has a near-
normal language comprehension but Patient 2 has moderately severe
comprehension deficits, based on the Token Test; right-left disorientation
and agraphia were more evident in Patient 2; and the performance on the
grammar test shows some differences, especially in the use of prepositions.

The defects found in our patients typifies the left posterior parietal
syndrome and illustrates the semantic aphasia described by Head (1920)
and analyzed by Luria (1970, 1976). Conversational language is adequate
and fluent, with only a discrete tendency to word forgetfulness. There are
no defects in articulation, phonological recognition, prosody, or the comprehension of isolated words, and agrammatism was not observed. However, language comprehension does not go beyond the limits of isolated
elements or simple sentences, and comprehension of logicogrammatical
structures is seriously compromised. Comprehension of the existing relationship between the different parts of a sentence is difficult or impossible, as is the simultaneous synthesis of the different parts of a sentence.
Thus, there is, to say, a "relationship agrammatism" or "impressive
agrammatism" (Luria, 1970). Aspects of a spatial or quasi-spatial nature
(preposition—e.g., to, from; passive sentences—e.g., from whom and to
whom the action is directed), in particular, show alterations.

It is interesting to compare the effects of posterior parietal lesions and
temporal-parietal-occipital lesions in both hemispheres. Above all, it
should be pointed out that in subhuman primates damage in this region in
either of the two hemispheres produces similar deficits: defects in the
perception of simultaneous stimuli, disorders in the visual control of
movements and in occulomotor control in general, errors in spatial orientation and in going through labyrinths and such (Lynch, 1980). In man,
the effects of equivalent lesions (as happens in the case of damage to any
area of cortical association) produce asymmetric defects that are in some
way parallel. Right posterior parietal lesions imply constructional aprax-

ia, difficulty in the performance of spatial tests, hemispatial neglect, hemiasomatognosia, topographic and spatial agnosia, and such (Ardila & Ostrosky-Solis, 1984). Lesions in the left homologous area produce semantic aphasia, which on occasion is associated with autotopagnosia, agraphia, anomic aphasia, disorders in visual exploration, and simultaneous agnosia (Botez, 1985; Hecaen & Albert, 1978; Luria, 1966).

LeDoux (1982, 1984), basing his observation on studies of patients with a divided brain, emphasizes that mechanisms of visuospatial perception are represented in both hemispheres. Also, the specialization of the posterior parietal region of the right hemisphere refers not to visuospatial perception per se but to the regulation of spatially guided behavior that can be observed in activities such as orientation in the medium according to spatial signals from the environment. It can be supposed that the acquisition of articulate language by man in some way modified the relative basic interhemispheric symmetry found in subhuman primates. Although the fundamental function continued to be the same (knowledge of space and one's own body with respect to external space), it began to suffer the intervention of language (spatial knowledge with the intervention of language), such as the use, for example, of logicogrammatical relationships of a spatial kind and arithmetical abilities.

Angular acalculia is a primary acalculia since it is considered not to be a consequence of other cerebral disturbances (e.g., attentional disorders, amnesia, aphasia; Boller & Grafman, 1985). On occasion it has been included within the so-called Gerstmann syndrome (1940), together with finger agnosia, agraphia, and right-left disorientation, a syndrome that Gerstmann considered to be a consequence of a disorder in the "body scheme."[1]

An extensive study of Hecaen, Angelergues, and Houiller (1961) represents a key point in the neuropsychological analysis of the acalculia. The authors distinguish three groups of acalculia: (1) alexia and agraphia for numbers (left temporal-occipital damage), (2) spatial acalculia (right parietal-temporal-occipital lesions), and (3) anarithmia (left retrolandic lesions). Other forms of acalculia have been mentioned in the literature; for example, Grewel (1960) speaks of frontal acalculia and is corroborated by Luria (1973). The acalculia that accompanies Gerstmann syndrome would be anarithmia (Boller & Grafman, 1985). Critchley (1953) emphasizes the spatial deficit in acalculia, which is especially apparent in writ-

---

[1]We should remember that the word *digit* comes from *digitus*, the Latin for "finger." Digits can be taken to be the fingers of the hand, and we can see that the act of calculating stems from counting the fingers of the hand. This association between fingers and counting seems to go back to the very origin of calculation (Cauty, 1984). The association between finger agnosia and acalculia would not then be fortuitous as far as cerebral organization is concerned, nor would the fact that both can be included simultaneously within the same syndrome.

ten calculations, and related it to the parietal damage. Kinsbourne and Warrington (1962) indicate the simultaneous presence of computational, spatial, and symbolic errors in acalculia. Luria (1966, 1973) observes that the difficulties with calculation in patients with left parietal damage are related to the deficits in grammatical structures of complex numbers.

The distinction between alexia and agraphia for numbers and anarithmia, although conceptually valid, is, in practice, sometimes difficult to establish. Damage topography is similar (Levin & Spiers, 1985), and if the existence of Gerstmann syndrome is accepted, it must be supposed that the anarithmia is associated with at least certain agraphia. Deloche and Seron (1984) emphasize the existence of a double code (alphabetic and numerical) in calculation. Using transcoding tasks between codes, they observed the presence of errors due to position in a series (130–140; lexical errors) in patients with Wernicke's aphasia (the opposite of what happens with Broca's aphasia). In Broca's aphasia, the errors are stack errors (140–104), and as a result, syntactic errors. In patients with Wernicke's aphasia, the errors would be more of a semantic type, and the deficits in calculation can be related to lexical-semantic errors in the reading and writing of numbers.

Boller and Grafman (1983, 1985) consider that ability in calculation can be altered in various ways as a result of (1) the inability to appreciate the meaning of the names of the numbers, (2) visuospatial deficits that interfere with the spatial arrangement of the numbers and also with the mechanical aspects of the operations, (3) inability to remember mathematical facts and to use them appropriately, and (4) defects in mathematical thinking and in the comprehension of the underlying operations. Perhaps, we could add the inability to conceptualize quantities (quantification) and reverse operations (e.g., add–subtract). Angular acalculia would correspond more to defects in the second and fourth points frequently associated with defects of the first type (alexic and agraphic acalculia). The spatial defect (point two) would be a consequence not of errors in the handling of the external space on performing calculation operations (spatial acalculia due to right lesions) but of a defect in the handling of the spatial concepts underlying the numbers and their permutations (like "carry" in arithmetical operations), as has been stated by some authors as previously observed.

Dahmen, Hartje, Bussing, and Sturm (1982) studied calculation disorders in patients with Broca's and Wernicke's aphasia. Using factor analysis, they were able to identify two different factors: numericosymbolic and visual-spatial. The slighter calculation defects found in patients with Broca's aphasia are derived from their linguistic alterations, while with Wernicke's aphasia defects in visual-spatial processing contribute to calculation difficulties.

The existence of Gerstmann syndrome has been widely debated and even questioned in the literature (Benton, 1977; Botez, 1985; Poeck & Orgass, 1966; Strub & Geschwind, 1983). Some authors have reported the presence of Gerstmann syndrome without aphasia (Roeltgen, Sevush, & Heilman, 1983; Strub & Geschwind, 1974; Varney, 1984), but the presence of a possible semantic aphasia has not been specifically explored in the evaluations used. According to Strub and Geschwind (1983), the localization would be angular, with the lesion extending not toward the occipital lobe (as Gerstmann proposed) but toward the supramarginal gyrus and inferior parietal. The associated agraphia would be an apraxic agraphia (and not aphasic), from which it is supposed that it need not necessarily be related to alexia (Benson & Cummings, 1985). The report of Morris, Luders, Lesser, Dimmer, and Hahn (1984) on the appearance of a Gerstmann syndrome with electrical stimulation of the cerebral cortex would affirm its angular localization. Finger agnosia could be interpreted as a restricted form of autotopagnosia, and the right-left disorientation implies difficulties in the application of spatial concepts in the body's lateral orientation.

Agrammatism in aphasia has classically been considered to be a component of Broca's aphasia (Benson, 1979; Hecaen & Albert, 1978; Kertesz, 1985). However, Luria (1970, 1976) refers to defects in the comprehension of the relationships between parts of a sentence found in semantic aphasia as a "relationship agrammatism" or "impressive agrammatism," thus opening the door to the existence of a second type of agrammatism, but this time at a different level (also different from the paragrammatism that, on occasion, was associated with the Wernicke's aphasias). This would correspond to a defect in the comprehension of the grammatical structure of the sentence or an error in the comprehension of the syntax (Hier et al., 1980).

Schwartz, Saffran, and Marin (1980) used tasks similar to those used in the assessment of semantic aphasia on agrammatical patients with Broca's aphasia: comprehension of active and passive structures, locative statements, and transitive verbs. The aphasics made mistakes on all of these tasks, which, from the point of view of the performance, would make them equivalent to patients with semantic aphasia. However, the authors find that their defects are the result of a different underlying factor: errors in the comprehension of word order within a sentence. Thus, they conclude that agrammatic patients have a syntactical mapping defect such that they are unable to utilize a fixed and principal set of procedures to recover the relational structure of spoken sentences. Broca's aphasics are capable of processing the semantic features of spatial prepositions (Goodglass, Gleason, & Hyde, 1970), but they fail to decode the syntax of words even in simple, active declarative sentences. In semantic aphasia the difficulty would depend more exactly on the semantics of the spatial relationships underlying passive sentences (from whom and to whom the action is directed), locative statements, and transitive verbs.

It would seem, then, that it is possible to distinguish basic cognitive defects that in some way could underlie the diversity of neuropsychological alterations found in the case of left posterior parietal and parietal-temporal-occipital damage: defects in spatial conceptualization, spatial through which language intervenes, knowledge of the external spatial environment (and the spatial dimensions of one's own body and in the spatial organization and sequencing of its movements) by means of verbal symbols and such. In other words, Gerstmann syndrome (left angular syndrome) and the so-called semantic aphasia are manifestations of the same underlying cognitive deficits. They would conform a unified neuropsychological syndrome.

REFERENCES

Ardila, A. (1981). Las afasias. Bogota: Instituto Neurologico de Colombia.

Ardila, A. (1984). Neurolinguistica. Mexico: Trillas.

Ardila, A., & Ostrosky-Solis, F. (1984). The right hemisphere and behavior. In A. Ardila & F. Ostrosky-Solis (Eds.), The right hemisphere: Neurology and neuropsychology pp. 3–50). New York: Gordon and Breach.

Benson, B. F. (1979). Aphasia, alexia and agraphia. New York: Churchill Livingstone.

Benson, B. F., & Cummings, J. L. (1985). Agraphia. In J. A. M. Frederiks (Ed.), Handbook of clinical neurology, Vol. 45: Clinical Neuropsychology (pp. 457–472). Amsterdam: Elsevier.

Benton, A. L. (1977). Reflection on the Gerstmann syndrome. Brain and Language, 4, 45–62.

Boller, F., & Grafman, J. (1983). Acalculia: Historical development and current significance. Brain and Cognition, 2, 205–223.

Boller, F., & Grafman, J. (1985). Acalculia. In J. A. M. Frederiks (Ed.), Handbook of clinical neurology, Vol. 45: Clinical neuropsychology (pp. 473–482). Amsterdam: Elsevier.

Botez, M. I. (1985). Parietal lobe syndromes. In J. A. M. Frederiks (Ed.), Handbook of clinical neurology, Vol. 45: Clinical neuropsychology (pp. 63–86). Amsterdam: Elsevier.

Brown, J. W. (1972). Aphasia, apraxia and agnosia. Springfield, IL: Thomas.

Cauty, A. (1984). Taxonomie, syntaxe et économie des numerations parlées. Amerindia, 9, 111–146.

Conrad, K. (1932). Versuch einer psychologischen Analyse des parietal syndromes. Monatschrift für Psychiatrie und Neurologie, 34.

Critchley, M. (1953). The parietal lobes. London: Arnold.

Dahmen, W., Hartje, W., Bussing, A., & Sturm, W. (1982). Disorders of calculation in aphasic patients—Spatial and verbal components. Neuropsychologia, 20, 145–153.

Deloche, G., & Seron, X. (1984). Some linguistic components of acalculia. In F. C. Rose (Ed.), Advances in neurology, Vol. 42: Progress in aphasiology (pp. 215–222). New York: Raven Press.

De Renzi, E., & Faglioni, P. (1978). Normative data and screening power of a shortened version of the Token Test. Cortex, 14, 41–49.

Gerstmann, J. (1940). The syndrome of finger agnosia, disorientation for right and left, agraphia and acalculia. Archives of Neurology, Neurosurgery and Psychiatry, 44, 398–408.

Goldstein, K. (1948). Language and language disorders. New York: Grune & Stratton.

Goodglass, H., Gleason, J. G., & Hyde, M. R. (1970). Some dimensions of language comprehension in aphasia. Journal of Speech and Hearing Research, 13, 595–606.

Goodglass, H., & Kaplan, E. (1972). Assessment of aphasia and related disorders. Philadelphia: Lea Febiger.

Grewel, F. (1969). The acalculia. In P. J. Vinken & G. W. Bruyn (Eds.), Handbook of clinical neurology (pp. 181–196). (Vol. 4). Amsterdam: North-Holland.

Head, H. (1920). Aphasia and kindred disorders of speech. Brain, 43, 87–165.

Hecaen, H., & Albert, M. L. (1978). Human neuropsychology. New York: Wiley.

Hecaen, H., Angelergues, T., & Houillier, S. (1961). Les variétés cliniques des acalculies au cours des lesions retrorolandiques: Approche statistique du problème. Revue Neurologique, 105, 85–103.

Hier, D. B., Mogil, S. I., Rubin, N. P., & Komros, G. R. (1980). Semantic aphasia: A neglected entity. Brain and Language, 10, 120–131.

Kertesz, A. (1979). Aphasia and associated disorders. New York: Grune and Stratton.

Kertesz, A. (1985). Aphasia. In J. A. M. Frederiks (Ed.), Handbook of clinical neurology, Vol. 45: Clinical neuropsychology (pp. 287–332). Amsterdam: Elsevier.

Kinsbourne, M., & Warrington, E. K. (1962). A study of finger agnosia. Brain, 85, 47–66.

LeDoux, J. E. (1982). Neuroevolutionary mechanism of several asymmetry. Brain, Behavior and Evolution, 20, 197–213.

LeDoux, J. E. (1984). Cognitive evolution: Clues from brain asymmetry. In A. Ardila & F. Ostrosky-Solis (Eds.), The right hemisphere: Neurology and neuropsychology pp. 51–60). New York: Gordon and Breach.

Levin, H., & Spiers, P. A. (1985). Acalculia. In K. M. Heilman & E. Valenstein (Eds.), Clinical neuropsychology (2nd ed., pp. 97–115). New York: Oxford University Press.

Luria, A. R. (1966). Higher cortical functions in man. New York: Basic Books.

Luria, A. R. (1970). Traumatic aphasia. The Hague: Mouton.

Luria, A. R. (1973). The working brain. New York: Basic Books.

Luria, A. R. (1976). Basic problems of neurolinguistics. The Hague: Mouton.

Lynch, J. (1980). The functional organization of posterior parietal association cortex. Behavioral and Brain Sciences, 3, 485–634.

Morris, H. H., Luders, H., Lesser, R. P., Dinner, D. S., & Hahn, J. (1984). Transient neuropsychological abnormalities (including Gerstmann's syndrome) during cortical stimulation. Neurology, 34, 877–883.

Poeck, K., & Orgass, B. (1966). Gerstmann's syndrome and aphasia. Cortex, 2, 421–437.

Roeltgen, D. P., Sevush, S., & Heilman, K. M. (1983). Pure Gerstmann's syndrome from a focal lesion. Archives of Neurology, 40, 46–47.

Schwartz, M. F., Saffran, E. M., & Marin, O. S. M. (1980). The word order problem in agrammatism: Comprehension. Brain and Language, 10, 249–262.

Strub, R., & Geschwind, N. (1974). Gerstmann's syndrome without aphasia. Cortex, 10, 378–387.

Strub, R., & Geschwind, N. (1983). Localization in Gerstmann syndrome. In A. Kertesz (Ed.), Localization in neuropsychology (pp. 295–322). New York: Academic Press.

Varney, N. R. (1984). Gerstmann syndrome without aphasia: A longitudinal study. Brain and Cognition, 3, 1–9.

Wechsler, D. (1955). Wechsler Adult Intelligence Scale: Manual. New York: Psychological Corporation.

Zucker, K. (1934). An analysis of disturbed function in aphasia. Brain, 57.

Basal Ganglia and Cognitive Activity

Cognitive Effects of Adrenal Autografting in Parkinson's Disease

FEGGY OSTROSKY-SOLIS, IGNACIO MADRAZO,
RENE DRUCKER-COLIN, and LUIS QUINTANAR

The microsurgical autografting of adrenal medullary tissue to the caudate nucleus has recently been implemented to treat patients with Parkinson's disease (PD) who are no longer satisfactorily responding to pharmacological treatment. Initial results show significant improvement in the motor symptomatology of these patients (Drucker-Colin et al., 1988; Madrazo et al., 1987).

Clinical studies have indicated that some degree of cognitive impairment is as much a feature of PD as the classical motor symptoms. In fact, a spectrum of cognitive disorders have been reported in PD patients. In some patients, specific deficits in areas such as memory (Pirozzolo, Hansch, & Mortimer, 1982), language (Matison, Mayeux, Rosen, & Fahn, 1982), visual perception (Villardita, Smirni, Le Pera, Zappala, & Nicoletti, 1982), visuospatial processing (Mortimer, Pirozzolo, Hansch, & Webster, 1982), and behavioral programming under novel conditions (Taylor, Saint-Cyr, & Lang, 1986, 1987) have been reported, whereas in others, global dementia has been found (Boller et al., 1980; Elizan, Sroka, Maker, Smith, & Yahr, 1986; Gaspar & Gray, 1984; Lieberman et al., 1979). Dementia or the irreversible deterioration of intellectual functions, including memory, cogni-

FEGGY OSTROSKY-SOLIS • Department of Psychophysiology, Faculty of Psychology, National University of Mexico, Mexico D. F. 4510, Mexico.   IGNACIO MADRAZO • Department of Neurosurgery, Specialties Hospital, Centro Medico "La Raza," IMSS, Mexico D.F. 02990, Mexico.   RENE DRUCKER-COLIN • Department of Neurosciences, Institute of Cellular Physiology, National University of Mexico, Mexico D.F. 4510, Mexico.   LUIS QUINTANAR • Department of Psychophysiology, Faculty of Psychology, National University of Mexico, Mexico D.F. 4510, Mexico.

tion, and perception, have been observed in approximately 30% of the PD patients (Elizan et al., 1986; Lieberman et al., 1979).

PD is a chronic neurodegenerative disease in which neural death is progressive and so motor signs and cognitive deterioration are a slow, inexorable process. There is at present no pharmacological treatment for the progressive deterioration of these patients.

PATHOLOGY AND PATHOGENESIS

In 1817, Parkinson described the clinical characteristics of the illness nowadays known as idiopathic PD, but it was not until 1912 that Lewy described a pathological abnormality known as the "Lewy body" (eosinophilic cytoplasmic inclusion bodies), which is necessary to confirm the PD diagnosis. In 1919 Tretiakoff showed that the cell loss is located in the substantia nigra, thus giving rise to the anatomoclinical concept of PD that distinguishes idiopathic PD from other parkinsonic syndromes (see Agid, Javoy-Agid, & Ruberg, 1987, for a review).

In 1960 the analysis of the biochemistry underlying PD was initiated. Carlsson showed that the administration of reserpine to rats caused catatonia associated with a decrease in the concentration of dopamine, which could be reversed by reestablishing the normal concentration of dopamine with L-dopa, a precursor of dopamine (Carlsson, Lindquest, & Magnusson, 1957). Ehringer and Hornykiewicz (Ehringer, Hornykiewicz, & Verteilung, 1960) showed that the concentration of dopamine had decreased in the basal ganglia of PD patients. These findings led to the administration of a precursor of dopamine (Cotzias, Papavasiliov, & Gellene, 1969).

It has been shown that patients with PD show loss of nerve cells and depigmentation in the substantia nigra and in other pigmented subcortical nuclei (e.g., the locus coeruleus). The severity of the changes in the substantia nigra parallels the reduction of dopamine in the striatum. Given that the pars compacta of the substantia nigra contains most of the brain's dopaminergic cell bodies, these observations suggested that the nigrostriatal dopaminergic pathway is involved in this disease.

Dopamine normally is synthesized in the striatum, in the nerve endings of the dopaminergic neurons whose cellular bodies lie in the substantia nigra; at these nerve endings, the neurotransmitter is taken up into the vesicles and released in the synaptic cleft when the cells fire.

Neuroanatomically, the denervation of the striatum affects the output from the striatum to the cortex via the striato-pallido-thalamo-cortical (motor cortex) system and the nigro (pars reticulata) thalamo-cortical (premotor and prefrontal cortex) system. The concept of "motor" and "complex" loops has been proposed in the relationship between basal ganglia and frontal lobes (Delong, 1974; Delong, Georgopulos, & Crutcher, 1983).

In this model, the motor loop is devoted to the control of motor parameters and involves the agranular sensorimotor and premotor cortical areas, the putamen, the caudal portions of the basal ganglia efferent system, and a diencephalic relay through the ventral lateral nucleus to the supplementary motor area. The complex loop has a topographically organized input from all cortical association areas to the caudate nucleus; it transmits information to the rostral portion of the basal ganglia efferent system with diencephalic relays via the ventral anterior nucleus and centromedian nucleus to the frontal eye fields and frontal association areas that are involved in cognitive operations (see Taylor et al., 1986, for a review). Figure 1 shows a schematic representation of the motor and complex loops.

Functionally, the basal ganglia show a segregation between motor and nonmotor functions. Thus, the differences in connectivity between the putamen and the caudate nucleus have led to the notion that the decrease in dopaminergic activity in the putamen causes the motor symptomatology (tremor, rigidity, and akinesia). Within the motor loop there is also segregation of functions; for example, it has been speculated that the loss of pallido-cortical fibers is important in the genesis of the tremor and that rigidity is related to the loss of putamino-pallidal fibers. The symptoms of akinesia and the postural and equilibrium defects are symptoms derived from the degeneration of the cellular bodies in the substantia nigra (Selby, 1967). The caudate nucleus seems to be involved in complex cognitive functions. Symptoms reminiscent of frontal lobe dysfunction have been reported among PD patients. These frontal lobe type symptoms are expressed by an impaired ability to order and maintain cognitive (goal-directed) programs and by frontal type motor signs, such as the inability to maintain repetitive gestual sequences. In visuoperceptual and visuospatial tasks, segmentation and loss of figure-ground perspective are observed (Agid, Ruberg, & Dubois, 1986; Ostrosky-Solis et al., 1988; Taylor et al., 1986).

As Taylor et al. (1987) point out, the normal distribution of dopamine within the caudate nucleus becomes critical to cognitive functions in terms of the ability to affect fronto-caudate circuits within the complex loop that ultimately return information processed in the caudate nucleus to the prefrontal cortex.

It has also been found that the ventral area adjacent to the pars compacta of the substantia nigra shows a loss of dopaminergic cells in PD (Javoy-Agid et al., 1984; Uhl, Hedreen, & Price, 1985). This area gives origin to the meso-limbic-cortical pathway that projects primarily to the medial frontal area and the limbic areas (nucleus accumbens, amygdala, cingulate cortex, hippocampus, paraolfactory gyrus, and septum) (Javoy-Agid & Agid, 1980; Javoy-Agid et al., 1984). Reduction of dopamine in the frontal cortex areas of PD patients (Scatton, Rouquier, Javoy-Agid, Agid, 1982) seems to be related to the cognitive disorders observed (Agid et al.,

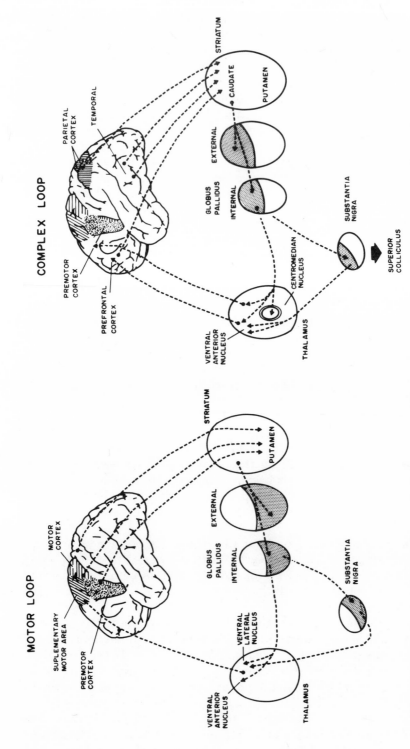

FIGURE 1. Schematic diagram of the motor and complex anatomical circuits. Motor loop: cortico-putamino-pallido-thalamo-cortical (motor cortex). Complex loop: cortico-caudato-nigro-thalamo-cortical (premotor and prefrontal cortex). (Adapted from DeLong, Georgopulos, & Crutcher, 1983.)

1986; Brozoski, Brown, Rosvold, & Goldman, 1979; Lees & Smith, 1983; Stern & Langston, 1985; Taylor et al., 1986, 1987).

In spite of the fact that the primary pathology of PD is the degeneration of the dopaminergic projection to the striatum, not all these patients' symptoms can be attributed to loss of nigrostriatal dopamine. There are other neurochemical systems that are found to be affected in PD, such as the noradrenergic cells in the locus coeruleus, serotoninergic neurons in the dorsal raphé nucleus, and acethylcholine due to lesions in the septohippocampal system and the substantia innominata. At the cortical level, a reduction in somatostatine has been reported (see review in Agid et al., 1987).

The reduction of acethylcholine and its enzymes in the nucleus basalis of Meynert has been associated with demential disturbances (Gaspar & Gray, 1984). As for the other neurotransmitters, no clear relation has yet been established between the biochemical changes and the clinical symptomatology. However, in light of data obtained from animal research, it has been hypothesized that the selective alteration in the noradrenergic systems could cause attentional disturbances; the reduction of serotoninergic metabolism has been associated with depression, and the decrease in somatostatine at the cortical level has been correlated with intellectual deterioration (Agid et al., 1987).

It would appear that the lesions in the different neuronal systems do not evolve in parallel but may be additives or potentiate one another in terms of functional expression. From the biochemical point of view, it has been found that the cholinergic activity in striatum and cortical areas is related to the quantity of dopamine receptors. In PD patients with a low number of dopamine receptors, labeling of cholinergic muscarinic receptors revealed decreased numbers in both the caudate nucleus and the cortex. Individuals with an increased number of dopamine receptors displayed evidence of a corresponding increase in cholinergic receptors (Rinne, 1982). The variety in the extension and the degree of lesions that has been found among PD patients could be the pathological substratum for the wide variety of motor and cognitive symptoms that have been observed.

TREATMENT

On the basis of the physiopathological description of PD, multiple pharmacological and surgical treatments have been tried.

The motor disturbances can be grouped in two types of deficits: primary functional deficits directly attributed to the loss of function subserved by specific neurons, and secondary deficits that may be caused by the appearance of an abnormal pattern of action in neurons when part of this controlling input (usually inhibitory) is destroyed as a result of the illness.

Neurosurgical Treatment

The tremor and rigidity of Parkinson's disease have been attributed to a loss of an inhibitory influence within the basal ganglia, which leads to the release of the inhibition and to an abnormal outflow of the internal portion of the globus pallidus to the ventral anterior and lateral nuclei of the thalamus and finally to the motor cortex. Neurosurgical treatment of PD began in 1930 (Selby, 1967) and involves stereotaxic lesions in the globus pallidus or in the ventro-lateral thalamus contralateral to the side of the body that is most affected. This technique apparently decreases the abnormal activity (disinhibited) and relieves the tremor and rigidity. The bradykinesia of the patients does not improve, however (possibly because it is a primary deficit), and for this reason the performance of daily activities remains affected. It has been reported that the tremor and rigidity reappear 1 to 3 years after surgery. In the cognitive area, different disturbances appear as a result of the surgery (especially when performed bilaterally), such as deterioration in language and in visuoperceptual functions, and severe conceptual and emotional disturbances (Darley, Brown, & Swenson, 1975; Riklan & Levita, 1970). The success of pharmacological therapy has decreased the need for this type of surgery.

Pharmacological Treatment

The cornerstone of pharmacological treatment in PD is the use of the precursor of dopamine, levodopa, a substance that is able to cross the hematoencephalic barrier and be transformed into dopamine by the dopaminergic system and, more recently, the use of dopaminergic agonist agents.

When PD patients are treated with levodopa, an initial improvement is observed, and then gradually, over the years, the improvement decreases. A large number of patients present secondary effects to the action of the drug, including dyskinesias or abnormal involuntary movements, "on-off" phenomena characterized by the presence of severe akinesia and periods of relative mobility, "wearing-off" or "end of dose" phenomena characterized by an accelerated deterioration in the beneficial effects, and psychiatric disorders. These side effects are on occasion more severe than the disease itself.

The conventional treatments used do not alter the course of the illness since they produce only a temporal symptomatic relief. Currently, the need exists to develop new therapeutic approaches that will produce the medication or appropriate procedure that can supply dopamine in *situ* and in an adequate concentration for the individual physiological demands.

Tissue Transplants

It is in this context that a line of research arose within the basic neurosciences in which the treatment of experimental models of Parkinson's disease with transplanted dopaminergic neurons has been explored. That is, an attempt has been made to fulfill all the theoretical assumptions of the ideal drug, infusing dopamine through the neurons or cells that synthesize it (i.e., the substantia nigra or adrenal medulla) into portions of the brain deficient in this neurotransmitter.

The capacity of several tissues to survive and grow when they are transplanted within the central nervous system has been known since Ramón y Cajal (1938). The central nervous system is an immunologically privileged organ with a low capacity for rejection and an ideal place to transplant autologous or fetal tissue (Barker & Billingham, 1977). It is thought that in the brain the access to the immune system to foreign tissues is limited for two reasons: (1) The brain lacks lymphatic vessels and lymph nodes from which many of the cells of the immune system are deployed, and (2) the walls of the blood vessels in the central nervous system are specialized in creating a "blood–brain barrier." The absence of rejection in the neuronal transplants can also reflect the suitable characteristics possessed by the nervous cells. Many cells on their surface bear large molecules known as Class I major histocompatibility antigens. Different in each animal, the antigens are molecules that the immune system recognizes as foreign when it rejects grafted tissue. Few of these antigens are found in neurons.

The development of experimental models of Parkinson's disease and the verification of the viability of the monoaminergic neurons on being transplanted within the central nervous system produced a wide field for research in neurobiology. In 1971 Ungerstedt (1971a,b) described an experimental model for Parkinson's disease that consists in the destruction of neurons from the nigrostriatal system with a selective-6-hydroxidopamine neurotoxin. This substance selectively destroys the neurons, fibers, and terminals that contain catecholamines (for example, dopamine). When the dopamine pathways on both sides of the brain are destroyed, a generalized akinetic syndrome is produced that is reminiscent of the hypokinesia of Parkinsonism and includes interruption of eating and drinking habits and death of the animal if it is not given intensive care. Unilateral lesions of the nigrostriatal pathway result in turning movements away from the side of the lesions that can be measured quantitatively by a rotometer. Following unilateral lesions of the substantia nigra, the ipsilateral striatum responds to denervation by becoming supersensitive to dopamine. If the lesions spare more than 5% of the dopamine-containing fibers, the animal can recover within 1 or 2 weeks, and rats do not exhibit abnormal turning unless they are challenged with drugs. Amphetamine releases dopamine from the intact side, causing ipsilateral rotation. Apomorphine, which is a postsynaptic dopamine agonist, produces a greater effect on the denervated striatum, resulting in rotation of the animal away from the side of the lesion.

Another experimental model of PD is provoked using a neurotoxic chemical (MPTP). In the course of a few days, the animal develops some of the characteristics of PD, especially hypokinesia, rigidity, and postural instability (Forno, Langston, Delanney, Irwin, & Ricaurte, 1986; Langston, Ballard, Tetrud, & Irwin, 1983). MPTP damages the dopaminergic neurons that are found in the pars compacta of the substantia nigra and results in a degeneration of the fibers of the nigrostriatal system and in a loss of striatal dopamine and its metabolites.

Recent studies employing the above animal models of PD have shown that grafting of fetal substantia nigra cells to the lateral ventricle adjacent to the denervated neostratum reverses most of the behavioral, biochemical, and anatomical abnormalities induced by the dopamine-denervating lesions. Biochemically, the transplants restored up to 50% of the lost caudate dopamine. Anatomically, the transplanted dopaminergic cells appeared normal and sprouted in a limited manner into the substance of the caudate, and, behaviorally, all the abnormalities except adipsia and aphagia could be reversed (Bjorklund, Dunnett, Stenevi, Lewis, & Iversen, 1980; Dunnett, Bjorklund, & Stenevi, 1983; Dunnett, Bjorklund, Stenevi, & Iversen, 1981a,b; Freed, 1983; Perlow, 1987; Perlow et al., 1979).

Since transplanting embryonic human tissue for clinical trials raises ethical difficulties, investigators began to examine alternative sources of catecholaminergic tissue for grafting to the brain, specifically adrenal medullary cells. These cells have the same embryonic origin as neurons; that is, both develop in the ectoderm. They contain large amounts of catecholamines: adrenaline, noradrenaline, and dopamine. Moreover, chromaffin cells possess a high degree of phenotypic plasticity. When they are surrounded by adrenal cortex, they become rounded and absorb large amounts of epinephrine, but when they are removed from the gland, placed in culture, and incubated with nerve growth factor, they change morphologically and biochemically, simulating catecholaminergic cells (Unsicker, Rieffert, & Ziegler, 1980; Wurtman, Pohorecky, & Baliga, 1972).

In 1981 Freed et al. began a series of studies in which adrenal medullary allografts were transplanted in the lateral ventricle adjacent to the denerved striatum and found that apomorphine-induced rotation was induced by the grafts. These and further studies (Freed, 1983) suggested that behavioral recovery was related to the release of catecholamines, adrenaline, noradrenaline, and dopamine and their diffusion to hypersensitive dopamine receptors in the striatum.

A different mechanism of action of the transplant has been suggested by recent experiments carried out by Bohn, Marciano, Cupit, and Gash (1987) in rats and by Gash et al. (1987) in cebus monkeys. Both groups have found that adrenal medullary grafts into the caudate nucleus promoted rapid recovery of tyrosine hydroxylase immunoreactive fibers that appear to be from the host rather than from the graft itself. The authors postulated that adrenal medullary exert a neurotrophic action in the host brain, promoting recovery of dopaminergic neurons damaged by MPTP.

ADRENAL MEDULLARY GRAFTS IN PD PATIENTS

In 1982, researchers in Sweden made the first attempt to transplant adrenal medullary tissue into the striatum of PD patients. Using a stereotaxic technique, they transplanted suspensions of autologous adrenal medullary tissue into four PD patients. The tissue was contained in a steel spiral to mark its position in the brain. The implants were placed in the parenchyma of the caudate nucleus in two patients (Backlund et al., 1985), and in two others the tissue was placed in the putamen (Lindvall et al., 1987). With this technique, the patients presented a modest clinical improvement during short periods of time. As reviewed in Drucker et al. (1988), the question arises as to whether placement of adrenal medullary tissue in the parenchyma is an appropriate procedure, or whether better survival of this tissue is obtained when it is placed within the ventricle. Animal work has strongly suggested that the latter is more appropriate since it appears that survival of adrenal medulla grafts placed within the striatum is limited, regardless of whether they are introduced as solid blocks or as dissociated cells. As a result, such grafts do not effectively induce recovery of apomorphine rotational behavior, although, with the injection of nerve growth factor at the site of transplantation, the graft then becomes much more effective. On the other hand, when grafts are placed within the lateral ventricle, rotational behavior is significantly reduced without need of nerve growth factor. The fact that the cerebral ventricles provide a fluid-filled cavity that may act as a nourishing medium for the maintenance of grafted tissue prior to vascularization, and also provide a medium for transport of neuroactive substances released from grafts, may explain in part the better results obtained in counteracting rotational behavior of lesioned animals.

In view of this difference between intraparenchymal and intraventricular placements of grafts in animals, and in view of the very modest improvement reported by the Swedish team, Madrazo et al. (1987) modified the procedure and transplanted adrenal medullary tissue in two young (35- and 39-year-old) PD patients. The adrenal medullary fragments were grafted within the lateral ventricle with partial inclusion within the head of the caudate nucleus.

Surgical Technique

The surgical procedure involved simultaneous adrenalectomy and frontal craniotomy. Upon extraction of the adrenal gland under a dissecting microscope, six to eight fragments of adrenal tissue were obtained (0.8 g in total approximately) and placed on a wet surface. Simultaneously, the caudate nucleus was approached, with the aid of a surgical microscope, through the lateral ventricle by means of a nontraumatic transcortical (second frontal gyrus F2). In the head of the caudate nucleus, a 3 × 3 × 3-mm bed was constructed and the adrenal medullary fragments were placed within the cavity. Initially, six small fragments were inserted in the cavity, and then the last two fragments, which were slightly larger, were anchored to the ependyma of the caudate nucleus with a couple of stainless-steel miniature staples. In this manner, the inner fragments cannot dislodge themselves from the cavity, but the cerebrospinal fluid can bathe all the grafted tissue. In both patients, clinical improvement was noted at 15 and 6 days (respectively) after implantation and has been maintained 24 months in the first patient and 18 months in the second. Rigidity and akinesia were significantly reduced, and functionally both patients are completely independent in their daily activities and are working, the first as a farmer and the second as a civil engineer.

Since these results appeared, the autologous graft of adrenal medulla to the caudate nucleus has been carried out in a larger number of PD patients who presented severe symptoms of rigidity, tremor, akinesia, and pronounced on-off effects. Patients have been studied with video, spectrophotography, electromyography, neurophysiological, and neuropsychological studies.

NEUROPSYCHOLOGICAL FINDINGS

The technique of autologous graft of adrenal medulla implanted in the ventricle surface of the caudate nucleus is performed by means of a right frontal craniotomy, and in order to implant the fragments of adrenal medulla a cavity is made in the caudate nucleus; for this reason one of the objectives of the neuropsychological evaluation of the patients subjected to this surgery is to monitor if any negative effects appear as a result of the surgery.

The chromaffin cells of the adrenal medulla secrete a large quantity of substances such as encephalines, somatostatine, neuropeptides, epinephrine, and norepinephrine, as well as dopamine. It has been reported that different cognitive disorders associated with deficiencies in dopamine and other neurotransmitters are present in the PD population. For this reason, another objective of the neuropsychological evaluation has been to study whether positive effects exist in the cognitive area as a result of the transplant. A group of operated and unoperated patients with PD (diagnosed at the Parkinson's Clinic at the Centro Médico "La Raza") were studied. The operated PD group comprised 18 patients who underwent autografting of adrenal medullary tissue to the caudate nucleus to treat PD as described above. They were 12 males and 6 females, whose ages ranged from 34 to 60 years (mean = 47.4 years). The duration of illness ranged from 3 to 16 years (mean = 9.5 years). Education ranged from 1 to 17 years (mean = 9.8 years). The unoperated PD group included 10 patients (6 males and 4 females) who were candidates for surgery. These patients were matched with the operated PD patients with respect to illness, severity of symptoms, and duration of treatment. The severity of the disease was evaluated using the Unified Parkinson Rating Scales, the Hoehn and Yahr Classification, and the Schwab England Scale, which measure disability expressed in the activities performed during daily living. Given the scores obtained, 5 patients were classified as mild to moderately affected, 7 as moderately to severely, and 6 as severely affected.

Before surgery, the patients had received L-dopa alone or in combination with other "antiparkinsonian" drugs. The initial response to the medication had been positive, but there was a gradual decrease of the beneficial effects, and all patients developed drug-related complications that included an "end of dose" deterioration phenomenon and disabling side effects (dyskinesias and/or on-off phenomena).

A series of neuropsychological tests based on Luria's diagnostic procedures and adapted for the Mexican population were also used (Ostrosky-Solis et al., 1985, 1986). These tests explore nine different areas, which are described in Table 1.

To obtain additional information on behavioral and cognitive functions reported to be at risk among PD patients, such as attention, memory, verbal fluency, depression, and global dementia, several other psychological instruments were applied. Details of the tests and procedure can be found in the paper by Ostrosky-Solis et al. (1988).

The preoperative neuropsychological testing was carried out 2 to 4 weeks prior to surgery. In the immediate postoperative period, behavior was evaluated on a day-to-day basis. Formal neuropsychological testing was carried out at 3 months and at 12 months after surgery. The control group was evaluated with the same battery and at the same time intervals as the operated PD patients.

The preoperative neuropsychological testing revealed specific cognitive deficits, which varied in degree. The patients showed frontal lobe

TABLE 1. Neuropsychological Scheme[a]

Motor functions	Includes tasks that require the coordination, reproduction, and repetition of simple and complex movements with the hand, the arm, and bucofacial movements. Series of alternating motor activities.
Somatosensory knowledge	Includes the discrimination of tactile stimuli, recognition of shapes, reproduction of hand positions, and tactile memory.
Visuoperceptual and visuospatial recognition	Explores recognition of simple and complex drawings, figure-ground discrimination, visual closure, visual analysis and synthesis, reproduction of drawings and designs, object assembly, and block designs.
Auditory knowledge and language	Assesses the detection and discrimination of phonemes, tap-out asymmetrical rhythms, retention and evocation of a list of 5 meaningless syllables, repetition of verbal sequences, and recognition of natural sounds.
Cognitive processes	Includes logical reasoning, classification of objects, understanding of analogies, picture completion, and picture arrangement.
Oral language	Explores the production of simple and complex words, comprehension of language, verbal learning curves for bysyllabic words, immediate and delayed memory for sentences, naming of objects and body parts, complex grammatical relations and passive constructions.
Reading	Includes recognition of letters, syllables, and words, oral and silent reading.
Writing	Assess automatic writing, copy, and dictation.
Basic calculus	Explores mathematical notion and basic arithmetic operations.

[a]Includes 95 items from which 195 scores can be obtained, and emphasizes two aspects: (1) quality of the mistakes—each item is scored according to one or several criteria and not simply according to whether the subject performed the task or not, and (2) a simple quantification is carried out under three categories for each criterion—namely, normal performance; regular performance, moderately anomalous; and impossible performance. Hence, the poorer the subject's performance, the higher his score.

type deficits with alterations in behavioral programming, leading to difficulties in the organization of motor sequences and alternating programs. Visuoperceptual and visuospatial tasks were also affected, reflecting a pattern of performance commonly observed after lesions of the frontal lobe, such as segmentation and loss of figure-ground perspective (see Figure 2). Verbal functions were better preserved, with slight reduction in fluency, but no aphasic symptomatology was found. Immediate memory was diminished, with marked difficulties in delay memory. Speech was hypophonic, dysarthric, and aprosodic. Facial expression was hypo-

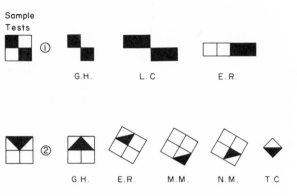

FIGURE 2. Preoperative performance on a block design task by
PD patients. Patients showed
segmentation and loss of figure–
ground perspective. Even in the
simplest design, they broke the 2
× 2 configuration and attended
only to the salient features of the
design.

mimic. No limb or bucofacial apraxia was observed. There was formal
perseveration of reading and writing, although motor problems and bradykinesia affected the quality of the written product, there was no
dyscalculia.

Figure 3 compares the neuropsychological test-retest evaluation profiles obtained from the unoperated PD with the pre- and post-operative
evaluation profiles obtained from the operated PD groups. The test-retest
profiles of the unoperated PD control group overlapped, whereas the profiles of the operated PD group did not. A median difference analysis
(using the Mann-Whitney U test), which compared the scores obtained in
each section of the neuropsychological diagnostic scheme in the test-
retests condition by the unoperated control group and in the pre/postop-
erative condition by the operated PD group, revealed a significant ($p <$
.05) postoperative improvement in I (motor functions) and III (visuoperceptual and visuospatial recognition).

Individual analysis revealed that preoperatively 7 (39%) of the patients showed a normal cognitive profile and 11 (61%) patients presented
specific cognitive deficits. In 7 of the 11 patients with abnormal preoperative profiles, the postoperative evaluation revealed a significant
amelioration of the frontal lobe type symptoms, and visuospatial deficits
(see Figure 4) as well as an improvement in memory tasks that require an
active organization of the response. Immediate and delay memory difficulties remained unchanged. The improvements were unrelated to improved increased alertness or sustained attention. Three patients with
abnormal preoperative profiles did not show a significant amelioration of
the frontal lobe signs. Patients with a normal preoperative neuropsychological profile showed no postoperative deficiencies, and their profiles
proved to be very similar to their preoperative performance. Changes were
shown to be sustained in the second evaluation carried out at 12 months.

In two patients there were neurological complications as a result of

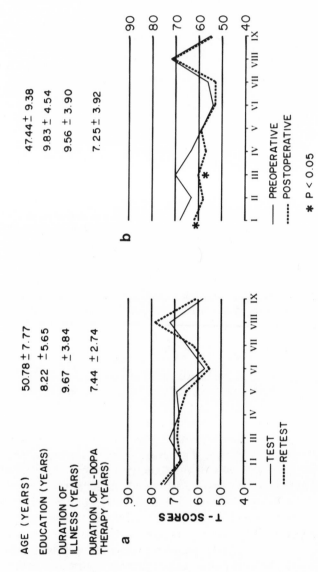

FIGURE 3. Mean scores of the neuropsychological diagnostic scheme obtained by (a) the control unoperated PD group ($n = 10$) in the test–retest condition and by (b) the operated PD group ($n = 16$) in the pre- and postoperative evaluation. The dark lines show the mean and the limits of 2 standard deviations. Higher scores reflect greater number of errors than average and lower scores reflect fewer numbers of errors. Level of significance of postoperative improvement is indicated, as well as mean values and standard deviations for the descriptive characteristics for the two groups. I, Motor functions; II, somatosensory knowledge; III, visuoperceptual and visuospatial recognition; IV, auditory knowledge and language; V, cognitive processes; VI, oral language; VII, reading; VIII, writing; IX, calculus.

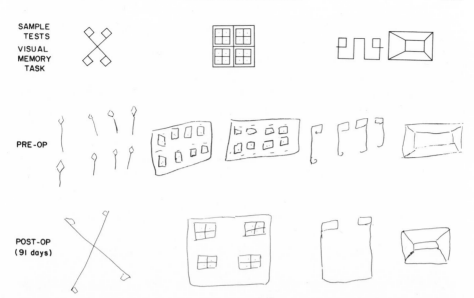

FIGURE 4. Pre- and postoperative (3 months) performance on an immediate visual memory task by a 60-year-old writer with 10 years of evolution of PD. In the preoperative evaluation he was able to copy designs but presented fragmentation and perseveration on visual memory tasks. Three months after surgery he shows integration and lack of perseveration. Before surgery the patient was dependent on others for most of his daily living activities. He was being treated with 750 mg of levodopa. Three months after surgery the patient is completely independent in most chores, although it takes him twice as long and he is aware of his difficulties. He has returned to work. He is on 600 mg of levodopa.

the surgery. One of the patients had permanent damage in the septum, causing an accentuation of cognitive difficulties, and the patient's disorientation, inattention inertia, and lack of initiative increased. In another case, after several postsurgical complications, the patient developed an encephalopathy that severely affected all cognitive functions.

In the immediate postoperative period, six patients presented visual and one auditory hallucinations that cleared spontaneously within 72 hours after the operation. Patients were aware of these hallucinations, in general were not frightened by them, and could speak about them without anxiety. The content of the hallucination varied in each patient. For example, one patient with hallucinations saw insects on the wall and another often heard the telephone ringing. Mental confusion was observed in five cases and perseveration in motor and verbal tasks in six. This behavior disappeared gradually within 2 to 4 weeks after surgery.

GENERAL CONSIDERATIONS

Neuropsychological evaluation has revealed that in a high percentage of the PD patients with an abnormal preoperative neuropsychological profile, autografting of adrenal medullary tissue to the caudate nucleus has positive effects on specific cognitive symptoms.

The neuroanatomical basis of the cognitive alterations in PD is still a matter of controversy. Some authors have suggested that cognitive changes are secondary to a dysfunction of the basal ganglia (Albert, Feldman, & Willis, 1974; Freeman & Albert, 1985; Mortimer et al., 1982). Others believe that a cortical abnormality is primary and that the coexistence of an Alzheimer-type dementia in PD is responsible for the mental deterioration (Boller et al., 1980; Hakim & Mathieson, 1979; Lieberman et al., 1979). Several studies have reported that the frontal-type symptoms appear early in the evolution of the disease and are observed in all patients who deteriorate progressively (Agid et al., 1986; Lees & Smith, 1983; Taylor et al., 1986). Our results agree with this since they show that the tasks sensitive to frontal deficits are precisely the ones that are most affected and that show an important improvement after transplantation. Thus, apparently in our patients, the frontal cortex is not damaged but only hypoactive, owing to the dysfunction of afferent fibers arising from the subcortical nuclei. Since immediate memory and retrieval processes remained unchanged after the autograft, these disorders might be due to the involvement of different cortico-subcortical structures, such as lesion of the septo-hippocampal cholinergic systems. Selective destruction of cholinergic neurons in the substantia innominata has been shown to induce complex mnemonic and cognitive disturbances (Dubois et al., 1983), and administration of subthreshold doses of anticholinergics in nondemented PD patients impairs performance in visual memory tasks (Dubois et al., 1987). In our study, memory tasks that require an active organization of the response, such as the recall of logic passages (WAIS Memory Scale subtest), did show an improvement. This is probably related to a frontal lobe involvement in the performance of these tasks (Luria, 1977).

Many of the cognitive and motor signs that improved after the autograft seem to be dopaminergic-dependent. Two of the main dopaminergic pathways are the nigrostriatal and the meso-limbic-cortical pathways (Bjorklund & Lindwall, 1978; Farley et al., 1978; Javoy-Agid et al., 1984). Current data seem to indicate that both dopaminergic pathways are involved for adequate cognitive processing.

The selective degeneration of the dopaminergic nigrostriatal pathway, as observed in patients intoxicated with MPTP, induced Parkinsonism with frontal-type cognitive impairment (Stern & Langston, 1985). As previously reviewed, anatomically, neural connections between the striatum and premotor and prefrontal cortex (complex loop) have been described.

A variable involvement of the dopaminergic system could be the basis of the heterogeneity in the motor signs and the cognitive profile obtained during the preoperative evaluation, as well as in the differential response to the autografting procedure.

Several investigators have reported a higher frequency of cognitive impairment in patients with more bradykinesia and rigidity. Mortimer et al. (1982) proposed two clinical forms of idiopathic PD—one with predominant bradykinesia and cognitive impairment, and the other with predominant tremor and relatively intact function. Lieberman (1974) reported less prominent tremor in PD patients with dementia, and Zetusky, Jankovic, and Pirozzolo (1985) reported a significant association between deterioration in mental status with bradykinesia, postural instability, and gait difficulty, whereas tremor was associated with a relative preservation of mental status and less functional impairment. Bernheimer, Birkmayer, Hornykiewiez, Jellinger, and Seitelberger (1973) found that regional chemical changes were correlated with the type and degree of clinical manifestations. For example, severity of akinesia correlates best with dopamine and HVA deficiency in the caudate nucleus, whereas the degree of tremor paralleled severity of HVA deficiency in the pallidum, and rigidity was not related to any specific regional distribution of dopamine or HVA deficiency.

Within the caudate, different cognitive functions are subserved by different regions. In PD, the maximal dopamine reduction is observed in the anterodorsal head of the caudate, which is the area that has greatest connection with the frontal cortex (Rosvold, 1972). In subhuman primates, experimental lesion in the anterodorsal and ventral part of the head of the caudate causes difficulties in tasks that require response-inhibition and produce perseveration, difficulty in shifting responses, and deficits in behavioral programming (Cools, 1980; Johnston, Rosvold, & Mishkin, 1968; Rosvold, 1972; Teuber & Proctor, 1964), and, in contrast, lesions in the tail of the caudate produced deficits in visual discrimination (Divac, Rosvold, & Szwarcbart, 1967). It could be that in our study, in the patients who show abnormal preoperative profiles, the disease affected the caudate nucleus, and thus the dopamine concentration in this structure is decreased. It is worth noting that the adrenal medullary fragments are grafted (within the lateral ventricle with partial inclusion) within the head of the caudate, and therefore the supply of dopamine to this region could explain the positive cognitive effects after the autograft. The possibility also exists that behavioral recovery is induced through the regeneration of fibers and dopamine-containing cells of the meso-cortical dopaminergic system.

One of the most fundamental questions to date in the study of transplants to the central nervous system is the identification of the basic mechanisms that are related to the clinical improvement observed in some of the patients affected by PD.

The transplant could exert functional effects through several mechanisms: (1) The grafted tissue could release dopamine. It has recently been demonstrated that the adrenal gland possesses a powerful dopamine-releasing factor that seems to be glycoprotein, whose activity is capable of inducing the release of high levels of dopamine from striatal tissue (Chang & Ramírez, personal communication). (2) The transplant and the lesion release specific neurotrophic factors that provoke the fragments of the adrenal medulla to regenerate and reinnervate the striatum. (3) The transplanted tissue enhances the recovery of the host dopaminergic neurons; that is, the improvement observed is due to the growth of the patient's own nigrostriatal and/or meso-cortico-limbic system.

It is possible, then, that a multitude of trophic, neurochemical, and synaptic mechanisms are involved in the recovery observed after transplant. These mechanisms permit the transplanted tissue to promote the functioning of the host brain and its recovery.

A large number of questions and perspectives have now arisen. Research into the interaction that exists between grafts and the host nervous system have suggested that the transplants may act as mediator to promote the production of growth factors or growth neuromechanisms leading to plasticity and recovery of damaged cells and pathways in the host, and this opens possibilities for the treatment of illnesses that have been incurable to date such as Huntington's corea or Alzheimer's disease.

A new, fascinating horizon full of questions and possibilities has opened up for the field of clinical and basic neurosciences.

REFERENCES

Agid, Y., Ruberg, M., Dubois, B., Pillon, B., Cusimano, G., Raisman, R., Cash, R., Lhermitte, F., & Javoy-Agid, F. (1986). Parkinson's disease and dementia. *Clinical Neuropharmacology, 9*, 522–536.

Agid, Y., Javoy-Agid, F., & Ruberg, M. (1987). Biochemistry of neurotransmitters in Parkinson's disease. In C. D. Marsden & S. Fhan (Eds.), *Movement disorders* (Vol. 2, pp. 166–230). London: Butterworths.

Albert, M. L., Feldman, R. G., & Willis, A. L. (1974). The subcortical dementia of progressive supranuclear palsy. *Journal of Neurology, Neurosurgery and Psychiatry, 371*, 121–130.

Backlund, E., Granberg, P., Hamberger, B., Knutson, E., Martenson, A., Sedvall, G., Seiger, A., & Olson, L. (1985). Transplantation of adrenal medullary tissue to the striatum in Parkinsonism. *Journal of Neurosurgery, 62*, 169–173.

Barker, C. F., & Billingham, R. E. (1977). Immunologically privileged sites. *Advances in Immunology, 25*, 1–54.

Bernheimer, H., Birkmayer, W., Hornykiewicz, O., Jellinger, K., & Seitelberger, F. (1973).

Brain dopamine and the syndromes of Parkinson and Huntington: Clinical, morphological and neurochemical correlations. *Journal of Neurological Science, 20*, 415–455.

Bjorklund, A., Dunnett, S. B., Stenevi, U., Lewis, M. E., & Iversen, S. D. (1980). Reinnervation of the denervated striatum by substantia nigra transplants: Functional consequences as revealed by pharmacological and sensoriomotor testing. *Brain Research, 199*, 307–333.

Bjorklund, A., & Lindwall, O. (1978). The meso-telencephalic dopamine system: A review of its anatomy. In K. Livingston & O. Hornykiewicz (Eds.), *Limbic mechanisms* (pp. 307–331). New York: Plenum Press.

Bohn, M. C., Marciano, F., Cupit, L., & Gash, D. M. (1987). Adrenal medulla grafts promote recovery of striatal dopaminergic fibers in MPTP treated mice. *Science, 247*, 913–915.

Boller, F., Passafiume, D., Keefe, N. C., Rogers, K., Morrow, L., & Kim, Y. (1980). Visuospatial impairment in Parkinson's disease. *Archives of Neurology, 41*, 485–490.

Brozoski, T. J., Brown, R. M., Rosvold, H. E., & Goldman, P. S. (1979). Cognitive deficit caused by regional depletion of dopamina in prefrontal cortex of rhesus monkey. *Science, 205*, 929–932.

Carlsson, A., Lindquest, M., & Magnusson, T. (1957). 3-4-dihydroxyphenylalanine and 5-hydroxytroptophan as reserpine antagonists. *Nature, 180*, 1200.

Cools, A. (1980). Role of the neostriatal dopaminergic activity in sequencing and selecting behavioral strategies: Facilitation of processes involved in selecting the best strategy in a stressful situation. *Behavioral Brain Research, 1*, 361–378.

Cotzias, G. C., Papavasiliov, P. S., & Gellene, R. (1969). Modification of Parkinson chronic treatment with L-dopa. *New England Journal of Medicine, 280*, 337–345.

Darley, F., Brown, J., & Swenson, W. (1975). Language changes after neurosurgery for Parkinsonism. *Brain and Language, 2*, 65–69.

DeLong, M. (1974). Motor functions of the basal ganglia single unit activity during movement. In F. D. Schmitt & F. G. Worden (Eds.), *The neurosciences* (pp. 319–325). Third study program. Cambridge, MA: M.I.T. Press.

DeLong, M. R., Georgopulos, A. P., & Crutcher, M. D. (1983). Cortico-basal ganglia relations and coding of motor performance. In *Neural coding of motor performance. Experimental brain research* (pp. 30–40). Berlin: Springer.

Divac, I., Rosvold, H., & Szwarcbart, M. (1967). Behavioral effects of selective ablation of the caudate nucleus. *Journal of Comparative Physiology and Psychology, 63*, 184–190.

Drucker-Colin, R., Madrazo, I., Ostrosky-Solis, F., Shkurovich, M., Franco, R., & Torres, C. (1988). Adrenal medullary tissue transplants in the caudate nucleus of Parkinson patients. In J. Sladek & D. Gash (Eds.), *Transplants in the central nervous system. Program in brain research.* Amsterdam: Elsevier.

Dubois, B., Danze, F., Pillon, B., Cusimano, J., Lhermitte, F., Agid, Y. (1987). Cholinergic dependent cognitive deficits in Parkinson's disease. *Annals of Neurology, 22*, 26–30.

Dubois, B., Ruberg, M., Javoy-Agid, F., Pluska, A., & Agid, Y. (1983). A subcortical cholinergic system is affected in Parkinson's disease. *Brain Research, 288*, 213–218.

Dunnett, S. B., Bjorklund, A., & Stenevi, U. (1983). Dopamine-rich transplants in experimental parkinsonism. *Trends in Neuroscience, 6*, 266–270.

Dunnett, S. B., Bjorklund, A., Stenevi, U., & Iversen, S. D. (1981a). Behavioral recovery following transplantation of substantia nigra in rats subjected to 6-OHDA lesions of the nigrostriatal pathway. *Brain Research, 215*, 147–161.

Dunnett, S. B., Bjorklund, A., Stenevi, U., & Iversen, S. D. (1981b). Grafts of embryonic substantia nigra reinnervating the ventrolateral striatum ameliorate sensoriomotor impairments and akinesia in rats with 6-OHDA lesions of the nigrostriatal pathway. *Brain Research, 229*, 209–207.

Ehringer, H., Hornykiewicz, O. (1960). Verteilung, Von. Noradrenalin und Dopamin (3-Hydroxytyramin) im Gehirn des Menschen und ihr Verhalten bei Erkrankungen des Extrapyramidalen Systems. *Klinische Wochenschrift, 38*, 1236–1239.

Elizan, T. S., Sroka, H., Maker, H., Smith, H., & Yahr, M. D. (1986). Dementia in idiophatic Parkinson's disease. *Journal of Neural Transmission, 65,* 285–302.

Farley, I. J., Price, K. S., & Hornykiewicz, O. (1978). Monominergic systems in the human limbic brain. In K. Livingston & O. Hornykiewicz (Eds.), *Limbic mechanisms* (pp. 333–349). New York: Plenum Press.

Forno, L. S., Langston, J. W., Delanney, L. E., Irwin, I., & Ricaurte, G. A. (1986). Locus ceruleus lesions and eosinophilic inclusions in MPTP-treated monkeys. *Annals of Neurology, 20,* 449–455.

Freed, W. J. (1983). Functional brain tissue transplantation: Reversal of lesion-induced rotation by intraventricular substantia nigra and adrenal medulla grafts with a note on intracranial retinal grafts. *Biology and Psychiatry, 18,* 1205–1267.

Freed, W. J., Morihisa, J. M., Spoor, E., Hoffer, B. J., Olson, L., Seiger, A., & Wyatt, R. J. (1981). Transplanted adrenal chromaffin cells in rat brain reduce lesion-induced rotational behavior. *Nature, 292,* 351–352.

Freeman, M., & Albert, M. L. (1985). Subcortical dementia. In J. A. M. Frederiks (Ed.), *Handbook of clinical neurology. Vol. 46: Clinical neuropsychology* (pp. 1049–1052). Amsterdam: Elsevier.

Gash, D., Bohn, M., Jiao, S., Fiandaca, M., Okawara, S., Kordower, J., Hansen, J., Notter, M., Snyder, J., Marciano, F., Schwarz, H., & Shoulson, I. (1987, October 18). *Adrenal medullary implantation promotes recovery of tyrosine hydroxylase immunoreactivity in host striatum of MPTP animal models of parkinsonism.* Paper presented at the Symposium on Etiology, Pathogenesis and Prevention of Parkinson's Disease, San Francisco.

Gasar, P., & Gray, F. (1984). Dementia in idiopathic Parkinson's disease. *Acta Neuropathologica, 64,* 43–54.

Hakim, A. H., & Mathieson, G. (1979). Dementia in Parkinson's disease: A neuropathological study. *Neurology, 29,* 1209–1214.

Javoy-Agid, F., & Agid, Y. (1980). Is the mesocortical dopaminergic system involved in Parkinson disease? *Neurology, 30,* 1326–1330.

Javoy-Agid, F., Ruberg, M., Taquet, H., Bukobza, B., Agid, Y., & Gaspar, P. (1984). Biochemical neuropathology of Parkinson's disease. *Advances in Neurology, 40,* 189–198.

Johnston, T. N., Rosvold, H. E., & Mishkin, M. (1968). Proyections from behaviorally defined sectors of the prefrontal cortex to the basal ganglia, septum and diencephalon of the monkeys. *Experimental Neurology, 21,* 20–30.

Langston, J. W., Ballard, P., Tetrud, J. W., & Irwin, I. (1983). Chronic parkinsonism in human due to a product of meperidine-analog synthesis. *Science, 219,* 979–980.

Lees, A. J., & Smith, E. (1983). Cognitive deficits in the early stages of Parkinson's disease. *Brain, 106,* 257–270.

Lieberman, A. N. (1974). Parkinson's disease: A clinical review. *American Journal of Medical Science, 267,* 66–80.

Lieberman, A., Dziatolowski, M., Kupersmith, M., Serby, M., Goodgold, A., Korein, J., & Goldstein, M. (1979). Dementia in Parkinson's disease. *Annals of Neurology, 6,* 355–359.

Lindvall, O., Backlund, E., Farde, L., Freedman, R., Hoffer, B., & Seiger, A. (1987). Transplantation in Parkinson's disease: Two cases of adrenal medullary grafts to the putamen. *Annals of Neurology, 22,* 457–468.

Luria, A. R. (1977). Las funciones corticales superiores en el hombre. La Habana: Orbe.

Madrazo, I., Drucker-Colin, R., Diaz, V., Martinez-Mata, J., Torres, C., & Becerril, J. (1987). Open microsurgical autograft of adrenal medulla to the right caudate nucleus in two patients with intractable Parkinson's disease. *New England Journal of Medicine, 316,* 831–834.

Matison, R., Mayeux, R., Rosen, J., & Fahn, S. (1982). Tip of the tongue phenomenon in Parkinson's disease. *Neurology, 32,* 567–570.

Mortimer, J. A., Pirozzolo, F. J., Hansch, E. C., & Webster, D. D. (1982). Relationship of motor symptoms to intellectual deficits in Parkinson's disease. *Neurology, 32*, 133–137.

Ostrosky-Solis, F., Canseco, E., Quintanar, L., Navarro, E., Meneses, S., & Ardila, A. (1985). Sociocultural effects in neuropsychological assessment. *International Journal of Neuroscience, 27*, 53–66.

Ostrosky-Solis, F., Quintanar, L., Madrazo, I., Drucker-Colin, R., Franco-Bourland, R., & Leon-Meza, V. (1988). Neuropsychological effects of brain autograft of adrenal medullary tissue for the treatment of Parkinson's disease. *Neurology, 38*, 1442–1450.

Ostrosky-Solis, F., Quintanar, L., Meneses, S., Canseco, E., Navarro, E., & Ardila, A. (1986). Actividad cognoscitiva y nivel sociocultural. *Revista de Investigacion Clinica, 38*, 37–42.

Perlow, M. J. (1987). Brain grafting as a treatment for Parkinson's disease. *Neurosurgery, 20*, 335–342.

Perlow, M. J., Freed, W. J., Haffer, B. J., Seiger, A., Olson, L., & Wyatt, R. J. (1979). Brain grafts reduce motor abnormalities produced by destruction of nigrostriatal dopamine system. *Science, 204*, 635–645.

Pirozzolo, F. J., Hansch, C., & Mortimer, J. A. (1982). Dementia in Parkinson's disease: Neuropsychological analysis. *Brain and Cognition, 1*, 71–83.

Ramon y Cajal, S. (1938). *Degeneration and regeneration of the nervous system*. London: Oxford University Press.

Riklan, M., & Levita, E. (1970). Psychological studies of thalamic lesions in humans. *Journal of Nervous and Mental Disease, 150*, 251–265.

Rinne, U. K. (1982). Brain neurotransmitter receptors in Parkinson's disease. In C. D. Marsden & S. Pahn (Eds.), *Movement disorders* (pp. 59–74). London: Butterworths.

Rosvold, H. E. (1972). The frontal lobe system: Cortical subcortical interrelationships. *Acta Neurobiologica Experimentalis, Warsaw, 32*, 439–460.

Scatton, B., Rouquier, L., Javoy-Agid, F., & Agid, Y. (1982). Dopamine deficiency in the cerebral cortex in Parkinson disease. *Neurology, 32*, 1039–1040.

Selby, G. (1967). Stereotactic surgery for the relief of Parkinson's disease. Part I. A critical review. *Journal of the Neurological Sciences, 5*, 315–342.

Stern, Y., & Langston, J. W. (1985). Intellectual changes in patients with MPTP induced Parkinsonism. *Neurology, 35*, 1506–1509.

Taylor, A. E., Saint-Cyr, J. A., & Lang, A. E. (1986). Frontal lobe dysfunction in Parkinson's disease. The cortical focus of neostriatal outflow. *Brain, 109*, 845–883.

Taylor, A. E., Saint-Cyr, J. A., & Lang, A. E. (1987). Parkinson's disease: Cognitive changes in relation to treatment response. *Brain, 110*, 35–51.

Teuber, H., & Proctor, F. (1964). Some effects of basal ganglia lesions in subhuman primates and man. *Neuropsychologia, 2*, 85–93.

Uhl, G. R., Hedreen, J. C., & Price, D. L. (1985). Parkinson's disease: Loss of neurons from the ventral tegmental area contralateral to therapeutic surgical lesions. *Neurology, 35*, 1215–1218.

Ungerstedt, U. (1971a). Adipsia and aphagia after 6-hydroxydopamine induced degeneration of the nigro-striatal dopamine system. *Acta Physiologica Scandinavica Supplementum, 367*, 95–122.

Ungerstedt, U. (1971b). Striatal dopamine release after amphetamine or nerve degeneration revealed by rotational behavior. *Acta Physiologica Scandinavica Supplementum, 367*, 49–68.

Unsicker, K., Rieffert, B., & Ziegler, W. (1980). Effects of cell culture condition, nerve growth factor, dexamethasone and cyclic AMP on adrenal chromaffin cells in vitro. In O. Eranko, S. Soinila, & H. Paivarento (Eds.), *Histochemistry and cell biology of autonomic neurons, SIF cells, and paraneurons* (pp. 51–59). New York: Raven Press.

Villardita, T., Smirni, P., Le Pera, F., Zappala, G., & Nicoletti, F. (1982). Mental deterioration, visuoperceptive disability and constructional apraxia in Parkinson's disease. *Acta Neurologica Scandinavica, 66,* 112–120.

Wurtman, R. J., Pohorecky, L. A., & Baliga, B. S. (1972). Adrenocortical control of the biosynthesis of epinephrine and protein in the adrenal medulla. *Pharmacological Review, 24,* 411–426.

Zetusky, W., Jankovic, J., & Pirozzolo, F. (1985). The heterogeneity of Parkinson's disease: Clinical and prognostic implications. *Neurology, 35,* 522–526.

11

The Striatum as a Temporary Memory Store

ROBERTO A. PRADO-ALCALÁ

The search for the mechanisms involved in memory storage has yielded an enormous amount of experimental data. To date, however, we are far from understanding how the nervous system integrates the relevant information derived from experience, and how that information is channeled to effector systems when the same, or a similar, experience occurs.

Recent work has provided evidence strongly suggesting that memory storage depends not upon the workings of a single neuroanatomical/neurochemical system but, rather, upon sequential activation of different systems (for a review, see Prado-Alcalá, 1985). What follows is a brief account of the experimental data that have given support to this hypothesis.

INVOLVEMENT OF THE NEOSTRIATUM IN MEMORY

A wealth of information concerning the involvement of the caudate nucleus (CN) or neostriatum in memory processes has accumulated. Strong support to the hypothesis that the caudate is critically involved in associative processes (Divac & Oberg, 1979) has been given by the demonstration that almost every type of conditioned behavior that has been studied is impaired after disrupting the functional integrity of this structure, with the use of a variety of lesioning techniques (Dunnet & Iversen, 1985; Glick & Greenstein, 1973; Glick, Marsanico, & Greenstein, 1974; Kirkby & Kimble, 1968; Mitcham & Thomas, 1972; Prado-Alcalá et al., 1975; Sanberg, Lehmann, & Fibiger, 1978; Sanberg, Pisa, & Fibiger, 1979;

ROBERTO A. PRADO-ALCALÁ • Department of Physiology, Faculty of Medicine, National University of Mexico, Mexico D. F. 4510, Mexico.

Winocur, 1974), as well as other methods that interfere with its neuronal activity, such as electric stimulation and topical application of potassium chloride (Le Piane & Phillips, 1978; Prado-Alcalá & Cobos-Zapiain, 1979; Prado-Alcalá, Grinberg, Alvarez-Leefmans, & Brust-Cammona, 1973; Prado-Alcalá et al., 1975; Prado-Alcalá, Kaufmann, & Moscona, 1980; Wyers & Deadwyler, 1971; Wyers, Deadwyler, Hirasuna, & Montgomery, 1973; Wyers, Peeke, Elliston, & Herz, 1968).

Although those studies indicated that normal functioning of the CN is important for the establishment of memory, they did not provide clues about the nature of the mechanisms implicated in such function, but were instrumental in the designing of experiments aimed at defining the neurochemical events that may occur during learning and performance of conditioned behaviors. Thus, it was shown that alterations in the activity of striatal dopamine (Kim & Routtenberg, 1976a; Phillips & Clouston, 1978; Stabuli & Huston, 1978), GABA (Salado-Castillo & Prado-Alcalá, 1987), and acetylcholine (Haycock, Deadwyler, Sideroff, & McGaugh, 1973; Neill & Grossman, 1970; Prado-Alcalá et al., 1972) also produce significant memory impairments.

Since dopamine, GABA, and acetylcholine are the main neurotransmitters regulating the activity of the nigro-neostriatal system, the data suggested that the nigro-neostriatal system is critically involved in memory functions. Several lines of evidence give support to this idea: Blockade of GABAergic activity of the substantia nigra (Cobos-Zapiain & Prado-Alcalá, 1986; Kim & Routtenberg, 1976b) and combined treatment of a dopaminergic blocker with intrastriatal atropine (Rivas-Arancibia & Prado-Alcalá, 1986) result in amnesia.

THE OVERTRAINING EFFECT

The effects of injections of ACh-receptor blockers into the anterodorsal aspect of the CN have been tested on the acquisition and maintenance of positively rewarded bar-pressing and alley-running tasks (Bermúdez-Rattoni, Mujica-González, & Prado-Alcalá, 1986; Prado-Alcalá & Cobos-Zapiain, 1977; Prado-Alcalá et al., 1972; Prado-Alcalá, Kaufmann & Moscona, 1980). In all cases a strong amnesic state was induced. These deficits were seen using two different muscarinic blockers (atropine and scopolamine) and two animal species (cats and rats). When the same treatments that induced amnesia were applied to other cerebral regions, such as the lateral ventricles (Prado-Alcalá et al., 1972), amygdala (Prado-Alcalá & Cobos-Zapiain, 1977), and parietal cortex (Bermúdez-Rattoni et al., 1986), no significant deficits were found.

The involvement of the CN in passive avoidance has been extensively studied (Polgar, Sanberg, & Kirkby, 1981) and, with few exceptions

(Olmstead & Villablanca, 1980), it is accepted that this behavior is dependent upon the functional integrity of this structure. Likewise, it has been consistently found that the application of atropine or scopolamine into the anterodorsal striatum shortly after training of passive avoidance produces a marked amnesic state when retention is tested 24 hours later (Giordano & Prado-Alcalá, 1986; Haycock et al., 1973; Prado-Alcalá, Cruz-Morales, & Lopez-Miro, 1980; Prado-Alcalá, Fernández-Samblancat, & Solodkin-Herrera, 1985; Prado-Alcalá, Signoret, & Figueroa, 1981; Prado-Alcalá, Signoret-Edward, Figueroa, & Barrientos, 1984).

In contrast, blockade of cholinergic activity of the posterior CN (Prado-Alcalá, Cruz-Morales, & López-Miro, 1980) or hippocampus (Haycock et al., 1973) does not produce such effect. The application of anticholinergic drugs to the cerebral cortex produces a retention deficit that is significantly smaller than that produced by the same treatments applied to the CN (Prado-Alcalá et al., 1985).

The amnesic effect produced by atropine injections into the CN is both dose- and time-dependent. In two related studies it was found that, as expected, when the dose of the anticholinergic is larger, so is the retention deficit (Giordano & Prado-Alcalá, 1986; Prado-Alcalá et al., 1985). In another experiment it was shown that when posttrial injections of atropine into the CN were closer in time to the time of training (2 min), a greater amnesic state was produced; no retention deficits were observed when the injections were made 15 or 30 minutes after training (Prado-Alcalá et al., 1981).

An unexpected finding, which seemed to contradict the reported detrimental effects of cholinergic blockade of the caudate nucleus on the maintenance of positively motivated behaviors, gave origin to a new hypothesis about the way in the caudate nucleus is involved in memory processes (Prado-Alcalá & Cobos-Zapiain, 1977). The injections of atropine into the CN did not alter the performance of cats that had been trained to press a bar in order to obtain milk. A previous study showed that this treatment produced an amnesic state in the same species trained in the same task (Prado-Alcalá et al., 1972). The only procedural difference was that the animals of the former study had been overtrained; i.e., they had been trained for 30 sessions instead of the usual 10 to 15 sessions.

Subsequent experiments have confirmed the protective effect of overtraining. When independent groups of rats are trained to bar-press during 5, 15, or 25 sessions and are then injected with scopolamine into the striatum, a significant deficit in retention is found in the 5- and 15-session groups, but no deterioration of the learned response in the 25-session group (Prado-Alcalá, Kaufmann, & Moscona, 1980). Equivalent results were found when a more complex task (spatial alternation) was studied (Prado-Alcalá, Bermúdez-Rattoni, Velázquez-Martínez, & Bacha, 1978).

In related studies it has been shown that when rats and cats are trained to bar-press until they reach asymptotic performance and then injected into the CN with a high concentration of potassium chloride, they show a significant retention deficit. Again, when training is extended, the same treatment does not produce retention deficits (Prado-Alcalá & Cobos-Zapiain, 1979; Prado-Alcalá, Kaufmann, & Moscona, 1980).

The results reported above strongly indicated that the CN is critically involved in the acquisition and early maintenance stages of positively reinforced instrumental conditioning, and that this structure is not engaged in memory after overtraining. It was reasoned that if this represents a general way of functioning of the striatum, equivalent effects should be produced when animals are trained in other types of tasks.

As stated above, the striatum plays a very important role in the consolidation of memory of one-trial passive avoidance, a negatively reinforced task. This task was used to determine whether the overtraining effect could be generalized further.

Overtraining, as studied in prior experiments, involved multiple training sessions, a high number of positive reinforcers, and a prolonged exposure to the experimental situation. In the case of one-trial passive avoidance there is only one training session and application of only one reinforcer, and the duration of the trial is brief. For the designing of the experiments to be described below, it was decided to vary the magnitude of only one of these parameters (the reinforcer), testing different intensities of the foot shock. This manipulation is equivalent to having different amounts of positive reinforcers.

In one experiment, the effects of posttraining injection of atropine into the anterodorsal aspect of the striatum on retention of passive avoidance were assessed. Independent groups of rats were given different levels of foot shock (0.25, 0.50, or 1.00 mA) during training. As expected, retrograde amnesia was seen only in the 0.25-mA group (Giordano & Prado-Alcalá, 1986).

In order to determine whether some striatal neurochemical system, other than cholinergic, became engaged in consolidating memory after overtraining, groups of rats were trained, using also low, medium, and high foot shock intensities, and then given intrastriatal injections of Xilocaine, thus arresting all normal neural activity of the injected area. It was reasoned that if consolidation was dependent upon the integrative functions of the striatum, an amnesic state would be produced, regardless of the intensity of the foot shock—i.e., regardless of overtraining. In agreement with the studies reported above, those rats that were submitted to overtraining had as good retention scores as intact animals (Pérez-Ruiz & Prado-Alcalá, 1986).

With regard to active avoidance, there are only a few relevant studies that could bear on this problem; however, these studies were not designed to study the overtraining effect, and interpretation of these results should be made cautiously. Briefly, when acetylcholine receptor-blockers are applied to the anterior aspect of the striatum of animals that are still learning the task (Neill & Grossman, 1970), have just learned it (Prado-Alcalá, Cepeda, Verduzco, Jimenez, & Vargas-Ortega, 1984), or are "overtrained" (Prado-Alcalá, Cruz-Morales, & López-Miro, 1980), a performance deficit is observed only in the former group.

In a recent study (Cobos-Zapiain & Prado-Alcalá, 1986), it was shown that injections of picrotoxin into the substantia nigra produced a profound amnesic state of passive avoidance; again, when the same treatment was given to overtrained rats, no deficits in learning were observed.

CONCLUSIONS

From the studies reviewed here it can be concluded that cholinergic activity of the caudate nucleus plays a major role in the acquisition and early maintenance stages of instrumental learning. The experimental evidence also points to the conclusion that striatal cholinergic activity is not involved in the performance of tasks that have become overtrained. The results obtained after the application of picrotoxin into the nigra of overtrained animals also point to the same conclusion. Taken together, the studies here reviewed suggest that activity of the acetylcholine-containing interneurons of the caudate nucleus and the striatonigral GABA neurons are critically involved in the processes underlying recent memory, while long-term storage of information is mediated by a different neurochemical system, which very probably is located outside the nigro-neostriatal system.

Along these lines, Miller (1981) has recently proposed a two-stage storage model of memory. According to this model, the caudate nucleus would constitute the first memory store for operant tasks, which then would be transferred to the cerebral cortex.

To date there has not been a single published study demonstrating unequivocally that the activity of a particular brain structure in the mammal is necessary for the maintenance (long-term memory) of instrumental behaviors. It seems that the failure to find such structure, or set of structures, simply reflects a misleading theoretical approach to this problem— i.e., trying to find an all-purpose single memory store (supposedly located in one structure or a system of structures). It is suggested that the search for the "engram" should be guided by a search for neuroanatomical and neurochemical systems that may be sequentially involved in such complex function. Very probably we will find multiple systems, each subserving different types of learned behaviors, which become operative, one after the other, depending on the relative age and degree of mastery of the learned response.

ACKNOWLEDGMENTS

This work was supported by Fundacion Miguel Aleman, A. C. and Fondo Ricardo J. Zevada.

REFERENCES

Bermúdez-Rattoni, F., Mujica-González, M., & Prado-Alcalá, R. A. (1986). Is cholinergic activity of the striatum involved in the acquisition of positively-motivated behaviors? *Pharmacology, Biochemistry and Behavior, 24*, 715–719.

Cobos Zapiain, G., & Prado-Alcalá, R. A. (1986). *Aplicación de picrotoxina en la substancia nigra reticulada: Efectos sobre la memoria de largo plazo, en una tarea sobreentrenada,* XXIX Congreso Nacional de Ciencias Fisiológicas, Mexico.

Divac, I., & Oberg, R. G. E. (1979). *The neostriatum.* Oxford: Pergamon Press.

Dunnett, S. B., & Iversen, S. D. (1981). Learning impairments following selective kainic acid-induced lesions within the neostriatum of rats. *Behavioral Brain Research, 2*, 189–209.

Giordano, M., & Prado-Alcalá, R. A. (1986). Retrograde amnesia induced by post-trial injection of atropine into the caudate-putamen. Protective effect of the negative reinforcer. *Pharmacology, Biochemistry and Behavior, 24*, 905–909.

Glick, S. D., & Greenstein, S. (1973). Comparative learning and memory deficits following hippocampal and caudate lesions in mice. *Journal of Comparative and Physiological Psychology, 82*, 188–194.

Glick, S. D., Marsanico, R. G., & Greenstein, S. (1974). Differential recovery of function following caudate, hippocampal, and septal lesions in mice. *Journal of Comparative and Physiological Psychology, 86*, 787–792.

Haycock, J. W., Deadwyler, S. A., Sideroff, S. I., & McGaugh, J. L. (1973). Retrograde amnesia and cholinergic systems in the caudate-putamen complex and dorsal hippocampus of the rat. *Experimental Neurology, 41*, 201–213.

Kim, H.-J., & Routtenberg, A. (1976a). Retention deficits following post-trial dopamine injection in rat neostriatum. *Society for Neuroscience Abstracts, 2*, 631.

Kim, H.-J., & Routtenberg, A. (1976b). Retention disruption following post-trial picrotoxin injection into the substantia nigra. *Brain Research, 113*, 620–625.

Kirkby, R. J., & Kimble, D. P. (1968). Avoidance and escape behavior following striatal lesions in the rat. *Experimental Neurology, 20*, 215–227.

Le Piane, F., & Phillips, A. G. (1978). Differential effects of electrical stimulation of amygdala, caudate-putamen or substantia nigra pars compacta on taste aversion and passive avoidance in rats. *Physiology and Behavior, 21*, 979–985.

Miller, R. (1981). *Meaning and purpose in the intact brain.* Oxford: Oxford University Press.

Mitcham, J. C., & Thomas, R. K. (1972). Effects of substantia nigra and caudate nucleus lesions on avoidance learning in rats. *Journal of Comparative and Physiological Psychology, 81*, 101–107.

Neill, D. B., & Grossman, P. S. (1970). Behavioral effects of lesions or cholinergic blockade of dorsal and ventral caudate of rats. *Journal of Comparative and Physiological Psychology, 71*, 311–317.

Olmstead, C. E., & Villablanca, J. R. (1980). Effects of caudate or frontal cortex ablations in cats and kittens: Passive avoidance. *Experimental Neurology, 68*, 335–345.

Pérez-Ruiz, C., & Prado-Alcalá, R. A. (1986). Differential effects of lidocaine injections into the striatum on short- and long-term retention of passive avoidance in overtrained rats. *Society for Neuroscience Abstracts, 12*, 714.

Phillips, A. G., & Clouston, R. (1978). Disruption of one-trial appetitive learning and passive avoidance following stimulation of the substantia nigra pars compacta. *Behavioral Biology, 23,* 388–394.

Polgar, S., Sanberg, P. R., & Kirkby, R. J. (1981). Is the striatum involved in passive avoidance behavior? A commentary. *Physiological Psychology, 9,* 354–358.

Prado-Alcalá, R. A. (1985). Is cholinergic activity of the caudate nucleus involved in memory? *Life Sciences, 37,* 2135–2142.

Prado-Alcalá, R. A., Bermúdez-Rattoni, F., Velázquez-Martínez, D., & Bacha, M. G. (1978). Cholinergic blockade of the caudate nucleus and spatial alternation performance in rats: Overtraining-induced protection against behavioral deficits. *Life Sciences, 23,* 889–896.

Prado-Alcalá, R. A., Cepeda, G., Verduzco, L., Jimenez, A., & Vargas-Ortega, E. (1984). Effects of cholinergic stimulation of the caudate nucleus on active avoidance. *Neuroscience Letters, 51,* 31–36.

Prado-Alcalá, R. A., & Cobos-Zapiain, G. G. (1977). Learning deficits induced by cholinergic blockade of the caudate nucleus as a function of experience. *Brain Research, 138,* 190–196.

Prado-Alcalá, R. A., & Cobos Zapiain, G. G. (1979). Interference with caudate nucleus activity by potassium chloride. Evidence for a "moving" engram. *Brain Research, 172,* 577–583.

Prado-Alcalá, R. A., Cruz-Morales, S. E., & López-Miro, F. A. (1980). Differential effects of cholinergic blockade of anterior and posterior caudate nucleus on avoidance behaviors. *Neuroscience Letters 18,* 339–345.

Prado-Alcalá, R. A., Fernández-Samblancat, M., & Solodkin-Herrera, M. (1985). Injections of atropine into the caudate nucleus impair the acquisition and the maintenance of passive avoidance. *Pharmacology, Biochemistry and Behavior, 22,* 243–247.

Prado-Alcalá, R. A., Grinberg, Z. J., Alvarez-Leefmans, F. J., & Brust-Carmona, H. (1973). Suppression of motor conditioning by the injection of 3M KCl in the caudate nuclei of cats. *Physiology and Behavior, 10,* 59–64.

Prado-Alcalá, R. A., Grinberg, Z. J., Alvarez-Leefmans, F. J., Gómez, A., Singer, S., & Brust-Carmona, H. (1972). A possible caudate-cholinergic mechanism in two instrumental conditioned responses. *Psychopharmacologia (Berlin), 25,* 339–346.

Prado-Alcalá, R. A., Grinberg, Z. J., Arditii, Z. L., García, M. M., Prieto, H. G., & Brust-Carmona, H. (1975). Learning deficits produced by chronic and reversible lesions of the corpus striatum in rats. *Physiology and Behavior, 15,* 283–287.

Prado-Alcalá, R. A., Kaufmann, P., & Moscona, R. (1980). Scopolamine and KCl injections into the caudate-putamen. Overtraining-induced protection against deficits of learning. *Pharmacology, Biochemistry and Behavior, 12,* 249–253.

Prado-Alcalá, R. A., Signoret, L., & Figueroa, M. (1981). Time-dependent retention deficits induced by post-training injections of atropine into the caudate nucleus. *Pharmacology, Biochemistry and Behavior, 15,* 633–636.

Prado-Alcalá, R. A., Signoret-Edward, L., Figueroa, M., & Barrientos, M. A. (1984). Post-trial injection of atropine into the caudate nucleus interferes with long-term, but not with short-term retention of passive avoidance. *Behavioral and Neural Biology, 42,* 81–84.

Rivas-Arancibia, S., & Prado-Alcalá, R. A. (1986). *Núcleo caudado y aprendizaje. XXIV. Interacción entre los sistemas dopaminérgico y colinérgico en procesos de memoria.* XXIX Congreso Nacional de Ciencias Fisiológicas, México.

Salado-Castillo, R., & Prado-Alcalá, R. A. (1987). Effects of picrotoxin injections into different regions of the striatum on retention of passive avoidance. *Society for Neuroscience Abstracts, 13,* 657.

Sanberg, P. R., Lehmann, J., & Fibiger, H. C. (1978). Impaired learning and memory after kainic acid lesions of the striatum: A behavioral model of Huntington's disease. *Brain Research, 149,* 546–551.

Sanberg, P. R., Pisa, M., & Fibiger, H. C. (1979). Avoidance, operant and locomotor behavior in rats with neostriatal injections of kainic acid. *Pharmacology, Biochemistry and Behavior, 10,* 137–144.

Stabuli, U., & Huston, J. P. (1978). Effects of post-trial reinforcing vs. subreinforcing stimulation of the substantia nigra on passive avoidance learning. *Brain Research Bulletin, 3,* 519–524.

Winocur, G. J. (1974). Functional dissociation within the caudate nucleus of rats. *Journal of Comparative and Physiological Psychology, 86,* 432–439.

Wyers, E. J., & Deadwyler, S. A. (1971). Duration and nature of retrograde amnesia produced by stimulation of caudate nucleus. *Physiology and Behavior, 6,* 97–103.

Wyers, E. J., Deadwyler, S. A., Hirasuna, N., & Montgomery, D. (1973). Passive avoidance retention and caudate stimulation. *Physiology and Behavior, 11,* 809–819.

Wyers, E., J., Peeke, H. V. S., Elliston, J. S., & Herz, M. J. (1968). Retroactive impairment of passive avoidance learning by stimulation of the caudate nucleus. *Experimental Neurology, 22,* 350–366.

V

Recovery from Brain Damage

12

Development and Plasticity in the Central Nervous System

Organismic and Environmental Influences

DONALD G. STEIN

Throughout this chapter I will be talking about plasticity in the central nervous system. Although the concept is central to both biological and psychological development, the term *plasticity* has been used in so many different ways that it has lost much of its meaning. For example, almost any change in behavior or in an organism's response to stimuli can be taken as an example of plasticity. Here, I will try to define the term in a way that makes sense for people in the neurosciences as well as in psychology, then I will give some specific examples of the kinds of plasticity that can be seen in both the developing and mature nervous system. Over the last decade, despite the problem of how to define the term adequately, there has been a major revolution in ideas about how the nervous system functions, how it develops, and what actually represents "plasticity."

Kaplan (1983) has provided a broad definition of plasticity in development that fits very well with events taking place in the central nervous system. In general terms Kaplan describes plasticity as "an ability to modify organic systems and patterns of behavior. In this context different *means* can be used to obtain specific *goals*. Plasticity will also refer to the wide individual differences in response to external or internal environmental demands." Kaplan also characterizes development as "a special way of regarding, analyzing, describing, and ordering phenomena of systemic change." "Developmental analysis is oriented principally to the relations between forms and function, parts and wholes, means and ends.

DONALD G. STEIN • Dean of the Graduate School and Associate Provost for Research, Rutgers University, Newark, New Jersey 07102.

Development is also defined in terms of differentiation and hierarchic integration."

Kaplan stresses that plasticity cannot be defined without reference to the means that are used to achieve certain ends. Thus, "a developmental analysis of plastic phenomena will also require careful study of *means–ends relationships* and how such means change in a given person, or organism, or group of subjects." In this context plasticity in development is seen as a form of creativity or flexibility.

In another definition, Gollin (1981) refers to plasticity as "the possible range of variations that can occur in individual development or to systematic structural or functional changes in a process and may involve variations that lie on a continuum of variation around some hypothesized average value" (p. 231). For Gollin, plasticity is the potential for change, the capacity to modify one's behavior or function and to adapt to the demands of a particular context. Again, the role of context or environment will be given considerable attention in my discussion about recovery from brain injuries.

From my perspective, Gollin's key phrase is adaptation to a "particular context" because what might be seen as a constancy—for example, a specific syndrome or deficit following damage to a specific CNS region—might only be *relatively constant*—that is, the *development* of an outcome occurring in one very specific context but not in another.

In one sense, the topic of this essay is "What is reality?" In terms of prevailing scientific paradigms, we will be talking about different "realities," different ways of looking at central nervous system function, asking what is "constant" and what is contextual. I will argue, for example, that much of what we know about cerebral localization is based on the evaluation of brain-damaged patients and animal subjects who are studied in very limited and circumscribed situations that are *specifically* designed to yield a desired outcome.

To highlight this point, I would like to quote from the introductory chapter in what is thought to be the most widely read textbook in the neurosciences (Kandel & Schwartz, 1981). In the section titled "Cognitive functions can be localized within the cerebral cortex," the authors state that "much of what we know about the localization of normal language has come from the study of aphasia" (p. 7). In the same chapter, Kandel and Schwartz also argue that "affective and character traits also are anatomically localizable" (p. 10). They also state that "clinical studies and their counterparts in experimental animals suggest that *all behavior* (emphasis added), including higher (cognitive as well as affective) mental functions, is localizable to specific regions or constellations of regions within the brain. The role of descriptive neuroanatomy, therefore, is to provide us with a functional guide to localization within the three-dimensional neural space—*a map for behavior*" (p. 11) (emphasis added).

Given this set of beliefs and attitudes, it makes sense that, in many laboratories, experimental lesions are created, employed, and controlled in such a way as to *guarantee* that an observable deficit will occur. In fact, this would be the most reasonable approach for those concerned with the mapping of behavioral functions onto increasingly discrete brain regions, zones, or even specific "command or control" neurons. But what if experimental conditions can be manipulated in such a way that the same *extent* of injury, created in a different way, leads to behavioral sparing or marked reduction in the impairment? Thus, if such outcomes were possible, the "constancy" of the lesion effect would be challenged and a new set of "contextual" factors would have to be considered in determining the development of events that will follow the injury.

Workers with a heavily vested interest in cerebral mapping and neuronal specificity are not happy with such a conceptual (or contextual) approach to the study of cerebral organization, and one can readily understand why. If, as we shall try to show, the cerebral circuitry underlying behavioral events can shift as a function of environmental, hormonal, and other organismic events, map making becomes very difficult at best. Picture what it might be like to have a state map where the locations of cities and towns (and the highways to and from them) would shift from day to day as a function of economic conditions, the weather, population shifts, famine, and other factors. Yet, in geography, such realities do occur, albeit perhaps more slowly. Nonetheless, following a catastrophe (earthquake, war, flooding), rapid and massive change could occur as new "centers" and paths develop to replace those that were lost. Can such contextually induced plasticity occur at the level of the individual central nervous system following the equivalent catastrophe of stroke, trauma, or penetrating injury? Is the hard-wired nature of the nervous system an inherent characteristic of the brain itself, or is it more a characteristic of the particular beliefs and attitudes we have developed to study it? We will need to return to this point many times as we proceed with this essay.

When we talk about brain injury or plasticity, we must keep in mind that these events (or processes) do not occur in a static system. Injury and subsequent change can be seen as a dynamic series of events in which many different variables play a role in determining the outcome of injury. Table 1, taken from a recent paper by Geschwind (1985), shows a number of specific and nonspecific changes that occur after lesions of the nervous system. Any one of these parameters could be the subject of a lifetime of research. It is easy to understand why, in the face of so many variables, one would be tempted to focus upon one or two factors and ignore the others.

Most research in neuroscience takes the approach that given parts of the central nervous system have highly specific structure–function relationships. In this view, each neuron, each organ of the brain is presumed

TABLE 1. Changes after Lesions of the Nervous System

Mechanisms (listings are not necessarily exclusive)
  Biochemical
    Nonspecific
      Edema and disappearance of edema
      Ischemia without destruction
      Immune responses
      Scarring
      Pressure effects
    Specific
      Increase or decrease in number of receptors
      Induction or inactivation of enzymes
      Viral alterations of specific cell function
      Immune responses to specific neural components
      Alterations in transmitter release
      Transmitter reuptake by inactive neurons (Zigmond effect)
      Alterations in membrane properties
  Structural
    Disrupted organization
    Sprouting—colateral and terminal
    Anomalous connections
    Demyelination
    Transynaptic and transneuronal degeneration
    Diminished cell death in other areas (in fetal and possible early life)
  Physiological
    Changes in facilitation, inhibition, and occlusion
    Loss of feedback effects
    Pacemaker shifts
    Slowed conduction
    Changes in synchrony
    Opening of ineffective synapses
    Changes of spatial or temporal summation
    Kindling and epilepsy
  "Psychological"
    Perception of change by intact regions
    Alternate strategies
Factors influencing late change
  Age
  Species
  Previous learning
  Individual differences (type and size of structures, connections, bio-
      chemistry, individual talents, handedness)
  Previous exposure to drugs, hormones, etc. (pre- and postnatal)
  Serial lesions
  Epilepsy
  Stimulation (such as skin lesions or deliberate stimulation)
  Emotional effects—motivation, hormones, circulating transmitters, etc.
  Susceptibility to immune attack of areas formed abnormally in prenatal
      life

to have a genetically determined, specific role to play. It is not uncommon to see this mechanistic view translated to the molecular level in the neurosciences in talk about command neurons, analyzers, perceptors, and so forth. In the context of such a "hard-wired" nervous system, there is apparently little weight given to the environmental and organismic factors that can modify and shape CNS function in temporary as well as permanent fashion.

Here is a good example of "contextual plasticity" from our own laboratory (Attella, Nattinville, & Stein, 1988) examining the question of whether hormonal factors determine the outcome of brain injury. It is well documented that females have fluctuating levels of estrogen or progesterone in the central nervous system depending upon the particular phase of their estrous cycle. When estrogen is high, progesterone is low. When progesterone is high, estrogen is low. What possible role could these alterations in ovarian hormones play in determining whether cognitive impairment would occur following injury to the frontal cortex? In the traditional view of static structure–function relationships in the CNS, one would hardly expect ovarian hormones to affect the outcome of brain injury— yet this is exactly what we were able to observe.

Studies show that when fully intact adult female rats were examined on a delayed spatial alternation task, alterations in hormone levels had no effect on learning ability. On errors and perseverations in the T-maze, whether an intact animal was pseudopregnant (low estrogen, high progesterone) or was cycling did not change cognitive performance. In rats, at least, "daily learning skills" remained intact despite significant shifts in hormonal cycling.

Further study has demonstrated what happens to normal cycling or pseudopregnant rats after they have been subjected to bilateral removal of the frontal cortex. In the standard brain-injury paradigm, this lesion almost always produces severe impairments of spatial learning ability in rats, cats, and monkeys. The sham-operated animals (no cortical damage), pseudopregnant or normal cycling, showed completely normal retention of the learned alternation; there are few, if any, errors during this phase of the training. There exist some interesting data showing what happens to rats that were brain-injured during normal cycling and then compared with pseudo-pregnant conspecifics. These data provide a dramatic demonstration that normally cycling animals with relatively high CNS levels of estrogen at the time of brain injury will have *severely* impaired retention performance in comparison to rats who were first made pseudopregnant at the time of injury.

This finding provides clear evidence that the outcome of brain injury is very much dependent on the female's hormonal state, not just on the site of the injury itself. The performance deficits we observed were dramatic and persistent.

Hormonal factors may also be important in regulating the extent of injury-induced, synaptic sprouting in the brain. Recently, Scheff, Hoff, and Anderson (1986) used quantitative electron microscopy to measure synapse formation in adult rats given partial lesions of the hippocampus followed by treatment with corticosterone. These workers found that if the rats were maintained on high levels of corticosterones (often employed as an anti-inflammatory agent), there was a decrease both in the rate of removal of degenerating synapses and in the rate of synapse replacement. If regeneration of this type were involved in the mediation of functional recovery, then one might expect a negative prognosis if the subject happened to have high steroid levels at the time of injury.

If nothing else, the results of these two experiments reveal that there is a very complex interaction between organismic (i.e., hormonal) state and outcome of brain injury. It is not just a question of damaging a given "circuit" and expecting to observe a fixed outcome at a given time. The context in which the injury has occurred has rather dramatically altered the behavioral sequelae. How, then, do we draw the detailed "map of behavior" referred to earlier?

PLASTICITY AND LEVELS OF ANALYSIS OF CNS FUNCTIONS

One important and difficult problem for many of us working in contemporary neuroscience is that often there is a confusion about the "most appropriate" level of analysis required to define function in the central nervous system. With respect to "plasticity," we can expect that different levels of analysis and different ways of measuring "important" events will lead to a different construct about what is "really important" to understand the CNS. Each area or subdiscipline of the neurosciences looks at these different outcomes and then attempts to derive its own working definition of plasticity. For example, a neurochemist might look at "plastic" phenomena in terms of alterations in the flux of ions at the membrane level of an injured neuron. Here, at the site of the injury or at the synaptic end-foot, stable or changing rates of calcium inflow or impaired neuropeptide uptake, or the incorporation of neurotrophic factors might be defined as an example of plasticity (or lack of it). In other words, changes in neurotransmitter levels or ionic influx or changes in membrane structure can become the definition of dynamic, neuronal plasticity. One step up, at another level of analysis, one might look at how a given region of the brain releases or induces growth promoting (trophic) factors in response to injury. The specific circuits or pathways are not evaluated. For biochemical assay, the tissue itself is ground up and destroyed so that morphological detail is forever lost. At an anatomical level, researchers have discussed neuronal and synaptic plasticity in terms of growth or regeneration of neurons, and they carefully map the connections and pathways that are formed. And at yet another level there are investigators who focus upon alterations or changes in specific structures of the CNS in response to injury.

In this context, the analysis turns from neurochemical assay and fixed morphology to the evaluation of ongoing activity in the living tissue *in situ*. Such assays often employ electrophysiological recordings from brain areas as subjects perform various tasks (e.g., maze running in rats, problem solving in patients). More recently, functional analyses of cerebral blood flow or other measures of ongoing metabolic activity employing various types of autoradiographic assays (e.g., NMR, CAT scan, uptake of labeled glucose analogues) have been used to study what different brain regions might be doing (e.g., active, inhibited) during task performance. Following brain damage, for example, an investigation could employ these "functional" techniques to ask whether there is substitution of function, wherein one area of the brain is thought to take over the function of a damaged neighbor (Slavin, Laurence, & Stein, 1988). Finally, one can examine changes in the cognitive, emotional, or perceptual aspects of behavior after injury, bringing us to the psychological level of definition. Here, there are sometimes attempts to *correlate* behavioral deficits with the locus of the injury, but there is not much interest in specifying the underlying mechanism causing the actual deficits or the recovery that can sometimes follow."[1]

Is there one level of analysis that is more appropriate for understanding CNS plasticity than another? I believe that if we are to understand recovery of function, we will need to apply a number of different levels of analysis. It is very doubtful that we will find a simple, monolithic explanation for "recovery." In this context, we should not fall victim to the idea that our approach is the best or that only the latest in new technology (e.g., molecular biology) can provide the answer. Given the complexity of the problem and the need for understanding CNS function at multiple levels, I believe that the best approach is to develop cross-disciplinary collaborative efforts.

In my laboratory we emphasize the importance of behavioral change, but we try to relate those behavioral changes to the different structural, anatomical, and biochemical alterations that could account for the "plastic" events we study. Roger Sperry in his Nobel Prize-winning address

---

[1]Psychologists often criticize their colleagues in the neurosciences for what sometimes seems to be a highly demonstrable lack of interest in what the nervous system does with respect to behavior. However, in all fairness to those in the neurosciences, there are many psychologists who feel there is nothing to be learned by developing a better understanding of how the nervous system works. This "black box" approach to the brain is still very much with us in academic and clinical psychology. Neither level of parochialism can ultimately benefit our understanding and treatment of neural and behavioral pathologies.

commented about whether or not reductionistic or molar approaches are appropriate and said, "All approaches to the analysis of 'plasticity' are legitimate and useful. Analysis at one level does not obviate the usefulness of analysis at another level."

It is also worth mentioning the obvious, and that is that change at any one level of function has the potential to alter plasticity or determine it at another level. For example, there is now a growing body of evidence (see Nieto-Sampedro, 1988) that growth-promoting and survival-promoting factors are endogenously induced by brain injury in adult subjects. These trophic substances that are produced at the site of injury increase the survival of neurons that would ordinarily die after injury. The surviving cells then maintain their projections (contacts) with the damaged zone and thus permit sparing or more rapid recovery of *behavior*. After a CNS injury there is a cascade of effects, over time, represented by alterations in brain biochemistry on up to significant behavioral changes. Thus, chemical factors that promote the survival of neurons are critical for morphological survival and reinnervation, which, in turn, might be essential to maintain behavior.

ENVIRONMENTAL AND BEHAVIORAL FACTORS "SHAPE" CNS MORPHOLOGY

It is also important to point out that behavioral activity can be used to promote neuronal activity that stimulates the growth of dendrites and synapses. In other words, how an organism responds to its environment can have structural (morphological/biochemical) effects on the central nervous system.

In one program of research, Greenough and Chang (1985) exposed rats to either isolated environments (in which animals live alone), social environments (in which there are several animals in a cage), or complex "condominiums" in which the animals are exposed to "enriched" stimulation, where they have an opportunity to interact vocally, play, and be exposed to many objects that are changed daily. After the rats were chronically exposed to the different environments, Greenough and his students employed the Golgi technique of staining entirely a select number of neurons, which could then be examined in three dimensions for the extent of dendritic branching and the number of spines (the processes along the dendrite where synaptic end-feet form the synapse and maintain contact with the afferent neuron). The number of dendritic branches and the number of spines are painstakingly counted to determine if exposure to different environments can "feed back" on the brain to produce structural alterations in the neurons themselves.

It was shown that chronic exposure to a "complex" environment can increase the length of dendritic fields in several classes of neurons found in the visual cortex. Exposure to complex environments and maze-learning experience also contributed to increasing the number of synaptic vesicles (the structures within the synaptic end-feet that contain neurotransmitters). Greenough and Chang (1985) have repeated and reviewed many other structural changes in brain morphology that are related to specific experience. In summary, the environment-induced changes in morphology and ultrastructure of neurons is important because these changes are directly related to the ability of the animal to process, store, and retrieve information.

The incredible amount of time required to perform both light- and electron-microscopic evaluations of the qualitative characteristics of dendrites and synapses in response to environmental stimulation forces investigators to focus on only a few brain regions. But if behavioral manipulation can, in fact, alter CNS morphology, we cannot assume that only the limited areas under study are changed. Can one assume that all other nuclei and their connections (pathways) remain fixed in function and activity, that the pathways are immutable? Or is it likely that many structures are in a state of structural flux in response to environmental pressures? If so, then what is the appropriate "time" to measure a constant aspect of CNS morphology?

The belief in fixed elements in the CNS can be considered as a philosophical statement that derives from the kinds of methods that are employed in the study of brain hodology. Even in the face of the newer, metabolic (functional) techniques, most neuroanatomical studies of the brain are made in dead tissue that is prepared at a single time, using highly toxic preservatives (or deep freezing) to permit cutting and mounting on slides. Geoffrey Raisman (1978), an electron-microscopist, known for his seminal work demonstrating injury-induced growth in the adult CNS, said that "it is this very feature of anatomical methodology that has tended to give anatomical observations the appearance of permanence and rigidity. The fact that a synapse exists and can be photographed in a form in which it appeared at the moment when the animal was killed gives no indication of how long that particular synapse had existed before the moment of death or how long it would have remained had the animal survived" (p. 102).

Raisman's observations are consistent with the results of an elaborate electron-microscopic investigation of serotinergic (5-HT) nerve terminals in the frontal cortex of adult rats conducted by Descarries, Baudet, and Watkins (1975). They used ^{3}H-5HT labeling to mark the nerve terminals and then sampled 50,000 photomicrographs to determine that only about 5% of the nerve terminals had formed "synaptic contacts" with "postsynaptic" membranes. Yet the presynaptic "knobs" had all the characteristics and morphology of normal terminals. The authors suggested that the presence of so many "free" terminals are not compatible with the view that the frontal circuitry is fixed and static. Instead they suggested that in living tissue there is an ongoing process of synaptic shifting and relocation that cannot be seen when tissue is examined postmortem.

If this type of plasticity does occur in the adult CNS, then it is possible to think that synaptic morphology and function will be altered by the organism's experience.[2]

If we can agree that behavioral manipulation can have a direct effect on CNS morphology, can such manipulations alter the outcome of brain injury? If, for example, environmental "enrichment" can enhance recovery or sparing of function after injury, under what conditions, then, is it appropriate to "specify" structure–function relationships in the central nervous system? Here one might see environment or training as part of the developmental process contributing to the dynamic reorganization of CNS morphology and function. Anatomical measurements taken from animals exposed to different environments have shown that enriched conditions can result in greater cortical thickness and more complex synaptic profiles in comparison with those raised under isolated conditions. Kelche and Will (1982), in a follow-up to their observations of behavioral recovery, demonstrated that hippocampal lesions can produce a reduction in the number of dendritic spines of pyramidal neurons in the occipital cortex. However, the number of spines was increased if the operated rats were maintained in complex environments. A thorough review of the issues surrounding the effects of differential housing and outcome of brain injury has been prepared by Dalyrimple-Alford and Kelche (1985).

Here again, the summary point to be made is that the context in which injury (or any other ongoing event) occurs cannot be overlooked in developing a theory of nervous system specificity of plasticity.

TEMPORAL FACTORS ALSO IMPORTANT IN PREDICTING THE OUTCOME OF BRAIN DAMAGE

Now we have seen that organismic (hormonal) as well as environmental (differential housing) effects can alter the "specific" outcome of brain injury. But even these important variables are alone, not always sufficient to account for defining structure and function in the CNS. When we look at the effects or the outcome of brain injury in order to define recovery, plasticity, or deficit, very often we look at relatively restricted periods of time following the injury (or treatment). Yet investigators in clinical neuropsychology have long recognized that it is not sufficient to

[2]Indeed, some investigators concerned with the anatomical substrates of learning (e.g., Baudry & Lynch, 1984) are reevaluating the earlier notions of Hebb (1949) in this very context, but this discussion is beyond the scope of this chapter.

look at one fixed period of time to examine (and predict) the outcome of brain injury. In one of the last papers of Norman Geschwind (1985) discussing the mechanisms of change after brain injury, he said that "there must be many cases in which the capacity for recovery is latent and revealed only by some further manipulation, but *experimenters have only rarely been zealous in their search for the right maneuver*" (emphasis added). Geschwind argued that the time needed for recovery in adults may be much longer than in infants. He went on to say that "most neurologists are gloomy about the prognosis of severe adult aphasia after a few weeks, and pessimism is reinforced by lack of prolonged follow-up in most cases." He then said: "I have, however, seen patients severely aphasic for over a year who then made excellent recoveries: one patient returning to work as a salesman, the other as a psychiatrist. Furthermore, there are patients who continue to improve over many years. For example, a patient whose aphasia was still quite evident six years after onset cleared substantially by eighteen years. Change after damage may show great individual variation" (p. 3). The concept of delayed recovery is yet another example of the "plasticity" that needs to be explained in developing an appropriate conceptual model of nervous system organization. There is no rule saying that, if recovery is to occur, it has to be immediate! One of the tasks of our laboratory and of the many students who have worked in it with me is to find a way to promote recovery as rapidly as possible, to get it to occur in a shorter period of time than the 6 or 18 years mentioned by Geschwind. Very often, as Geschwind indicated, we tend not to look for recovery if it has not occurred for a very long period of time. Thus, we can often miss the fact that the processes that underlie central nervous system plasticity may take far longer than we have previously assumed. We should also not overlook the fact that the "potential for plasticity" may be present but blocked by ongoing processes inimical to its manifestation. The focus in research, then, is to unlock those neural events that can lead to functional recovery even though the time course may be far longer than we would like to imagine.

ADAPTIVE AND MALADAPTIVE ANOMALOUS GROWTH IN RESPONSE TO CNS INJURY

In summary, and with respect to the inherent *potential* for CNS reorganization, it should be kept in mind that whether or not recovery occurs depends upon the various interactions taking place around the time of the injury. When we try to make definitive statements, particularly about the determinative aspects of structure—function relationships, we have to recognize that they are primarily probabilistic statements. In other words, the outcome (i.e., a specific deficit), like the outcome of epigenesis or development itself, is not inevitable because one cannot specify all of the factors that determine or influence the organism in its environment. With respect to brain injury, the extent to which the processes we refer to as "plasticity" are successful in mediating *functional* recovery depends upon the coming together of the appropriate variables at the appropriate time.

In this same context we can also point to examples of "negative" plasticity. Here one can think about the anomalous growth of neurons in response to injury that sometimes results in maladaptive behavior.

About 15 years ago, Gerald Schneider and his students at M.I.T. began a series of studies designed to study the anatomical basis for restoration of visual function following lesions of the optic tectum in neonatal hamsters (e.g., Schneider & Jhaveri, 1974). The hamster is a good model for this type of research because at birth the cortex has not yet grown over the superior colliculus, so the structure is easy to visualize and remove surgically. In response to this injury, Schneider found that fibers coming from the optic nerve do not simply die off. Instead, there is considerable, redirected growth that could be systematically studied and evaluated for its contributions to functional recovery—in this case restoration of vision.

If one were to examine the normal pathway of neurons from the eye crossing over at the optic chiasm and entering the superior colliculus (SC), one would see that most of the fibers terminate in the superficial layer of the SC. If, however, the SC is removed, the growing fibers end up by entering into the posterior portion of the lateral posterior nucleus, which does not, in normal animals, receive a heavy innervation from the optic nerve. Some of the fibers even terminate in the medial geniculate body, a part of the auditory system that does not receive such projections in normal animals. In addition, if one eye that normally has its terminations in the opposite hemisphere in the superior colliculus is removed, the fibers from the intact eye cross to the opposite hemisphere, but in the absence of an intact superior colliculus, *they grow back across the midline* of the brain to reinnervate the contralateral tectum, where they should not be.

What do these findings show? First, Schneider's data demonstrate a clear example of injury-induced neuronal plasticity, unequivocal evidence of neural regeneration and regrowth in the developing hamster. What of the behavioral correlates?

First, it does appear that the anomalous growth forms "structurally normal-looking synapses in abnormal places after neonatal lesions of the SC" (Kalil & Schneider, 1975), and single-cell electrophysiological recordings have been used to demonstrate that the new synapses are functionally active.

Second, when sunflower seeds were presented in various parts of the visual field, the hamsters would turn in the direction *opposite* of (away from) the presentation. In these animals, it was later confirmed that the developing retinal projections grew to the "wrong" side of the brain as a result of the neonatal injury (see Schneider, 1979, for a detailed review).

Schneider (1979) pursued the role of the abnormal projections one step further by asking what would happen if the abnormally recrossing fibers were to be eliminated in the adult animal. First, he mapped the visual fields (with perimetry studies) where both correct turning and incorrect turning to the sight of a sunflower seed could be elicited. Next, microsurgery was employed to transect the recrossing bundle of optic fibers. In the animals whose anomalous fibers were surgically prevented from recrossing the midline, turning in the wrong direction was completely eliminated, while turning in the appropriate direction to obtain reinforcement remained completely intact!

Schneider's clever experiments clearly demonstrate that, at least in early life, there is considerable neuronal reorganization in response to brain injury. However, it is sometimes the case that the redirected growth of axons can result in significant behavioral abnormality as well as potential sparing of function. The task of experimenters working in this area is to determine under what conditions such growth might lead to enhanced recovery and what leads to impairment. Unfortunately, most investigators interested in neuromorphology rarely examine the *behavioral* consequences of the anatomical "plasticity" that they observe, so one does not often know whether the changes seen are beneficial, maladaptive, or of no consequence to the functioning organism.

Schneider's work highlights the importance of careful behavioral follow-up following neonatal brain injury. Even more important, his work shows that, in some instances, maladaptive behavior caused by anomalous growth can be eliminated by later surgery.

Recently, Earle (1987) reviewed some of the literature on lesion size and recovery following damage to a number of different neural systems and concluded that, under the *right conditions*, secondary lesions or expansion of lesion size could actually lead to better recovery than with more circumscribed injury. One might speculate that the more extensive injuries could remove some of the "neural noise" (e.g., inhibition, spasticity) created by anomalous growth resulting from the initial damage. This is an area of research that clearly needs more attention, despite the fact that it falls outside of the more "traditional" approaches to structure–function analyses in the CNS.

BEHAVIORAL CONSEQUENCES OF LESIONS EARLY IN LIFE VIS-À-VIS INJURIES AT MATURITY

To demonstrate further how "context" plays such an important role in determining the outcome of CNS injury, let me now turn to studies of functional recovery after spinal cord damage in newborn and adult cats. Over the last several years, Barbara Bregman and Michael Goldberger (1983a,b) have been examining both the behavioral and anatomical correlates of recovery in cats with spinal cord injuries inflicted early in life or at maturity. First, Bregman and Goldberger carefully analyzed motor pattern recovery after hemisections of the spinal cord in newborn or adult animals. The cats' movements were filmed and quantified, and, although both groups showed recovery of function, the results indicated that the recovery was not "uniform"; some motor behaviors were better after adult injury, while some recovered better when the damage was inflicted early in life (Bregman & Goldberger, 1983b).

For instance, tactile placing was completely abolished after spinal cord hemisection in adults, but no loss of hind limb placing occurred when the lesions were made in newborn animals. In contrast, accurate foot placement during locomotion was much better in adult operated animals, as was hopping with the foot opposite to the side of the lesion. Bregman and Goldberger suggested that recovery or sparing of function occur when the lesions are made *prior* to the time that the motor reflexes begin to develop in normal animals. The better recovery in cats damaged as adults is thought to be due to the possibility that there may be more (neural) sources (spinal and supraspinal) that could participate in the adjustments needed for good locomotion.

To support these speculations, Bregman and Goldberger (1982, 1983a,b) carefully examined the anatomical changes that might account for the sparing or failure of motor function they observed in their injured cats. As in the visual system, lesions in the immature spinal cord lead to the development of aberrant neuronal fiber paths, which could mediate some degree of recovery (or maladaptive behavior).

Using retrograde neuronal marker techniques (HRP), the authors examined histopathology in cats with spinal lesions at 1 day of birth or as adults. The anatomical results supported the complexity of their behavioral data. First, whether lesions were made in neonates or adults had no effect on sparing of brainstem-spinal fibers—there was no "plasticity" here. In addition, neonatal lesions led to much greater retrograde degeneration in this path than did similar lesions created in adult cats. In contrast, corticospinal projections were dramatically spared, but "only in the neonatal group." There were also anomalous projections in the latter group that were not seen in the former (corticospinal neurons reached lumbar segments of the cord by an alternate course). Bregman and Goldberger emphasize that tactile placing is completely *abolished* after adult lesions, but completely spared after neonatal injury. One can infer, then, that the functional sparing is the result of the "anatomical plasticity of (this new) corticospinal projection." The sparing and development of the anomalous path is likely due to the relatively late arrival of this pathway during the normal course of development. Thus, since the fibers are not really present at the site at the time of the injury, they can grow past the site and reroute themselves to their appropriate targets (Bregman & Goldberger, 1982).

In summary, the work on early versus late injury and anomalous growth highlights yet again the importance of the context; in this case, stage of maturation can determine the outcome of traumatic brain injury. The factors that lead to survival and growth on the one hand, or loss of neurons on the other, are not well understood. Nonetheless, there is considerable progress being made to unlock the appropriate conditions or factors that lead to consistent recovery of function where none is expected.

Especially when attempts are made to facilitate recovery with drugs or experimental agents, the specific context, experience, or "background" of the subject will interact with the "treatment" to determine the outcome of the brain injury. In adult organisms, the potential for plasticity in the form of reorganization (or deblocking) of function is also present, but different rehabilitative strategies may be required to activate the mechanisms underlying the recovery itself.

One last example taken from the work of Dennis Feeney and his students will suffice. Feeney, Gonzalez, and Law (1982) found that injections of amphetamine can enhance the levels of the neurotransmitter norepinephrine in adult animals who have been depleted of this substance by lesions of the catecholaminergic system. Injuries in the motor cortex often block or eliminate visual, postural, proprioceptive, righting, and tactile placing reflexes. Amphetamine administration can apparently restore these reflexes and restore motor and visual performance, even after *acute bilateral* injury. In the face of a considerable amount of literature, it would seem that such a finding would lead to the development of an effective clinical treatment for brain injury, but the question is more complex.

First, in reviewing the literature, Feeney and Sutton (1987) found that recovery could not be maintained if animals did not receive *repeated testing* (general visual experience in the home cage was not sufficient). In cats, many tests of the specific placing response had to be administered for the drug to be effective in inducing recovery. To test the importance of experience in amphetamine-induced recovery from brain injury, Feeney and his students restrained rats with motor cortex lesions in a small box during amphetamine intoxication and compared them with counterparts allowed to roam freely or who were given beam-walking experience. Blocking ballistic movements eliminated the beneficial amphetamine effects entirely (Hovda & Feeney, 1984).

In reviewing their work, Feeney and Sutton (1987) suggest that "drug therapy alone may not be efficacious for inducing recovery. Rather a combination of drug plus *appropriate behavioral training and testing* (emphasis added) is required for induction of recovery. Importantly, these studies suggest that the capabilities (and neural pathways) for behavioral recovery may be present in brain-injured patients, but may never function or be expressed *unless appropriate treatments are provided*" (p. 142).

IMPORTANT INDIVIDUAL DIFFERENCES IN RESPONSE TO BRAIN INJURY THAT ARE NOT ADEQUATELY STUDIED

For the most part, the prognosis for recovery from brain damage in humans is poor. When it does occur, it is often characterized as an interesting anomaly, and there is little in the way of systematic inquiry into either the historical or present conditions that led to the patients' unique outcome in comparison with those who seem to be less fortunate. Yet individual differences in response to the same type or extent of injury could provide important clues as to some of the mechanisms underlying functional recovery. As early as 1902, two developmental neurologists, Baldwin and Polton, said that "apart from plasticity in general, the facts of *individual accommodation* make the nature and limits of brain plasticity a matter of great interest." They may have been among the first to talk about individual differences in response to brain injury.

Unfortunately, in the laboratory setting, our own empiricist orientations and the social conditions in neuroscience do not often permit the thorough study of individual accommodation to trauma. We are forced to employ statistical averaging methods to seek the mean case, and we are taught that deviation from the average is due to error in measurement. In the final analysis, we will need to address the question of whether there are effective tools to pursue our understanding of why there is so much individual variability in response to brain injury and what that variability can tell us about mechanisms of CNS plasticity.

Let me illustrate this point further by referring to work by R. Thompson (1978). In *A Behavioral Atlas of the Rat Brain* Thompson plotted all of the different areas reported by researchers to affect different behavioral functions. The ostensible purpose of the atlas was to provide the reader with a visually easy way to determine where one could create a specific lesion to produce a specific deficit. In illustrations, Thompson showed where damage to the brain results in maze-learning deficits. In examining all of the areas that appear to produce deficits in learning ability, it is hard for me to conceive of the fact that behavior as complex as maze learning could be localized in a single given structure or pathway in the central nervous system. Yet this atlas represents the results of many studies that have attempted to do just this. For the sake of argument one could say that with respect to a phenomenon as amorphous as learning, the processes involved should be relatively distributed throughout "higher" regions in the central nervous system. In contrast, consummatory or regulatory behaviors would be expected to be controlled by more "premature" subcortical structures, and there would be much less plasticity when the "centers" controlling innate behaviors such as eating and drinking are destroyed.

Thompson's work contains another map showing where damage results in aphasia and adipsia. Damage to the areas of the brain demarcated there results in failure to eat and drink. Animals who suffer lesions of this type will usually die if there is no forced feeding or drinking. Earlier research on consummatory behavior had localized these functions to the lateral and ventromedial hypothalamus. However, it can be demonstrated that even behavior as basic as eating and drinking can be affected by damage to a wide variety of cerebral "centers." Conversely, one may look first for one type of behavior while ignoring many other changes because that is what the person is interested in studying. The point that I wish to make here is that any given lesion will have widespread effects in the CNS. These effects (anatomical, biochemical, electrophysiological, behavioral) will be tempered or modulated by the *individual* history of the organism as well as the contemporary context in which the injury has occurred.

For example, Valenstein, Cox, and Kakolewski (1968) implanted bilateral electrodes into the lateral hypothalamus of adult rats. Electrical stimulation of this area was thought to activate the "excitatory" areas controlling eating (while lesions resulted in aphagia and adipsia). In the presence of food, Valenstein and colleagues stimulated the rats through the electrodes, and they observed that even though the rats were sated, they would begin to eat. This would certainly seem to confirm the hypothesis of an excitatory center for eating, except that the researchers carried their experiment several steps further.

The food was removed and either water or wood shavings were placed in the animals' cages. When the electrical stimulation was turned on in the presence of these "stimuli," the rats drank or gnawed on the chips, depending on what was available. When nothing was present, some of the rats simply picked up their tails and carried them around. It would seem from these data that the "context" or environment plays a major role in determining the behavioral outcome during *activation* of a CNS region. The different behaviors could have resulted from the ever-changing interplay of CNS regions rather than the specific "output" of a singular region.

In a similar experiment, Gazzaniga (1974) made rats severely adipsic by creating large lateral hypothalamic lesions. Such animals will not spontaneously drink and will eventually die unless forcibly fed water. Rats with these lesions will, however, try to run in an activity wheel. Taking advantage of this fact, Gazzaniga made running in the wheel (through behavioral shaping) contingent upon drinking first from a water spout for increasing amounts of time. The adipsic rats quickly learned to drink in order to be able to run.

Had Gazzaniga not manipulated the environment appropriately, he would have obtained the "classic" syndrome and confirmed the "principle" that the lateral hypothalamus controls drinking and eating. Instead, he, too, was able to show that the outcome of injury depends on the context in which the damage occurs rather than just the site itself.

It is appropriate that in experimental situations we try to control, as much as possible, the history and current context of the organism so that we can explain how our various manipulations might work. Nonetheless, in the clinic situation, carefully examining, rather than ignoring or downplaying variability, may be the key to understanding why some individuals seem to miraculously escape the effects of CNS injury while others are so devastated.

Work has been done showing what happens when a lesion is made in the rat's motor cortex. Results have shown the extent of change in the CNS that can occur from a focal lesion. The degeneration does not take into account transneuronal degeneration or retrograde degeneration where neurons that project to the lesion site also die off over time. Even though the degeneration represents monosynaptic changes, one can see how many different structures in the central nervous system, including visual areas, motor areas, and nuclei that are involved in consummatory behavior, are altered by loss of afferent inputs as a result of this lesion. The organism as a whole will change as the "outputs" of the different structures begin to adapt (or fail to adapt) to the brain injury.

Given the greater complexity of the human brain, would we expect less, or even more, variability in people? A composite map taken from Kertesz (1983) shows that direct electrical stimulation of the brain tested prior to surgery for excision of epileptogenic foci produces alterations in naming and sentence reading throughout a wide area of the cortical mantle, and not just in Wernicke's or Broca's area.

Once again the clash of concepts of plasticity, adaptability, and individual variability in the central nervous system and that of the concept of trying to localize functions by ever finer units of analysis (e.g., command neurons, pontifical cells) comes from the fact that there are really deep-rooted preempirical ideas about the nature of "neural" reality. Basic paradigms that scientists hold determine the methodologies they select and what interpretations they impose on the data that they collect. Stephen Jay Gould called this social phenomenon the "presupposition of limits." These presuppositions of limits, spoken or unspoken, certainly affect our views of how we conceive of the development of plasticity in both adult and young animals and what should or should not be studied.

An eloquent example of an explicit presupposition of limits was stated by a distinguished visitor to the United States early in this century. That visitor, a Nobel Prize winner in neuroanatomy, was Santiago Ramon y Cajal, who said: "Once development is ended, the fonts of growth and regeneration of the axons and dendrites dry up irrevocably. In adult centers the nerve paths are something fixed and immutable. Everything may die; nothing may be regenerated" (Cajal, 1928, p. 750). That is one very good example of a "presupposition of limits."

Another, more modern example of the presupposition is taken from the work of R. F. Thompson (1986), who made the following statement about memory, "*All* evidence to date indicates that the mechanisms of memory storage are local and do not involve the formation of new projection pathways. Furthermore, to the extent that they have been identified, essential memory trace circuits in the vertebrate brain are localized" (p. 944). Thompson's statement clearly implies that there is a very limited path (or set of methodologies that one should follow in defining the memory process or, by inference, in trying to develop a proper scientific measure of brain injury outcome or the process of recovery.

Contrast Thompson's statement with another that was made a month later in the same journal by John, Tang, Brill, Young, and Ono (1986). John, who is also interested in the physiological basis of learning, first trained cats to perform a maze-learning task. He then used radioactive uptake of a glucose analogue to measure changes in metabolic activity in a large number of brain structures as the animals tried to learn visual discrimination tasks. In light of his results, John concluded (and remember this follows 1 month after Richard Thompson's remarks):

> Our results do not fit well with the general computer-like model of the brain with information stored in discrete registers, no matter how many in number. A radically different model is necessary. Our data, like data from diverse electrophysiological and anatomical studies, better support notions of cooperative processes in which the nonrandom behavior of huge ensembles of neural elements mediate the integration and processing of information and the retrieval of memory. In view of the large number of neurons involved the question of how information represented in these neurons can be evaluated and appreciated by the brain becomes of critical theoretical importance. No conceivable neuron or set of neurons, no matter how diffuse its synaptic input, can evaluate the enormous amount of neural activity here shown to be involved in retrieval of even a simple form discrimination. Memory and awareness in complex neural systems may depend upon presently unrecognized properties of the system as a whole and not upon any of the elements that constitute the system. (p. 1174)

What we have here is a clear clash of paradigms. The question becomes what is the most appropriate way of analyzing and looking at brain function? (What is the best paradigm?) John uses the same scientifically

accepted *methodologies* employed by Thompson (single-cell electrophysiology, brain biochemistry, behavioral analysis) but comes to very
different conclusions and interpretations about how the brain works.

Kuhn, writing in *The Essential Tension* (1977), says:

> A paradigm is *a set of beliefs and attitudes* shared by a group of people that are
> committed to the same rules and standards of scientific practice. This commit-
> ment is a prerequisite for normal science, that is, the genesis and continuation
> of a particular research tradition. Without this commitment, any set of beliefs,
> attitudes, and techniques could serve as acceptable approaches to research.
> And that research would basically be a random activity with no unifying
> theme. Almost anything would be equally relevant. (p. 294)

I believe that basically what we need to do is to establish a different
paradigm relevant to the study of recovery from brain injury. Kuhn (1970)
also says the following:

> Normal science, the activity in which most scientists invariably spend almost
> all of their time, is predicated on the assumption that the scientific community
> knows what the world is like. Much of the success of the enterprise derives
> from the community's willingness to defend that assumption, if necessary, at
> considerable cost. Normal science, for example, often suppresses fundamental
> novelty because they are necessarily subversive of its basic commitment.
> Nevertheless, so long as those commitments retain an element of the arbitrary,
> the very nature of normal research ensures that novelty shall not be suppressed
> for very long. (p. 5)

In summary, the examples that I have provided show that there is still
turmoil in neuroscience that is being generated by dramatically different
ways of looking at nervous system functions. It is an important conflict
that spills over even into the more clinical areas of human neuropsychology. Let me again repeat the quote I gave earlier from the neuroscience
texts of Kandel and Schwartz (1981), here describing the clinical psychopathology of temporal lobe function. They claim that both cognitive functions and character traits are anatomically localizable. Thus, "their
clinical studies and their counterparts in experimental animals suggest
that *all behavior,* including higher mental functions, is *localizable to
specific regions* or constellations of regions within the brain. The role of
descriptive neuroanatomy is, therefore, to provide us with a functional
guide to the localization within the three-dimensional neurospace, a map
for behavior" (p. 11). Given the data presented so far, perhaps the reader
should draw his or her own conclusions about which of the competing
paradigms might be most appropriate for the study of physiological and
organismic plasticity.

Finally, I present here the summary statements taken from a recent
book on cortical localization in clinical neuropsychology (Kertesz, 1983).
Kertesz argues that "the *function* of an area is related to the lesion if: (1)
The same functional deficit always follows the lesion. (2) The same deficit

is not produced by other independent lesions. (3) The deficit is measured according to standardized and meaningful methods. (4) The lesion location is determined objectively and accurately. (5) Biological variables, such as time from onset, age, etiology and so forth, are controlled" (p. 294).

If one takes the contextual and organismic view that I have presented in this chapter, it seems to me that none of the criteria described by Kertesz can be used to infer "the function" of a given area. If the paradigm that I am proposing has merit, then one must begin to question whether traditional neuropsychological testing can provide meaningful answers to the questions about the physiological substrates of behavior in normal and brain-damaged subjects.

As Nottebohm (1985) recently stated in the preface to his book on CNS plasticity, new frontiers in the neurosciences are constantly being discovered. "However, even as we bow to the powers of reductionism and to the promise that molecular approaches hold for brain repair, we should remember that brains are also more than vast arrays of molecules" (p. ii).

SUMMARY AND CONCLUDING REMARKS

As we come to the end of this essay, I think it is safe to say that the neurosciences are undergoing a dramatic shift in ideas about the "limits of plasticity" in the central nervous system. We have seen that there are a variety of developmental processes leading to recovery or change that must be considered in describing or predicting the outcome of brain injury. It is no longer possible to describe or report symptoms simply in terms of damage to a specific path or circuit because those paths or circuits may not be constant. The conditions under which damage occurs at a given moment in the cumulative history of the organism must now be taken into account in our attempts to define structure–function relationships in the CNS. In this context, we must also be more aware of the fact that environmental influences can also modulate and sculpt neuronal morphology, such that the functional demands made on morphology may determine the output of a given neural area; thus, function (environment) may play some role in determining structure.

Mapping of neuronal circuits in fixed tissue is an important and useful endeavor in that it may give us the conditions by which we can begin to explore the more dynamic aspects of nervous system function. However, when such mapping becomes an end in itself, or when it becomes merely the demonstration of technique without any reference to behavior, then the science of understanding the function of the nervous system will not really progress. The fashion now is toward an ever-increasing, mechanical and ideological "reductionism" where behavior is often seen as an almost unwanted by-product that complicates the process(es) of studying neuronal tissue just for its own sake.

It may be time to move away from the concept of the brain as a colony of neurons that, when all the maps are done and all the circuits plotted, will give us a complete "understanding: of complex phenomena like learning, memory, and emotion. This view has been with us for almost a century and is probably one of the reasons why so little has been done to help the victims of brain and spinal cord injury (i.e., it is obvious that removal or damage of fixed and hard-wired circuits must lead to permanent impairment once the cortical component is gone). Now there is beginning to emerge a hope for a new neurology, as Nottebohm claimed in the title of his recent volume. There is a beginning (and maybe even grudging) acceptance of the multitude of factors that can shape and modulate nervous system function in normal organisms and alter the outcome of recovery in brain-damaged patients.

We have made great strides in our understanding of many operations of the nervous system at the molecular level through the employment of reductionistic research strategies. Now we have to begin to ask whether the collective properties of the nervous system may display novel features that are not discernible in the detailed observation of its component parts. Paul Weiss recognized this when he repeatedly emphasized that the dynamic interaction between neurons may not be more than the sum of the parts, but, surely, it could be very different!

ACKNOWLEDGMENTS

A fuller version of this chapter was published in the Heinz Werner Lecture Series-Clark University Press. This chapter is published with permission from Clark University Press.

REFERENCES

Attella, M., Nattinville, A., & Stein, D. G. (1987). Hormonal state affects recovery from frontal cortex lesions in adults females rats. *Behavioral and Neural Biology, 48,* 352–367.

Baudry, M., & Lynch, G. W. (1984). Glutamate receptor regulation and the substrates of memory. In G. Lynch, J. L. McGaugh, & N. M. Weinberger (Eds.), *Neurobiology of learning and memory* (pp. 431–450). New York: Guilford Press.

Bregman, B., & Goldberger, M. (1982). Anatomical plasticity and sparing of function after spinal cord damage in neonatal cats. *Science, 237,* 553–555.

Bregman, E., & Goldberger, M. (1983a). Infant lesion effect: II. Sparing and recovery of function after spinal cord damage in newborn and adult cats. *Developmental Brain Research, 8,* 119–135.

Bregman, B. S., & Goldberger, M. E. (1983b). Infant lesion effect: III. Anatomical correlates of sparing and recovery of function after spinal cord damage in newborn and adult cats. *Developmental Brain Research, 9,* 137–154.

Cajal, S. (1928). *Degeneration and regeneration of the central nervous system* (R. M. May, Trans.). London: Oxford University Press.
Dalyrimple-Alford, J. D., & Kelche, C. (1985). Behavioral effects of pre-operative—post-operative differential housing in rats with brain lesions: A review. In B. E. Will, P. Schmitt, D. C. Dalyrimple-Alford (Eds.), *Brain plasticity, learning and memory. Advances in behavioral biology* (Vol. 28, pp. 441–458). New York: Plenum Press.
Descarries, L., Baudet, A., & Watkins, K. C. (1975). Serotonin nerve terminals in adult rat neocortex. *Brain Research, 100,* 563–588.
Earle, E. (1987). Lesion size and recovery of function: Some new perspectives. *Brain Research Reviews, 12,* 307–320.
Feeney, D. M., Gonzalez, A., & Law, W. A. (1982). Amphetamine, haloperidal and experience interact to affect rate of recovery after motor cortex injury. *Science, 217,* 885–857.
Feeney, D. M., & Sutton, R. (1987). Pharmacotherapy for recovery of function after brain injury. *Critical Reviews in Neurobiology, 3,* 135–197.
Gazzaniga, M. (1974). Determinants of cerebral recovery. In D. G. Stein, J. J. Rosen, & N. Butters (Eds.), *Plasticity and recovery of function in the CNS* (pp. 203–216). New York: Academic Press.
Geschwind, N. (1985). Mechanisms of change after brain lesions. In R. Nottebohm (Ed.), Hope for a new neurology, *Annals of the New York Academy of Sciences, 457,* 1–11.
Gollin, E. S. (1981). Development and plasticity. In B. S. Gollin (Ed.), *Developmental plasticity: Behavioral and biological aspects of variation in development.* New York: Academic Press.
Greenough, W., & Chang, P. F. (1985). Synaptic structural correlates of information storage in mammalian nervous system. In C. W. Cotman (Ed.), *Synaptic plasticity* (pp. 335–374). New York: Guilford Press.
Hebb, D. O. (1949). The organization of Behavior. New York: Wiley Press.
Hovda, D. A., & Feeney D. M. (1984). Amphetamine with experience promotes recovery of locomotor function after unilateral frontal cortex injury in the cat. *Brain Research, 298,* 358.
John, E. R., Tang, Y., Brill, A. B., Young, R., & Ono, H. (1986). Double-labeled metabolic maps of memory. *Science, 233,* 1167–1175.
Kalil, R. E., & Schneider, G. E. (1975). Abnormal synaptic connections of the optic tract in the thalamus after midbrain lesions in newborn hamsters. *Brain Research, 100,* 690–698.
Kandel, E. R., & Schwartz, J. H. (1981). *Principles of neuroscience.* Amsterdam: Elsevier North-Holland.
Kaplan, B. (1983). A trio of trials. In R. M. Lerner (Ed.), *Developmental psychology: Historical and philosophical perspectives* (pp. 185–228). Hillsdale, NJ: Erlbaum.
Kelche, C., & Will, B. (1982). Effects of postoperative environments following dorsal hippocampal lesion on dendritic branching and spines in rat occipital cortex. *Brain Research, 245,* 107–115.
Kertesz, A. (1983). *Localization in neuropsychology* (p. 18). New York: Academic Press.
Kuhn, T. (1970). *The structure of scientific revolutions.* Chicago: University of Chicago Press.
Kuhn, T. (1977). *The essential tension.* Chicago: University of Chicago Press.
Nieto-Sampedro, M. (1988). Growth factor induction and order of events in CNS repair. In D. G. Stein & B. A. Sabel (Eds.), *Pharmacological approaches to the treatment of brain and spinal cord injury* (pp. 301–338). New York: Plenum Press.
Nottebohm, F. (1985). Neuronal replacement in adulthood. In F. Nottebohm (Ed.), *Hope for a new neurology* (pp. 143–162). Annals of the New York Academy of Sciences, 457.
Raisman, G. (1978). What hope for repair of the brain? *Annals of Neurology, 3,* 101–106.
Scheff, S. W., Hoff, S. F., & Anderson, N. J. (1986). Altered regulation of lesion-induced synaptogenesis by adrenalectomy and corticosterone in young adult rats. *Experimental Neurology, 93,* 456–470.

Schneider, G. (1979). Is it really better to have your brain damage early? A revision of the "Kennard Principle." *Neuropsychologia, 17,* 557–583.

Schneider, G., & Jhaveri, S. (1974). Neuroanatomical correlates of spared or altered function after brain lesions in the newborn hamster. In D. G. Stein, J. J. Rosen, & N. Butters (Eds.), *Plasticity and recovery of function in the CNS* (pp. 65–110). New York: Academic Press.

Slavin, M. D., Laurence, S., & Stein, D. G. (1988). Another look at vicariation. In S. Finger, T. E. LeVere, C. R. Almli, & D. G. Stein (Eds.), *Brain injury and recovery: Theoretical and controversial issues* (pp. 165–180). New York: Plenum Press.

Thompson, R. F. (1986). The neurobiology of learning and memory. *Science, 223,* 941–947.

Thompson, R. (1978). *A behavioral atlas of the rat brain.* New York: Oxford University Press.

Valenstein, E. S., Cox, V. C., & Kakolewski, J. W. (1968). Modification of motivated behavior elicited by electrical stimulation of the hypothalamus. *Science, 158,* 1118–1121.

Index